Not the F——ing Gilmore Girls

COURTNEY CANNON

Copyright © 2024 Courtney Cannon
All rights reserved
First Edition

PAGE PUBLISHING
Conneaut Lake, PA

First originally published by Page Publishing 2024

Any resemblance to real people or places is purely coincidental. Psych. But I did change the last names.

ISBN 979-8-89315-131-2 (pbk)
ISBN 979-8-89315-168-8 (hc)
ISBN 979-8-89315-142-8 (digital)

Printed in the United States of America

To my aunt and fairy godmother, Katherine, you are the only person who has always supported me. Thank you for being a believer in dreams, a believer in love, and above all, a believer in me. To my old friend Maria, for giving me the idea to go on TikTok. To my mother, without whom this book—and the writer of it—would not exist.

And to you, Sir. You are my one regret.

Dear readers,

If there's anything I know, it's that I wouldn't be anything without y'all. Literally, if I don't have people to love or help or smile at, my life is empty. So if this book ends up reaching twenty people or 20 million, it doesn't matter as long as you love it.

Please find me on TikTok @CocoPhoenix1313 and come chat about anything you love or that resonates with you. Together, we can make things happen. What is your dream?

With endless love,
Coco

Prologue

October 23, 1981

I never doubted that my mother loved me—until she started getting sick. Now understanding mental illness the way I do, I wonder if she didn't try to kill me when I was an infant. The story is a dramatic one. I was born into this world with a giant head that didn't want to come through, but after twenty-six hours of laboring, she finally won. It wouldn't be the only time I relented for her betterment.

I liked to imagine the giant, ugly baby that came out as the first version. I was not an attractive newborn. I know it's hard to believe when you look at the ravishing beauty that became me. But as mentioned above, my head is giant, not to mention I am stubborn as a mule, another trait I can thank my mother for since she's more stubborn than me and all the mules put together. However, have you ever seen an attractive newborn anything? Be honest.

If you asked my mother, she would probably have told you I was not an easy baby. As a matter of fact, she would probably tell you I'm not an easy adult too, and that's simply a lie. So now that I know myself so well, I wonder just how much of my existence she exaggerated, especially the bit where as a two-month-old I threw myself over the counter with such gusto that my entire car seat upended on top of me, shattering my skull and beginning my life of feeling like the problem child.

Follow that experience with the other traumas of infanthood: teething, colic, and various baby diseases, including seventeen cases of tonsillitis resulting in surgery to have the offending organs removed. Suffice it to say, I didn't enjoy life at a young age. My mother enjoyed it less, and of course, hers was the opinion that mattered. The tales of terror were used for humor at family gatherings, but when they were about you, they started to take a toll. In a way, I began to believe it. Something was wrong with me. I was too much—too loud, too bossy, too stubborn, too independent, too dependent, too emotional, too everything. I suppose everyone had an extra close eye on me because of my mother's mental illness, and that was to be expected since they were often hereditary. But it feels good to finally, definitively be able to say, it was not me.

Of course I have no real memory of my childhood before Jimmy, but I imagine it was a lot of my mother reading to me and my father traveling for work, possibly a screaming fight thrown in for good measure. But they did have sex at least one more time, and it resulted in my little brother. I don't know if my obsession with babies began with him or if it was instilled in me, but he was my everything. To look at pictures of us together is often hilarious, because even as an infant, you can see when I was overwhelming him. There are pictures of me with my arms slung around him, squeezing the air out of him. There are also pictures of him gazing back at me just as adoringly. He was my pal and my confidant.

It was right around when he would have started going through puberty that I started keeping a diary. I probably sensed that I was bugging him with word vomit (I can certainly sense it now). However, whether the suggestion to journal was mine, my mother's, or my therapist's, I cannot recall. I'm thankful I kept them, as thankful as I am that I've lugged several boxes of pictures around with me every time I move. Even if no one ever reads this book, even if I never make a dime off publishing, I'll consider it a win, because it will have given me a sense of putting all my memories in one place. If you struggle with any kind of mental illness, you might understand what I mean. I like the idea of being able to access something with ease. The same reason I have prayed for, worked for, and hoped for all my favorite people to be in one place all my life: ease of access.

So that being said (long-windedly), I'll start the story with my first journal entry, with a synopsis of the first fifteen years of my life as follows: I remember it being mostly happy. I was a moody AF kid, no doubt. Hormones and all that. But we had awesome holidays, went on amazing vacations, and generally had anything we wanted or needed, even love. Were there dark spots? Sure. No family is perfect no matter what social media pictures convey. Some people's spots might be darker than others, and it's all relative in my opinion. One man's trash and all that.

Darkness exists everywhere. This isn't that story. This is the story of rising above, the story of Coco Phoenix, aptly nicknamed as a teenager, drawn constantly toward the "neon light at the end of the tunnel"—name that song!—and finally breaking through. Won't you hold on to my wings?

(Y'all, I'm already laughing, because it's 1996, and I'm still talking about losing weight. *My entire life* is a record on repeat.)

The Teenage Years

December 30, 1996

> *Today I weigh 177 on the dot. That means I've lost 5 pounds, 3 oz exactly. No matter what my mom says, I don't eat when I'm not hungry. Then, when I get hungry, I try and eat healthy, but it's hard. When you try so hard not to eat junk, you start to crave it. But I'm going to lose more, than Chad will want me. I'm depressed, I think. 2 days till the new year. I'm going to change, be beautiful & gentle & thin. Well, more later. Bye.*
>
> *Courtney*

Reading this is equal parts hilarious and sad. This little girl's anxiety was already strong, and I want to give her a hug. Another reprieve I've always had: I don't eat when I'm not hungry. What I've learned as an adult is, there are different types of hunger, and I used to eat for all of them.

I am laughing at the spelling errors, which were not many, even at fifteen, and hearing my teenage tone. I wonder when I came into the "If a guy's worth it, he won't care what I weigh" mindset. My mother was among others, I'm sure, but hers were the words that mattered most: "If you'd just lose a little weight, boys would come running."

Even at forty-two and single my entire life, I scoff. You should see some of the men who like me just the way I am. (Does your body type have an entire porn genre devoted to it? I didn't think so!) But that's never been enough for me. I need to connect intellectually with someone to even consider having them be a part of my life. I'm thankful I have never given in to society's norms. I'm thankful I proudly love rainbows despite not being gay. I'm thankful I didn't marry the first guy to say he loved me. (What a dumb experience that was, by the way!) However, I am thankful I've learned to be more gentle. I would have driven myself crazy if I had to be around me at this age. (If I end up alone for the rest of my life, at least there will be a lot more rescued dogs.)

January 3, 1997

> I'm not depressed anymore. I started medicine on the 31st, and so far I lost 4 1/2 lbs. I weigh 172.5. Yea! I will change! Yeaaaaa! Well, gotta pack. Going to dad's. Oh, boy. The kids won't be there & my uncle Gene will. I don't wanna go! Bye.
>
> Courtney

I wonder what medicine I started at fifteen. Weight loss medicine? I doubt I thought that was a good idea then, because I certainly don't now. But when I look back to the other events of this year, I do wonder about my mother's stability. There's a triggering event coming up, but I wonder if something else had already started her downslide. There was a lot that happened in that house that I didn't know of—call it naivete, blissful ignorance, whatever you want—so I wouldn't be surprised, but it does make me think. I do remember being put on lithium at one point and my stepdad having to draw my blood regularly, but for some reason, I didn't think that would be this late in my teenagehood.

Listen to the difference in my tone when I'm with people versus alone.

January 10–11, 1997

> Yesterday & today were the absolute best days of my life. Last night was the dance and Chili's. That was awesome, after we started mingling. Chad, Chad, Chad. Then this morning was tilt. That was a blast too. Chad played w/ my hair. Then @ 5 we went to B&B Do America. I almost fell asleep.
>
> Then Suz had to go home & me, Jennifer, Chad, Michael Har, and Michael Hom went to Cici's. We talked a long time. Then Jenn went home & I was left w/ 3 guys!! They opened doors for me. Michael Har put his feet in my lap & played w/ my hair & kept staring @ me.
>
> Chad opened the door & said, "I'm going to walk you to the door, if you don't mind." I was like, sure! Then I said can I call you tomorrow, he said sure, I said I had something to ask him & that he probably knew what it was. He nodded & said bye & left. To make this the perfect weekend, Chad will have to say yes to the dance. Please-oh-please-oh-

> *please-oh-please-oh-please Lord, let him say yes! I ♥ U & him. Please!*
>
> ♥ *Me*

I'm sitting here wondering if there's actually a winner for the Guinness World Records for most dramatic kid and cackling because I do the same thing now in different fashion—underlines, bold prints, italics, lots of begging God (it still amazes me that my faith was instilled in me), and the heart to end the entry since I was happy (with myself) at the time. Who thinks he said yes? (If you raised your hand, sorry, but you're wrong this time! And spoiler alert: I got very used to rejection!)

January 20, 1997

> *Well, he didn't say yes, but that's okay. We're still friends. He told me something that I can never tell anyone. I'm glad he trusts me that much. I've lost 14 lbs in 3 weeks. I weigh 169.0. Yea! Well, nothing else to say. Bye.*
>
> *Me*

The sadness in my tone when I said, "We're still friends." That phrase would be my best friend over the years. "As long as I still have you as a friend. Don't let me push you away."

January 31, 1997

> *Chad likes Sara. When I first found out, (he told me; we talked for 3 hours) I was okay w/ it. I was happy, & I thought I was over him. Boy, was I ever wrong. It sunk in today. 3 days later, & I cried so hard my stomach hurt.*
>
> *You can't fall out of love that easily. And I am in love. How I know is, I think about him all the time. I make up stories about him, I dream about him, & I still like him no matter what he does. The Ryan thing, Sara, everything.*
>
> *He wrote her a song. I almost cried. But I'm going to help him get her, if that'll make him happy. I think she's scared of him. Or scared*

> *of boys all together? He's one of my best friends, & I wouldn't hurt him for anything. I wonder if he thinks that about me? And if he does, if he realizes how much this is hurting me?*
>
> 💔 *A (broken-hearted) person*

Do we love that hard from birth? Who teaches us to allow our hearts to be so open we fall in love with people who don't return the favor? I won't say I've never been loved before; that's silly. I've had lots of people love me. But have I ever (that I know of) inspired in someone that passion that always gets lit in me? Nope. It hardly seems fair.

February 8, 1997

> *Well, nothing has changed about my love for Chad. Hell, if anything, I love him more. I also, however, like Josh Peoples too. But unfortunately he's going out with Audrey. He's cheating on her w/ me! Next Friday's the Valentine's Dance. Suzie's going to talk to Michael & Michael to Chad. I hope he likes me. But that's wishful thinking. Anyway, I have nothing else to say. G-G!*
>
> ♥ *Me*

So somehow, in the space of a week, I managed to convince myself that his love for Sara was fleeting. A week later and I was willing to put my heart on the line for the same guy, the same person, who rejected me mere days before. I sure do view life through rose-colored glasses sometimes.

February 23, 1997

> *Sorry I haven't written in so long. Yesterday Suzie & I sang at UIL & we both got 2's. Then we delivered fertilizer with the Scouts. Chad & I got pulled off the pick-up & spent the rest of the day alone together. Everybody asked me if we were going out. I wish I could have said yes. Oh well. Then Reed Mudley took us home. My parents weren't home, so I went back to Chad's. His mom wouldn't let us be alone in his room w/ the door shut. I ate dinner*

there & we walked to Michael Harmony's & to Ryan Macaw's. Ryan has been sober for almost 2 months. Yea!

Okay, on to a way diff. subj. The reason no one was home was b/c they were out at my mother's b-day dinner. I feel so awful. I had no way of getting in touch w/ them though. I didn't have my pager, & we were driving all day w/o a phone. My mother is so mad at me. She has a right, though. I think she hates me. I'm going to kill myself. But I can't. It would hurt too many people, & after seeing how much Neal South hurt people, I couldn't do that. I think I'm going to spend a few days at Suzanne's. Bye.

♥ *Me*

This was the roller coaster of moods that alarmed people when I was a kid. I read this and hurt so much for this kid, this teenager who lived solely for other people, even when she was young. That would be the only time you'll see me write something like "I want to kill myself" down. (I hope beyond hope I never spoke the words out loud to anyone.)

If you want to know the truth, this entry is crossed out and edited in several places. The two most notable are a "not true" written in red ink above "We were driving all day without a phone," and "going to" is scratched out heavily, and "want to" is written above it. I couldn't even lie to myself without making amends. It got to the point, as an adult, where I wouldn't even try to lie.

This isn't an easy thing, reading these journals with the knowledge I have now. It actually makes me angry, and I spent enough time being angry, which even makes me angrier. I look at these entries, the one above, written the day after my mother's birthday, and the next one, nearly three months later. Coming off the heels of a depression spell that ate six months of my forty-first year, I ache for the Coco who hid in her bedroom for ten weeks because her mother was likely giving her the silent treatment for making a (somewhat honest) mistake and choosing herself over someone else. I understand her anger; I'd be angry if my mother missed my birthday dinner too. Oh, wait. She did, many of them, sometimes because she was holding a grudge. And how silly is that?

By May, I had forgiven myself even if she hadn't fully forgiven me. (She never did fully forgive.)

COURTNEY CANNON

May 9, 1997

> *Wow, I sounded depressed. Life is going much better. Tonight was the last dance of 9th grade, besides the 9th grade party. Chad was there, writing. He seemed depressed. Brandon said I was going to be the next dance, but Erin got to him first, that bitch! God! I cried. Then we went to Chili's. Brad's not really that bad. Anyway, g-g.*
>
> ♥ *Me*

And there, finally, is the first mention of my first real boyfriend, Brandon. I'm sad I wasn't journaling when we dated, because his story is the one real first I feel like I got to experience, so much so that I created *Diary of a Stranger*, which was the first version of this book, based on my relationship with him. I'd even go so far as to say I compared every relationship I had in the future to him. I suppose everyone feels like that about their first love, but I still believe that Brandon *is* a good man. I got lucky at least once.

Because there are nearly six months where I don't write again, including what would have been my sixteenth birthday and a pretty remarkable experience, in my opinion, I'll use these pages to tell what I do remember about that time in my life.

For most of my life, I've thought of myself as someone who likes younger men because of both Brandon, who was a year and a half younger, though only a grade below, and all my brother's gorgeous friends, who ranged in ages from eighteen months to three years younger than me. I was insanely boy crazy, as we used to call it. (Do they still say that?) The walls of my room were *covered* in pictures from *Tiger Beat* and the likes, and I constantly had crushes. I daydreamed and imagined and hoped and planned and prayed for the one person who would eventually be mine. It was all I ever wanted out of life: someone to love who would love me back.

I knew Brandon as a sevvie when he came to Forest Meadow. My friend Erin dated him before I did, and I say dated because I don't remember much of the details. Erin was as boy crazy as I was, but I didn't like her particular way of going about it, and I remember feeling sorry for Brandon before I even really knew him. (Erin, if you read this, forgive me. Teenage silliness!) But it fizzled out as quickly as I expected it to, to the point where when I saw him at summer camp many months later and as an introduction said "Didn't you use to date Erin J——," his answer was a firm no.

My sister Audrey was also a huge flirt, and despite not enjoying girl competition even then, it was strong with my sister when it came to Brandon. I knew without a doubt he liked me, so I asked her one night not to flirt with him. She said snottily, "He flirts with me too," and all I could think was, "That's not the point." But I simply moved on, because even if it was true, I knew he wasn't into her like that. It felt good to finally have a boy's attention, and having the added bonus of him looking like Brandon did? I will say it again: I got lucky at least once.

That entire week at camp, we cuddled while watching the movies at the end of a hard workday, and I'd fall asleep on his shoulder. I was there for two weeks; Brandon and his sister were there for one. I was so sad when they went home that I didn't stay for the rest of the summer with my brother and sister. I went home so I could see Brandon. I got to hang out with him a few times, my favorite of which was when two other friends from camp, Scot and Chrysta, came over, and we watched *The Shining*. I had already seen it, so I slyly used it to my advantage.

"There's a scary part coming up," I said demurely. "I need a hand to hold."

(By this time, Chrysta and Scot were making out.)

Brandon held up both hands and said, "Which one do you want?"

I resisted the urge to smile and seriously answered, "The one closest to me."

He gave me his right hand and twined his fingers in mine, then wrapped his left hand over mine.

To this day, it was the safest I felt when holding someone's hand. Possibly because I hadn't had my heart broken yet? Possibly because I was still young enough to truly trust love when it was offered? Who knows? I know someday, I'll get back there, because I finally believe I'm worth it. I love freely and without strings, so I know there are truly people in the world who do.

I can't say for sure how long we were together. I remember tricking my parents into letting him spend the night by getting my brother to ask them. I remember my sister asking him once—clearly, we got over the competition—why he never put his arm around me and then him draping it around my shoulders just as quickly. I remember him talking about the difference between boxers and briefs when it came to sweaty balls with my brother as they ran laps around the track and my being so thrilled when they were honest about what I had overheard.

I remember him breaking up with me about a week into the ninth grade, saying he wasn't ready for a girlfriend, and then getting together with Sara what felt like mere days later. Was that when I started to crush on Chad? I remember almost failing world geography, which Chad and I had together, because I spent the entire class learning *him*. What did I care about Russia or New Zealand when this beautiful, interesting creature cared about *me*?

So then came my sixteenth birthday. I remember taking driver's ed with Kelly at Valley View Mall, where we learned to drive on Camaros. My mother hates that I say that, because she says she taught me to drive on the van. I neither remember that nor care if it's true. I also took driver's education at Valley View Mall and learned to drive on a Camaro.

(It was during this time that I believe my mother was at her sickest that we knew about as kids. Princess Diana died in August of this year, and I vividly remember my mother getting the news, nearly falling down the stairs in dramatics, and retreating to her bedroom for weeks. As an adult, I relayed this memory to my brother, and he added that he remembered being the one who delivered the news to her.)

For my sweet sixteen, I invited three girlfriends to spend the night in the Westin Galleria Hotel at the Galleria Mall. We also went to dinner and a movie, which Chad got to come to. We saw *My Best Friend's Wedding*, which made me cry like a freaking baby and surely made Chad hugely uncomfortable, yet he stayed my friend. He still cared about me. We continued to get closer until I considered myself in love with him, and despite sharing a few amazing firsts with him too, he was never my boyfriend or my first kiss. (For the record, I asked him to another dance as a sophomore, when I was at a different school from him. He accepted, and we had a really great time, including my first slow dance with my head on a boy's shoulder.)

So there we were. I was a driving sophomore at Richardson High School, filled with teenage angst that drove me to do insane things that only hurt myself. A pro self-sabotager—that was me.

November 11, 1997

> It's funny (more ironic) to think that I've had this book for a year & I don't have more than 10 entries, despite all the turmoil I endure in life. I'm sitting here writing rather than doing my homework, which is just one of the many, many things wrong with me right now. I've begun letting Chad go. It's unhealthy for me to like him so much, even though I ♥ other guys too. He will always remain my second best friend in the world, but that's gonna be it, if I can ever let him go fully.
>
> I cheated on a chem test. Dumbest thing I ever did. Then I lied about it. And there have been a few other lying/cheating occurrences. And now I'm grounded a month. I'm gonna have to do volunteer

> work. There are gonna be a lot of entries between now & Dec. 8, when I get off. Please don't let them cancel the Europe trip.
>
> ♥ Me

Spoiler alert: they did cancel the Europe trip. I was supposed to be going to Europe with my best friend's Latin class. (Her mother was the teacher.) I don't blame them for doing that, in a way. As an adult, I have zero tolerance for lying. But grounding me for a month *and* the Europe trip? I've still never been to Europe. Did the punishment fit the crime for an otherwise pretty good kid? I don't know.

Fortunately, however, here was also where Suzanne and I did the school musical, *The Will Rogers Follies*. At Richardson, which was a magnet school for arts and sciences, you didn't have to audition if you just wanted to be in the chorus. And at the time, my audition fright was strong. So Suzie and I went to rehearsals, had fun getting to know other cast members, developed crushes—surprise, surprise!—and generally had a ball. The couple of months I disappeared this time, I imagine, were filled with a lot of love and light despite a possibly tense home environment due to endless hours of musical practice and cute boys.

January 23, 1998

> Hmm, there shore weren't a lot of entries. But now, the musical is almost over. Despite all my complaining, I've found I really will miss it. I will miss Chris Layla. Mark Skrilla & Chris Battalion don't have any classes w/ me, & I barely will see them. Mark, man, I will so miss Mark. I really really like him. He's darling, hot, sweet, & funny. Geez, I'm going to miss him.
>
> ♥ Me

January 24, 1998

> I really thought I was gonna cry. But I didn't. I got 2 hugs from TJ. I asked Mark if I could model a character after him. He said "go for it." He didn't show up at the party until 12:30, when it was over. That made me want to cry. I won't see him, like,

> ever! And I think he's scared of me now. But, hey, at least I have his permission. I really like him. I feel like I can't talk to Suzanne about him bcuz she doesn't think he's cute. She gets this far away look in her eyes when I talk about him. And it doesn't seem fair b/c she talks about Philip every single second! I can't really say I hate him anymore, but geez, I know him. She doesn't know Mark. I hate listening to her talk & talk & then she won't listen to me. Anyway, I really do like Skrilla. And I want to have a party.
>
> ♥ Me

Somehow, this must have been the beginning of the end of my friendship with Suzanne. I had come to find out that I intimidated her into a lot of things, like skipping school when she didn't want to, and it made me feel horrible. Reading this, where I felt like I could no longer talk to her, makes me think I began to pull away.

This next entry is where another big crush comes into play, and I met him through my Lake Highlands friends. Connecting the dots is weird. I wonder if you guys will even care about chronological order.

March 1, 1998

> Mark is still my fantasy, but now I like a true-in-life person named Josh Quacky. He's sweet & funny & flirty. I've only known him, went out w/ him, two times. But I really like him! I say that a lot. Anyway, I'mma go to bed!
>
> ♥ Me

March 22, 1998

> I am talking to Josh now. He can be a big jerk sometimes, but he is still really cute. Hmm, I don't know what to write. Today I went out with Josh. It would have been fun, but like I said... hehe. And Eddie & Chris & Laura were there. And Laura thinks Eddie is very cute. And that it's adorable when guys are shy. And we are going to see Grease next week-

end but Josh isn't b/c he doesn't like it. But I'm going to go do my chem. Buh bye!

♥ *Me*

Y'all, here come the dramatics again. It was the end of the school year, which meant I had to decide to stay at RHS or move to LHHS. In my entries, I made it sound like the decision was mine, but I do not remember that being the case. I ultimately think I lost RHS because I didn't maintain the grades necessary to remain in the magnet program. I wonder, if I'd graduated from there, would I have had a better chance at staying at Baylor or even choosing another path entirely? But you know my belief: no day but today. The decisions are made, my life is what it is, and I firmly believe I have control of the outcome. I somewhat hope God is working through my fingers, because it creeps me out a bit to think of having total control. Jesus, take the wheel, eh?

But these crushes! Good grief, these crushes.

May 31, 1998

> *Oh, God! Life is so hard. I want so much to go back to school, to RHS, my home away from home! God, I miss it. Where should I go? Preston... & Brandon... & Josh... oh my God! Preston, holy cow, it's back to Preston again. I don't think I've ever liked anyone more than Chad, but Preston is a close second. Why? He's an unreachable freshman! Oh, God, please let summer school bring relief... please let me lose weight & get a bf & make decisions. Do I really like Pres? Or am I anticipating a boyfriend? Help me!*

♥ *Me*

June 14, 1998

> *Wah! Cameron thinks I like Preston! She can't think that! I don't wanna lose her friendship. I'm going to start starving myself. It's got to work. Pleease! Oh, God, pleeease! I need a life! Pleaase!*

♥ *Me*

The desperation in my tone at the thought of losing a girlfriend because I had an uncontrollable crush on her boyfriend is tough. The older I got, the more I understood you couldn't help how you felt about someone, but you could help what you did about it.

These next few entries, all made over the summer before my junior year, are riddled with anxiety. I remember it being a good summer, with lots of church stuff, which I had just gotten into, hence meeting Cameron, who was our pastor's daughter. There was some drama, like wanting to tell someone not to look at me because it hurt, but I guess that's what makes a good story, right? I don't think anyone would want to read (or watch) if it is boring.

July 12, 1998

> *Cams still probably thinks I like Pres ♥ but she's nice to me again. Cams, Pres ♥, & Jim are leaving for camp 2morrow. So not fair. I want to go soooo bad. Stupid summer school. And I don't wanna go to Newport either. Oh, I'm going to cry. One more week of being grounded, then Calif, then 21 days (3 weeks) til school. Oh, yuck. Please let me go to RHS. Please! And please help me to lose weight in this last 1 month 1 week. Please God, give me the will.*
>
> ♥ *Me*

July 29, 1998

> *This was the first day I've seen Preston in 2 1/2 weeks. I caught him looking at me a couple of times. I wanted to tell him don't, this hurts. Tomorrow I really want to go to 6-Flags. I want to tell Preston I like him, but I don't want to hurt Cams. Oh, oh, oh, oh. Anyway Newport was the bomb. I wanted to stay forever. I should go. I ♥ Preston Vanderbilt so much. Oh, why can't he be my age?*
>
> ♥ *Me*

July 30, 1998

> *I went to 6-Flags with church today. It was awesome, basically. Headache now—more tomorrow.*
>
> ♥ *Me*

While the summer was fun, I did not get my wish to go back to RHS. I must have been sadder about it than I remembered—it wasn't like I was going to a whole new school, and I had tons of friends at LH!—because within the first few weeks, I was in depression mode. I know for a fact that by this time, my family thought I had bipolar. I had been on heavy medication already and taken to therapy. Mood swings I had, for sure.

The more I grew to understand my anxiety and depression, not to mention possible ADHD, the more I knew I didn't. The new crushes going as quickly as they came just proved my intense need to have people around me. It's a little sad actually. I hooked on to anyone who showed me attention, especially of the male species. It took me to until my very late thirties to understand my worth didn't directly hinge on whether a man appreciated my existence.

October 6, 1998

> Catch up time! I haven't talked to Preston in forever. At 6-Flags, we spent most of the day 2gether, then @ the end, we walked w/ Cams & Justin Conrad. Fun! Well, now I like another freshman in addition to Pres, Joey Jacobs, & Josh Q. His name's Russell. Why do I like younger guys? Sigh. Life's tough. All the freshmen are so cute. I wish Jimmy & all his friends were juniors (Jim & I twins)!
>
> PS. Today was Pres' & Cams' 8-month anniversary
>
> ♥ Me

October 8, 1998

> I think it's time for me to do a heart-spiller. I'm in one of my depressed modes—gaining weight, always wanting to cry, the works—I hate it. I just got grounded for my grades—meaning no social life until next report card—also meaning missing 4 of the potentially best weekends of my life: the RHS vs LHHS game this weekend, along w/ the retreat, HC game & HC next weekend, then my birthday weekend, & then Halloween. I could have had so much fun.
>
> Today I let Russ drive home & Jimmy got pissed & walked home. Truly, I rarely think about Pres

> *anymore cause of Russ. I mean, if I saw Pres again, I'd probably start liking him more. I don't think I'll ever fully stop liking him—I've liked him for 3 years, for heaven's sake. But Russell, man. I hate myself, truly. I know I'm pretty, but I'm fat. For some reason unbeknownst to me, guys are dense & can't see past that. I danced w/ Brandon Mars today. We hardly looked at each other, but it kinda loosened up. I'm thinking about RHS & the seniors (Cameron L. mainly) & Justin Conrad. I wish I was at college now. Maybe life would be easier. I hate high school, esp. being a junior. I can't wait to next year.*
>
> *My lowest grade w/ honors is an 87!*
> *I dislike my mom so much right now.*

I remember this entry vividly, because when I reread it as a young adult, I remember being horrified that she even grounded me for an 81, much less an 87 with my honors points. But now I'm also horrified that this was as a junior in high school. I thought maybe eighth grade? An 87 in high school seems awesome to me, especially for someone like me who could never take a test, whether I studied or not.

I joke a lot that I was lucky to graduate high school, but that was mainly because I skipped so many classes I was in danger of repeating just because of that. So I shaped up for the end of the semester, got some tutoring help from friends in computer sciences, and graduated. I also got into Baylor and had a partial scholarship based on my grades.

The next entry is about the retreat I so badly wanted to go on. It says, "My mom would have let me go anyway," which leads me to believe she was simply torturing me for my grades.

October 11, 1998

> *This weekend was basically one of those that you wish you could take a picture in every scene in every act—it was wonderful, awesome—oh, man! I was going to try to relive it hour by hour, but I will probably leave something out & have to come back & add it—so here goes.*
>
> *First I have to explain that I got ungrounded. My mom would have let me go anyway.*

NOT THE F——ING GILMORE GIRLS

Ok, I got up at about 7 to get ready. We got to the bus & we went to the camp—no sleep. It was boring 'coz I didn't have my CDs or anyone to talk to.

When we got to camp, it was about 10:15. I don't remember what we did after we got all settled (10-12 & 7-9). But after lunch, when Crystal told me (one out of like a thousand people) that I had really pretty eyes, we went hiking. Anna & I started talking & that's when we clicked. She's so sweet. Anyway, when we got back down the hill, we went to look at the haystacks & me, Cams, & Anna stayed for like 25 minutes, jumping on hay. When we went back, we went & played volleyball & nuke 'em. It was fun.

(I'm just going to outline the retreat & then tell the fun stuff.)

We had worship after dinner, I think. (Sorry, it all ran together.) At worship, I was sitting left ankle crossed over right & Jordan put his leg on mine. My left foot fell so fast asleep—I was moving my toe & I could see it, but I couldn't feel it. After worship, it was getting chilly by then. Anna & Amelia helped me move my stuff into their cabin. Then we went outside. Oh, no! We had worship late, I remember. Then we looked at stars & took a hike in the dark. Scary! Anna, my leader, my saver, lead me by the hand. Awesome kid, she is.

I think it was after the hike that me, Anna, Michael Chase, Austin, Spencer, Amelia, Lacey, Shannon?, & Marshall, got our sleeping bags & pillows & curled up on the boys' porch. First we had a massage party & I got possibly the best massage I've ever had from Michael. He definitely knows how to use his hands. Then Spencer suggested "Honey, I love you," but we only played one round before we switched to Truth or Dare. Marshall told me he wanted to ask Anna out & he wanted me to find out if she liked him.

Oh yeah, there was a dance also after the hike. It was basically boring. Rhett & I & a few other people walked out to the field where 5 peeps were in *a circle. Then Rhett & I walked over to Jordan & Greta. Jordan had his hands on her ass. Then Rhett left & John Chase came over & Greta & Jordan left. At about midnight, we were spose to watch a movie. My group was all together at the front in our blankets. But the TV didn't work, so we opted to talk—everyone else went outside. We were just chatting it up. Michael & I have a lot in common.*

Earlier Amelia & I were looking for gum, so we went to the guys' cabin. Someone said we couldn't go in. Marshall came out, gave me ten & a hug, & said I was awesome. Then Jordan came out & asked if he smelled good. All of a sudden A&F cologne hit me. Jordan & Marshall both had it on. So I had to tell them they had to sit on either side of me. They did & I was lovenly engulfed. Ahh! Yum!

I am now getting sleepy enough so that I can't remember. I was really excited when Adam got there. He's sweet too, & an awesome dancer, esp swing. I wish I could dance.

Marshall & Amelia were stuck to me, & I was attatched to Anna. As I remember it, I'll add more. It kicked such ass. I had a blast. Today was kinda worse cause we didn't have much free time—more if I can remember!

♥ *Me*

I was always more about the people than the places. It sounds like it was a magical time with a bunch of people who were (again) younger than me. Did I yearn to be Mama Coco even then? Was that even, possibly, what all the crushes were about? God surely works in me in mysterious ways, including making me tell my best friend's mom that I wanted to be a mom by the time I was sixteen. I even said "a young mom." I wonder if I would have thought that if *Teen Mom* had been on MTV yet.

I'm sad that I again neglected to write about my birthday. Despite—or possibly because of—being an October baby, October is my favorite month, and it's always held a rarer magic than the other months. I'm a birthday month girl now, and yet I barely mentioned it when I was a kid. My father moved out of our house on my seventh birthday. (I remember the U-Haul in the driveway getting in the way of us playing the piñata properly. I bashed my friend Patrick in the nose with the baseball bat while I was blindfolded!) Did that taint every birthday after that? Who knows? All I know is how important birthdays have become to me as an adult.

October 30, 1998

> I think I'm getting to the point if I don't back off from liking Russell, I'm going to get very hurt. Tonight Jimmy was spose to spend the night with Russ & AT, but then he called saying all they were going to do was drink—I almost burst into tears. Then I went to Court H's house & like a billion people got in the van—when Russ got in, all "get out y'all, I got a ride!" I almost said "no you don't!" Then I did burst into tears w/ Court & Alex & Jess standing at the window. I couldn't stop crying & Court hugged me. When I dropped Russ & AT off, Russ made me get out of the car & he hugged me for a long time. I started to cry on his shoulder when he said "I'm sorry" cause he didn't know what I was upset for!

November 9, 1998

> Man, I didn't write about the Halloween party. Oh well. Mom said if I have a failing grade on my report card, I had no social life until the end of the calendar year—oh, big woop, right. I have no social life! I'm so depressed! I'm not a brain person—I'm creative, not smart. My comp. sci. final's going to kill me. Anyway.
> I love Russell still—even though he threw up on my brother.

November 30–December 1, 1998

> It's midnight on a school day, but I just had to write so I could get some sleep. Russell gave Jimmy back my friendship bracelet. He's pissed b/c I wouldn't let him talk to Jimmy so he's mad forever now. I said that was fine—he'd just never get a ride. He said the Marses were quicker, smelled better, & comfy van—so I hung up on him. The Marses left him, so he walked home. We went to offer him a

ride & he said, "I'm not getting in the damn car!" I feel awful. I just indulged a whole box of chocolates. Blech! Everytime I look @ my right hand, I start crying for the bracelet—it's all stretched out. Please let him take it back!

♥ (t) me & ♥ Russell

I don't remember feeling particularly stronger about Russell than I did for anybody else in that particularly hormonal time of my life, but fighting with him brought forth an idea of passion I didn't get with anyone else, so that was fun. I might not have ever had the typical boyfriend experiences that I craved so desperately in high school, but I had more than my fair share of drama.

The frustrating part comes when I see the terrible decisions I made. Yes, I was young. Maybe that's the only excuse I need. I read over this next entry, and it sounds like a lie to me, much like the day I skipped my mother's birthday dinner. But I didn't edit it, so perhaps it wasn't a lie. Perhaps I just didn't think she'd mind.

January 14, 1999

> My life is pitiful. I borrowed $25 for a BSB shirt, using my mom's credit card w/ the full intention of paying it back. But she called it stealing & took Disciple Now away from me. I can't do that—I need DN so much! The threat is, if I go to DN, I have to move out. Move out! I'm 17! I don't have a job! I'm not a bad kid. I don't drink or do drugs or have sex! Geez. Audrey's done all of the above & my mother keeps forgiving her. My scalp is so bad & my hair is falling out. I need DN so much! This is my time to get to know Christ—my time away from my mother. This weekend will surely kill us both if I can't go. Surely.

January 19, 1999

> Well, needless to say, it didn't kill either of us. We're on good terms again. I went to the Sat night part of DN—but I missed all the best stuff. Regretted

muchly. I have to do my hw. Thought I needed to update.

♥ *(t) Courtney*

February 11, 1999

I went to see She's All That with Laura tonight. All through the movie, we were like "Oh my God" at Freddie Prinze Jr. I've never been that affected by an actor, performance or looks, since except maybe Ben Affleck. This guy was incredible. His eyes & smile hit me sooo hard. And Paul Walker, ooh! "Nothing compares...to you!" At the end, I was out of breath from awe. Laura & I laughed so much walking out! People must have thought we were crazy! But it felt good to laugh. Tomorrow's Favorites! Yikes! Oh, Zach was so beautiful! Paul Walker's smile is to die for as well!

♥ *Me*

February 14, 1999

It's 2:30 in the morning Valentine's Day. Last night was Favorites. It was fun. We went to Royal Tokyo & Mike loved it. Then we went to the dance & saw Brandon (♥) who looked incredible, Josh (♥) & Chloe, & Tyler Grantham, who looked great in a tux. Then at 12 we went to Denny's. Michael's really funny. But I gotta hit the sack coz I got to babysit tomorrow.

♥ *Me*

These are the moments I wish I recorded with more detail. What I wouldn't give to have this already written, ready-for-Netflix rom-com at my fingertips. I was cute, I was funny, I was dramatic, and I had boy drama. It's what movies are made of. But alas, the brain works in mysterious ways, and I believe mine has invented a very sparkly canopy to lay over the darkness. So I chat in between entries, and I tell you what I wish it had been, what I remember it being.

March 11, 1999

We got to Colorado Sunday night at about 5:15 their time, then to the condos at about 8:30, 8:45 after grocery shopping. The condos were very nice. Kelly & I roomed together, & Beth & Em, & Lauren & Mel slept on the fold-out couch. That night we had like sooo much trouble deciding what to do for dinner. Then we went to Darren's room, who was across the hall with Travis, Adam McCool, Alan, Robbie, Dimitri, & Nick Gillian. We were the only people w/o a chaperone. So we had the meeting & then the 6 of us watched Dazed and Confused. Then we went to bed.

At 8:30 the next morning, we were renting skis & lockers. I put my shoes in Jordan & Jimmy's & very much regretted it later. So me & Jimmy & Marshall were playing on the snow trying to get the hang of skiing. Marshall fell standing up. Then Jimmy went up w/ Mel, Lauren, Sarah Poppy, & Juli maybe? Marshall & I found Sarah Jasper & went to wait for ski lessons. Sarah had told me she saw Blake Exeter. Ooo-wie! Hot. So we had ski lessons, & Jimmy had come to his senses & come joined us. M. got sick & had to sit down, then I did.

I went to the top after I drank a lot & skied down slowly. The teacher said I was his favorite. There was this really cute guy named Ryan Fitzpatrick that goes to Fellowship in Waco or Plano. He was really sweet. Then me & Sarah & Jimmy & Marshall went to get pizza, then Marshall & I left w/ Carson. I was going to meet M. in the spa. In my room, I emptied my pockets & laid down. I thought I heard footsteps on the stairs, so I looked outside & the door locked behind me so I walked in bare feet to try & find the spa but I couldn't, so I went to M's, & he wasn't there. Then later I saw him, & he let me call the housekeeper. She never came, but Emily did.

So I went in & got into my swimsuit & me & M & Em went to the pool. Soon every1 was in there. Then we took showers & the senior guys, us, Juli, & Cams went to eat then Juli & I shopped. Then we went to a meeting. The next morning, I slept until 9, then I watched TV all day. My calves hurt like a bitch. Then we all went to the pool & the oldest girls decided to have a party. In the spa we met Stingle who had two broken arms. That night, we watched Face/Off w/ a lot of people & Carson fell asleep while I stroked his hair & his back. I am in love w/ Carson. Totally in love with him. The 7th grade boys really like me: Marshall, Spencer, Carson...all my babies.

Then everyone except Rachel Grateful went home. It was about one. Then Stingle called & we went down to their house. Stingle was crazy-ass drunk. He & his friend Cade were talking to us. Then Rachie went home & Stingle called & talked to me & Lauren who we woke up, & Kelly. We tried to get them upstairs & finally they snuck through their window & came up. Cade was getting sober. Stingle was still trashed.

We were laughing so hard at 2:30 that Lauren farted & we named her Mrs. Pooter. Stingle didn't even notice, but Cade's face was red with laughter. They finally went home at about 3:10. I finished packing & went to sleep.

Next morning we had to have our stuff out of the condo & into Darren's room. Then we went on the lift for our group picture. The lift scared the shit out of me. When we got on, Carson sat back on my arm & my poles were on his right side. Carson had to get them & they were tangled with his, & he thought they were gonna drop. My ski was also tangled w/ his. When we got off, I tripped & I swear Carson & I were both going to go down. But we didn't. We took the picture & of course I got scared going down & started to cry. Thankfully, Carson wasn't with me. Marshall & Cams & Sarah J. were with me & Mrs. Mathers.

But suddenly the hill went steep & I couldn't go any farther. Cams & them went to call ski patrol & Mrs. Mathers stayed with me. The snow mobile took me back to the lift & I got to ride it down. Kinda embarrassing, but fun. Then I went to return my skis & went to Darren's where Robbie & Dimitri were. I was freezing my ass off. So we watched TV a while. Then people came back. Carson fell asleep & he's so cute. Finally we got on the bus. Carson & Travis had an argument, heated. Then Marshall said something mean either to or about Carson & Travis totally changed gears & goes, "Shut up. If you ever say something bad about Carson again, I'll break your neck! Only I can talk mean about my brother!" Aww!

Then we did a massage & Carson told me I have great hands. Then we did that elbow thing. When we got to the airport, we got Mickey D's then went to the plane. We sat down & Darren borrowed my CD player. This girl behind me goes "I'm so nauseous," and me and Darren look behind us, then at each other & burst out laughing. That's like the only time we really talked. Then Cams took us home. We found out Ace died. I got a new camera & only got 5 pictures. It was a lot of fun.

♥ Courtney

March 15, 1999

There was one thing I left out. At the meeting on night 2, we got in groups to have prayer. It was like we were telling a story to God. Beth started to cry, then I did when Sarah J started talking about how sometimes one didn't believe God was there. Then Sarah P & Juli said they had done some stuff they couldn't forgive themselves for. Then Sarah J mentioned Neal South & I really started to cry. Then we sang Angel. It was sad but cool, if you know what I mean.

♥ Me

So what do ya know? There are a few good stories fully written for our (hopefully) mutual pleasure. I hope it's as fun for y'all to read as it is for me even if you don't know the people. Imagine the thrill of seeing real snow for the first time as an adult, which I didn't write of course. (Jordan and I dubbed ourselves the naked snow bunnies club.) Imagine the panic I had facing a hill with undiagnosed vertigo. Imagine the joy the seventeen-year-old heart got from being able to baby a bunch of boys. I have mostly happiness rereading all these memories, because it's clear I *knew* love and joy and delight from both children and men alike, which is what I have craved for my entire life. It makes me a little sad to think that may be all I ever get, but it won't stop me from searching for it at every turn.

March 19, 1999

> *I'm in such a good mood, & I don't know why. In 5th period we did Tae-bo & I think that has something to do w/ it. But today Russell came over & took a shower. He has a great body. We had a talk about Suzie & he might get back together w/ her. For his sake I hope they do. But I told him to treat her right. He said he definitely will & that he misses her so much. He knows how special she is. Jeremy Mars has a really good voice. I'm giddy for some reason. Let them all have a great night—Lisa & Jim, but most especially Russell & Suzie.*
>
> ♥ *Me*

March 24, 1999

> *Today was UIL. We (Choraliers & A Capella girls; 1st period guys & A Capella guys; A Capella) all got Sweepstakes. I'm sooo hyper. The day was all in all awesome. It is 10:00 and there is no way I can sleep. Kelly & I were acting drunk today—singing at the top of our lungs, making Laura mad.*
>
> *We talked to Doug for a while. He looked at me the entire time we were talking. I am in love with him. Oh sweetie. I am so excited. At the end, we, Kel, Laura, & me, were thanking God for good directors, then Kel said "And all the hot a Capella guys," then we both screamed as we were walking out: "and hot Espree guys!" to Jacob Wobbler. He heard us. Please let me see & talk to Doug more. Maybe he could be it for me, right?*
>
> ♥ *Me*

And there it is, a simple prayer—and yes, if you haven't picked up on that, all my entries are prayers—and one I said every time I clicked with a new guy. To start hoping at seventeen—and long before if my crush on Kurt from *The Sound of Music* was any indication at five!—but still never see it happen at nearly forty-two is tiring. I might have even considered myself done with hoping a couple of months ago. I am the *eternal optimist*, and hope I will forever.

March 26, 1999

> *I don't have anything special to say; I just need to write. I'm in a bad mood. I hate everything my mother has said to me since she's been back. I just want good grades, a life, and Doug. And a fair chance at Espree. Please let me bring up my grades & have Laura's party here. That would so kick ass. Sigh. Just let something in my life go right!*
>
> ♥ *Me*

Something I learned over the years: appreciate the small stuff, the in-between stuff, more. I try to find a reason to celebrate every day—there's an app for that!—and I make sure to do something I enjoy for at least an hour before bed every day. It makes it easier to say I have a good life despite the big, looming *but* that's been there since I was a kid. "But I don't have a boyfriend" transitioned into "But I have no one to share it with," which moved finally into "But you can't save everyone."

I began to focus on making sure I could save myself first and foremost. You hear it all your life: you won't find someone who will love you until you love yourself. I thought I had loved myself my entire life, so that statement always frustrated me. But I've learned as an adult that almost everything I do is a form of self-harm: overeating to the point of illness, picking at scabs or ingrown hairs until I bleed, and not showering for days at a time, which is not great for allergy-prone skin. It's a strange mirror to look in. Would you do that to a friend who is crying? Then why are you doing it to yourself?

I will also never not have dogs. They are the best of friends.

April 18, 1999

> *I went to see Anything Goes at Woodrow today. It was soooo good, mostly bc of Adam ♥ & Travis. After the end, I gave Adam a hug & he held me for so long. I was like "You did so great" & he was like*

> *"Thank you so much!" God he's sweet. I'm going to miss him so much next year. Sooo much. Anyway.*
>
> ♥ Me

May 7, 1999

> *Tonight was the choir banquet. I couldn't take my eyes off Doug. And Stuart was crying, which made me cry more. And Doug doesn't know I like him & he's leaving. I don't really have... I walked up to Stuart & put my hand on his arm & said, "You don't know my name, but you look so sad I had to come see if you're okay." He promised he was. Cry.*
>
> ♥ Me

Not to toot my own horn, but I wonder how he felt after I did that. I've learned from people who do know my name that my touch has somewhat of a healing property. Even writing this, I feel extraordinarily arrogant saying so, but it's because I haven't touched anyone in a while. When I do, especially if it's someone I'm close to, I feel powerful afterward—dogs, babies, and adult humans. I like to think it's God, but everybody has a different belief. Does it lessen your faith in me? It feels amazing to think that finally, I've learned what I was put on this earth to do: Touch. Feel. Heal. Love.

May 9, 1999

> *Today was Mom's Day. Last night we spent the night in the Fairmont Hotel. It was nice. We ate lobster bisque & dover sole in the Pyramid Room. Then we watched V Blues & At First Sight. Today we went to Scarborough Faire. I got a rainbow choker. A wrap to match, & a henna tatoo. It was fun. 19 more days!*
>
> ♥ & fear Court

The "19 more days" could only have been until end of school. But what was I fearing?

June 19, 1999

> Saw Never Been Kissed last night. I started crying & almost couldn't stop. It was so ♥-breakingly true-to-life! But it was sooo good. God, it was good. I want to have a church party. Can't wait til Tuesday!
>
> ♥ Me

June 29, 1999

> I'm in a strange mood—not exactly depressed, but on my way down. I was watching Hope Floats & she was dancing with her dad & I thought about when Russell hugged me. I was starting to cry. I am in Russ-withdrawal. And I was thinking about kissing Adam. I think we'll definitely be okay. I was stretching on Sunday night & he walked by & tickled my side. Just a small gesture, but...anyway.
>
> ♥ Me

So in the space of less than three months, I went from talking glowingly about Adam—he was a grade ahead of me and a total delight—to having some kind of falling out with him. I do not remember what caused that. I do remember (in the entry to come, you'll read it) making up with him. The magic of a hug laced with forgiveness is all-powerful.

July 11, 1999

> I was baptized today—I was quite nervous but very excited. I ♥ed seeing everyone stand up for me. We took 22 people out to lunch. I ♥ Dylan Prowler. He barely knows me. But on my card he wrote "you're very sweet" & after lunch hugged me from behind. What a great day! Camp tomorrow!
>
> ♥ T Me

July 12–July 17, 1999

> Camp started yesterday. We woke up at 6 am & got to the church at 6:30. At 7:00 we left. The bus ride was really fun. Derek sat next to me for a long

portion & Michael sat behind me. When we got here, we got settled then had lunch. After, me, Krystal, Kate, & Jennifer went to the ropes course. Krystal chickened out on both times. There were 3 hot guys there: Austin, Travis, & I think Greg? But we had fun. Derek joined us at one point & was telling us about the soccer game. He said "I got hit in the ball with a stomach." He had a ball print on his shirt. Dylan & Cable bleached their hair. We played volleyball. Took showers. Then I played volleyball again. Carson had his shirt off & every time he moved to hit the ball, his muscles flexed unbelievably well. I think he'll be better looking than Travis in five years. I-yi-yi.

Anyway. So we ate dinner & then had worship. At about 9:30, we watched Better Off Dead. I gave Carson a massage for like 30 minutes. He said, "Courtney, the hands of God are calling me." I laughed and said What, so he rephrased it, "the best hands in the world." Talk about a way to make a person feel good! So when I was done, John wanted me to play with his hair. It was sooo soft! Anyway, he was laying in my lap & then I had to move my legs, so he laid on one of my knees, & Carson laid on the other. I switched legs so much & then I didn't want to make John move, so my leg fell dead-asleep. I couldn't feel it. Ew.

Afterwards I started feeling like I was going to throw up. I was all shaky. Out of nowhere, Carson gave me this huge Carson-sized hug & I felt better. I like couldn't sleep at all. No pillow! So I like woke up every hour. I woke up for the last time at 5:45. It was still dark. I got up when it got light & went down—1st there—to the meeting room. Milton's show is pretty funny. We ate nasty eggs then came here. We're going horseback riding at 2:00. My stomach hurts. Marshall got sick last night from a bug bite. Cabin inspections are going on right now. Carson's getting his hair bleached on his bday. Yikes! More later.

Yesterday me & Kate hung out in the meeting room & listened to the DJs. We missed our 2:00 riding time so we went at 3. It was ok. The instructor had a nice butt. Let's see. We took showers, ate dinner... I was helping Greta make signs. We had bible study really late. There was a dance at 9:00 that would have been funner if I could have danced. Adam & Greta and Travis & Greta & Luke & Cams were all swinging. Adam drew a cool color tattoo on my wrist & Carson drew one on my arm & on my leg. Oh, & my foot. My feet feel dirty all the time. So far nothing has happened today. The 11th grade boys slept through breakfast except Boobs.

2 things from last night: Dylan said he sees life where when someone trips, you have 3 choices: (1) help them up & continue on the way, (2) step over them & don't bother, or (3) trip over them & make the same mistakes. And Adam: "Life is like a book. Those who don't travel read only one page."

Other words of wisdom:

"A true friend is the gift of God & he only who made hearts can unite them."

"A time we will always remember, a place we will never forget." —Indian summer.

Yesterday was pretty uneventful. After bible study & lunch, Kate & I went swimming in the lake. People were doing the blob. Carson's bday is today & I gave him a big hug. Yesterday I got quite sunburned. The VOL sang & I got sooo sleepy. It was kind of boring too because I didn't know any of the songs. I have a headache right now. I'm going to write some more notes. Tonight's date night.

"Living like there's no tomorrow means loving all you can today."

Yesterday was spent writing notes. And watching people warm up for talent show. I was going to sing 3AM with Marshall & Ronnie but it fell through. I really like Ronnie. Johanna came last night. I got Stevie for date night. I knew I would—mine was the 1st name called. He's so sweet! Then was the talent show. Jacob Champion amazes me, truly, he's

> *so good! After we went outside & me, Luke, Ryan, Jimmy, & Garrett beat the other team in volleyball. Then Jimmy switched sides, & Luke, Ryan, Garrett, & I still won twice. We made a major comeback on the 1st game. I got hit in the face with the ball & got sand everywhere. Luke had it everywhere too. Then we went to bed & my poor CD player dropped. String thing tonight!*
>
> *"You never really leave a place you love—part of it you take with you, leaving a part of yourself."*
>
> *Oh my goodness, morning worship was sooo X's 10 sad. Travis got up and started to speak & I started bawling. I cried for like an hour & a half while people talked. Derek gave me the string & I gave it to Cameron. We hugged for a long time. I only cried when Greg & Kate hugged then when Travis gave it to Carson who gave it to Greta. I guess I got all my tears out earlier. But Adam was crying and that broke my heart. I gave him a long hug, and it felt sooo good to hug him again. I got a lot of great hugs. Then I stayed up til 4:00 w/ Zack. More about that later.*

Sigh, just when you're getting into a story, the details stop. My hand must have gotten tired. Two days later, I was annoyed with another boy, so Zack must have fled my mind. I wonder what shenanigans we got into that night (I vaguely remember streaking, but I don't think I would have done that alone with another guy I barely knew. Maybe he did??). The thing about reading about church camp: the small miracles don't seem so out of place. Like *knowing* I was going to get Stevie for my date. I remember Darren calling my name and thinking "he's going to say Stevie." And if I remember correctly, Stevie had sensed it too. I wonder what little psychic moments like that are about? Like, if I'd been more aware back then, would I have dug deeper with Stevie that night? Probably. Is there a part of me who wants to reach out and ask Stevie if he remembers that too, and what it meant to him? Absolutely.

Stay tuned.

July 19, 1999

> *I'm pissed off. Derek & Marshall basically stood us up. We went to see Eyes Wide Shut & got kicked out*

so we went to Blockbuster. Derek said he & Marshall were going to rent a porn & go to Derek's. Krystal & I got very pissed & we couldn't understand why. They're dumbasses!

♥ Me

July 23, 1999

Went to see The Haunting. Sucked. Dave sucked. It wasn't loud. Preston just told me Dylan & Cameron have kissed. Yuck! I'm in a weird mood.

♥ Me

So the grown-up, been-through-therapy version of me sits here, again aching for this kid. So many feelings, so many crazy emotions, coursed through me that I had zero idea what to do with. All I knew to do was love so hard, I pushed people away over and over again. Derek and Marshall probably wanted a guys' night away from the females they had spent the last week with. I would be annoying me too. (And honestly, it's kind of flattering to think they spent a week with us at camp and wanted to cap it off by watching porn!)

August 1–August 2, 1999

After church we went to go pick up Pres. Long wait in airport—ate at Friday's—saw some familiar people. Boarded, slept all the way. Taxi to ship. Boarded. Went to dinner. Were in search of cute guys—saw one right next to us. Awesome jeans & shoes, yellow shirt (off to the side in another color is what looks like "fruit fish"). After dinner went to Galax-Z—boring. Found out et cost. Bingo $10. We met Alicia, Courtney, Jamie. Ping Pong shuffle board. Went to stores. Broke my foot. Pizza buffet 10:30. International food place 12:00. Went to the dock w/ Charles, guitar-playing singing cool jeans 14-yr-old. Pres & I played slots—got kicked out. Woosh. Don't feel like writing.

♥ Me

Y'all, there ain't no party like a Carnival party. Again, I'm disappointed in the details here, but I believe you'll get the gist. We went on a cruise (Disney's

Ocean Princess) when I was ten, and I fell hook, line and sinker (forgive the pun). But then you know, COVID happened, not to mention the horror stories you heard about people being trapped and vomiting all over one another. I'm not honestly sure if I'll ever be able to go on another one again, but I'd like to hope so. They're pretty insanely magical, and I love some good magic.

August 2–August 3, 1999

> *Woke up at 11:00. Audrey left w/o me. Went to pool. Met Matt. (lunch burger) Watched Pres do Olympics. Stayed in pool long time. Played volleyball. Went to get ready for dinner. Dinner was very long. Had lobster (& shrimp). Went to mocktail—boring. Aud & Charles went off to deck, me Court2, Jim, & Pres went to GalaxZ. Jim got pulled out by a security guard for his knife. Phillip confined him to his room so we played Cash. We went to the pasta buffet. More Cash. It. Matt came over.*

Here's the hard thing about reading these journals: sometimes, I have no idea what I was talking about. I'm enjoying the different-colored notes of what I ate all day. But otherwise, not only do details elude me, but I'm also left going, "Huh?" And that's not what one wants when trying to tell a story. So let me just assure you, I have no idea either.

August 3–August 4, 1999

> *Up at 11:00 again. Dressed to deck to lunch. Ate fishsticks ooh yuck. Matt was there. Went swimming. Boat was majorly rocking. 2:45 teen trivia game. Dumb. Matt shoved the guy who told on Jimmy for his knife. Asked to apologize. Said "fuck no." Got kicked out. Court Jim Pres & I went to play in a ping pong tournament. Court & I both lost. Played Cash more. Hehe, Court's dense. After was dinner—lobster bisque & nasty steak. I was queasy.*
>
> *After, we got lots of pictures taken. Went into the game show. After, GalaxZ. Boys stuck on gambling. Karaoke. J, P, me, & A sang Summer of '69! People were cheering for us. A sang Crazy. Ih. More Cash. Hit my head on the light. 2, Jimmy 1. Jim & Court kissed right in front of me & Preston. Court*

had a 12:00 bedtime. Us 3 went to Western buffet. Preston was being strange. More gambling. I lost like ten bucks. Sigh. I am addicted too. Jamaica tomorrow!

August 4–August 5, 1999

Up at 7:30—brecky omelet, milk, oj. Loaded off, on bus. Jamaicans drive maniacally. Scared me & nauseated me. Got to beach, got my hair braided. Meghan Munchky is here. In ocean & laying out about 2 hrs. Left went shopping. Lady wanted to rebraid my hair. Better much. Bracelet & anklet. Went to pool & laid out. Got quite burned. Came back, watched "Playing by the Heart." Aud fell asleep. I came close. At 5:20, put on make-up. Dinner—tiger shrimp leek in cream gross. Sole yummy usually but bad sauce. Salad w/ ranch. Did Macarena. Left, went to look at pix. Got caught trying to take them. Ping pong.

Court & I went to get cameras. Made pillow men in sexual positions in Jimmy's room. Took pictures pro & in the frog mouth. Bored. Ping-pong. Pres made Court & I chase him to his room. 9:00 went to boys' room. Had boy/girl trivia w/ Pres. He's good. Walked Court to bed at 10:00, went gambling! Won. Watched gay magic man & comedian w/ Sally & some other people. Left. More boring ping-pong. Met Natalie's sisters. (One girl played volleyball @ beach.) I hate it when Preston says things about Audrey's body. It's like, rub it in. He said, "Hey baby. Oh whoops, didn't know it was you" and said she had a good butt & didn't notice it was big. They flirted all day at the beach. Sting rays tomorrow!

August 5–August 6, 1999

Got up, went sting ray swimming. I got touched a few times, but mostly I ran from them. They're thick gross. Back on boat 2 ship. Ate pizza & ice cream @ 2:00. Came to the boys' room. Court was in there. Watched Simply Irresistible. Pres & I fell asleep. 4, took shower, dinner salad & shrimp &

Baked Alaska. Went hunting for Court. Found in casino with guys. Gambled.

Court & I walked around. Jim was being cold. Court was upset. Ping pong, they had a loooong talk. Jimmy went back on all that he told her. Played Cash w/ 2 other girls. Switched teams for them but wouldn't switch for us. Court & I screamed in the elevators. Buffet, Jimmy saved us seats & then the guys didn't even look at us. Left, came here. Court went to bed. I told Aud about et & Jimmy was listening at the door then they threw apples at our door. Put paper over the peep. Cleaned it up. Pissed.

August 6–August 7, 1999

Got up at 1. Went shopping at the strip in Cozumel. Came back, wandered. Wrote letters. Court came back at 4:30. Talked to her. Showered. Dinner—filet mignon, corn chowder, crab meat cocktail. Went to look at pix. Found 4 we liked. Jim was being nice again. We were playing Cash & watching trivia. Jimmy, "Don't give me mean looks." Preston, "I wasn't looking at you." Jimmy walked off, Preston called him an asshole. Curly girly came later, after C & I tried to spike P's hair. "Oh, Preston, smile, don't cry." Jim & P shook hands, girl's like, "Oh are we all friends now." No, bitch. Eek I hate her.

Met 2 hot guys: Sphinx & Matt. Talked with them. Went to dance. Lotta fun on video. Our blue plaid guy was there looking smoking in yellow. He was watching us. (Met Adam, ping pong.) Met up w/ Sphinx & Matt. Jim walked up & put his arm around Court. To casino. P & J left into GalaxZ. We 4 went too. We sat, curly-girly goes, "Jimmy, when are we going back to your room?" at the top of her curly lungs. Then, "Jimmy, let's dance." J walked to us, and "Jimmy, where you going?" Court & I both wondered if he had told them all Court's problems.

Talked to Sally. Came home got locked out. Audrey bitched at me for turning on the lights.

She's just pissed b/c she got in trouble for being a slutty bad seed again.

August 7–August 8, 1999

Awoke, ate, slept until 11:45 when Court called. Went to deck, yellow, blue-red plaid guy was sunning hot when he put his hands up, gorgeous when he smiles. Watched him rub oil…ah. Adam was tanning too. Not like he needs it. Sexy. Sphinx joined us, dropped a glass near a fat lady. Blue plaid guy was watching us. Went to look at Sphinx's Mexican stuff. Wore a kimono. Hot. Gift shop, teddy bears. Strawban daquiris. Showers. Dinner. Sunset pix. Gift shop w/ parents.

Court & I wandered around. Looked for hot guys. Adam thought we were following him. We kept bumping into each other. His little brother is so awesome. Craig. Danced. Got a lot of cute pictures. Lots of Adam. Danced, hunted for J. My knees started to hurt. Watched some karaoke.

Some girl had it out for Court. Thought she was a slut. Her bf said he'd protect Court. But then he wanted to beat up Adam. Very screwed up. She kept staring at Court, so I said, "Don't stare, bitch, it's rude." She confronted Court about it. Haha, I'd fight her. Then that guy (Russ & Nikki) had it out for Adam so he stopped protecting Court. Craig said Adam could take him. Hehe. Anyway. So we got Adam's address & Sally's. Good trip. Lots of fun.

♥ Me

So that was a cluster. I'm debating the fun in adding pictures for effect, because I'm not sure I would have felt like I was on the ship if my memory wasn't fueled by photos. To me, this reads like a jumble of words, and I wrote it. So.

I am wholly ashamed of several of the things in this entry, and this is the first time I think, "This girl needs some good parenting." First of all, why did I ever think it was okay to call other women sluts, especially my own sister? Second is my descriptions for some people—colors mostly but then *fat* and several times *bitch*. I hope beyond hope I meant it as nothing more than a descriptive word. But then I think, "Well, you were also seventeen and hadn't grown up yet." Forgive yourself and move on. Read that again. You too.

August 15, 1999

> *Ah, the start of a new school year is upon us. I'm very hyper. Just got back from church lunch. Greta made me xited about being seniors. Luke is awesome, I'm in* ♥ *again. But at least it's not with Dylan. I can't wait for school! I'm going to have an awesome year!*
>
> ♥ Me

Aww, check out that manifestation before I even learned what *The Secret* was. To be honest, I'm not sure it worked, but maybe my optimistic self saw only the best. Also, I wonder why I said, "At least it wasn't Dylan." Dylan is Luke's older brother, and super hot too. I wonder if I considered him off-limits after I found out he kissed Cameron. Hmm.

August 20, 1999

> *So far the year looks promising. I made a couple of new friends. Boring classes, but it's all good. Went out with K tonight. Met RiceGuy37 Matt. Icky. I should look thru the outside & see the guy on the inside...but.*
>
> ♥ Me

Observation number 912 along this journey: This has been something I've struggled with my entire life. Whether it was about myself or someone I was talking to, I always said, "Looks shouldn't matter. It's about the heart." But then I would feel hugely guilty if I wrote someone off because I wasn't physically attracted to them. What I have come to realize as an adult is, I wasn't judging their faces. I was judging their energies. My intuition, which has only gotten stronger over the years—or perhaps I've just started listening more closely—has rarely, if ever, failed. So I look back at this entry about poor Matt, who once we met in person just wasn't my cup of tea. I immediately wrote it off (literally) as being about his face. I can still picture what he looked like. I hope he found his tea drinker.

September 12, 1999

    Last night was our 2nd footb game. Lots of fun! I hung out w/ Chloe the whole time—saw Doug Mayo—man he looks gooder than good! Yikes. Kyle Wahlberg gave me high five & said what's up. Nick J kept flicking my arm. He's such a flirt. When we rushed the field, I got a huge, toothy white smile, a "Hey, Court!" and a hug from Brandon right in front of his gf! Then I hugged Joey. On the way to IHOP, Wanna be a Baller came on... Luke!!!!!! Then Chloe & I just talked at IHOP. Good night!

                                                             ♥ Me

September 25, 1999

    Last night was boring. I went to Chili's w/ Sarah & Michael. Sarah & I talked a lot about HC & Derek. I know now that he wants to go to HC... Anyway, tonight Senior Women. But I didn't go!

                                                              ♥ Me

October 10, 1999

    This weekend was the retreat. Check it out, I wrote about it last year too! In ways this one was better, but I liked last year's overall better, most likely because it was my first thing with the church. We had fun playing Mush, but then again we always do. I was giving Ryan a back rub & he started a train & we got in trouble for it. Now about Derek. I swear I don't think that boy has any brains sometimes. He's so dense & it's so obvious that I want him to ask me. Ryan & Krystal are both supposed to talk to him but it's not happening. Okay, Derek just came down here while I was writing about him.

    I have bug bites all over my right arm. Owch. Anyway. Me & Kate spent a lot of time together last night, per usual. It's hot where I'm sitting. Betcha my eyes look really green. Sex talk in 15 minutes. 5 hours til we go home. I hope when I get home I have something good to say about Derek. That would be *just too cool. Anyway, more tonight. Oh, we're trying to teach Bud our names. I think it's finally sticking. I think he & Peter are the cutest people. Bud was telling us about his gf moving to NY & he said he "couldn't be a freak without his freakette" at the Halloween Dance. He's sooo cute! Anyway! More tonight, really!*

Okay, nothing!! I'm so upset! Why won't this happen? Katie & I made it home really well on our own. Okay I'm like going crazy. This truly sucks. I have three weeks to find a date.

♥ *Me*

Okay, I'm going to get whiny for a mo. I remember the anticipation surrounding Derek asking me to homecoming. I made it about as clear as a bell on Christmas morning that I was interested. Homecoming weekend was always on my birthday weekend. It was incredibly important to me when I was younger (and still now, as much as I love football season and nostalgia).

I was a senior here; Derek was my last shot at a hoco I'd always remember. And it was, don't get me wrong. Lots of fun. But why did this boy choose to show up at my house to ask me on a night he knew I wouldn't be home? Why was I the girl who got the "So you wanna…" in the hallway the next morning? Why, I ask you, when all I wanted was the epic rom-com experience? I'm almost forty-two, and I've never been…grand-gestured.

But for once, I write about my birthday…and an epic rom-com episode of a different kind.

October 23, 1999

Okay, ketchup. Derek asked me. "I've been by your house like three times." "I know, I've heard." "So do you want to?" Cute.

Tonight was my party. Michael & I talked a lot. Chad gave me a hug. Joey came. Derek left—made me mad—came back. Marshall promised he wanted to go to HC with me…not just asking. He wants to read my story even though the last time he read it, he was all making fun of it. Anyway, pretty good night!

♥ *Me*

October 25, 1999

> *Saturday night, something weird happened.*
> *Hello?*
> *Hi, do you know who this is?*
> *No. Who?*
> *Jason. I just want to call and wish you a happy birthday.*
> *Thank you. Who is this?*
> *Jason.*
> *Jason who?*
> *Just Jason! Can I sing to you?*
> *Sure.*
> *Really? You're not going to hang up on me?*
> *No.*
> *I can't believe I'm talking to you!*
> *I promise not to hang up.*
> *(He starts stuttering.)*
> *I'm sorry, I stutter when I get excited or nervous.*
> *I just can't believe I'm talking to you! I'm sorry, I have to go! I love you, bye!*
> *It was sooo weird. I can't figure out who it was...*
> *Jason Barthalow.*
>
> ♥ Me

My first experience at feeling like a celebrity was thrilling but also a mystery that bugged me for a long time. I spent a lot of years as a young adult being told I was unapproachable or intimidating, and I could never understand why. Over the years of learning to truly love and enjoy myself—thank you, Snapchat—I started to understand a bit better: I am a giant. I am a puppy, a lover, no doubt. But I am a lot, and if you don't know me—or even if you do—I can be intimidating. I'm sorry.

October 29, 1999

> *Tonight was the game. We lost. Went to Snuffer's in a Mustang. Jennifer's really sweet. Brian's so funny & really cute. We had a lot of fun.*
>
> ♥ Me

NOT THE F——ING GILMORE GIRLS

Lake Highlands Homecoming had nothing on Richardson Homecoming, I'll tell you that. Themed instead of formal, we dressed in camo and fifties because no one could agree on a theme. It was a fun time, no doubt. I do wish (again) there was more detail here, because I'd love to rewatch the night.

January 21, 2000

> My first entry of the "new millenium." Last night I went to see Anything Goes at LH. WW was better. But the night was sooo good. I talked to Justin W, trying to explain how to email surveys. Got hugs from Natalie R and get this Adam Putnam. I swear that was soooo cool! Susan came up and hugged me & said, "You should go say hi to Adam, he'd like to see you."
>
> I saw Adam all of twice in the 4 years I was best friends w/ L. But he leaned on his mom's shoulder and said where, so I had to go say hi. He gave me a huge hug & a kiss on the cheek. We talked & he gave me another hug. God it was cool. Laura says he was gay. Then I went to buy cigs for Laura & the guy like read my mind. He was all "hard pack of Camel Lights" before I even got pack out. Weird. Great night!
>
> ♥ Me

Talk about feeling like a celebrity! The grown-up version of the silly best friend of his little sister got to see the man behind the myth, and he was as amazing as I expected him to be. I remember walking past his room once when I was spending the night and seeing a mural of the Marlboro man that Adam had done himself. I have no idea now if it was a painting on the wall—that's what I see in my mind's eye—or something much smaller, but I do know he was (and likely still is) insanely talented. I love seeing his pictures on Facebook, especially when they're posted by his mother, who adores him. I'm blessed to have been a part of that family in any way, but especially when I think of Susan (Mama) examining my scalp when my head wouldn't stop itching (diagnosis: psoriasis) or sharing with her that I wanted to be a teenage mom. (I'm real glad that didn't go as planned!) I may not have had the typical mother, but I had a lot of mothers who loved me.

February 29, 2000

It's actually March 2, but the 29 is when this happened. I got smart & asked Juan for a ride home... I was kind of scared that it'd be awkward cause he wouldn't talk, but he did. I met Gabbie, his Favorites date. On the way to his car, I told him my mom had a Porsche & he like stopped walking to stare at me with those pretty brown eyes... he was really shocked. He wanted to know if I could drive it & I said no. Then he said come over to my house so I can, but I thought he was going to say come over to my house so I can teach you.

Anyway so I told him he could take me to work in it if my mom would let him & he loved that idea! So he took me home & we talked the whole way. At home, Mom wasn't there, but he said, "If you need a ride to work, I'll give you one" so he came in and played with my animals. Bert really liked him. It was cute. Bert & guys, really?? But it was so cool having Juan in my house. He stayed for like 35 minutes then took me to work. Sigh.

♥ Me

March 6, 2000

So, Juan drove the Porsche. He kept saying thank you & I owe you one. I was like anytime. I went to BSB on Saturday. It was so awesome. I mean, the dancing was great, the singing ROCKED! and I could not believe I was looking at the BSB live. Damn, I screamed so long & loud. I sang every song. It was so much fun. Something I'll remember forever.

♥ Me

March 12, 2000

Today was good—not special, just good. Luke Prowler winked at me—so cute! David was bouncing off walls hyper. Rachel & I & Kate & I and Katie &

I all had good talks or hung out. YAC meeting was fun!

♥ Me

March 25, 2000

  Friday night was so fun! Spaghetti Supper: Mrs. Stefano was like picking on me. She jumped down my throat for something Mrs. Rose said was okay. I think she was picking on me cause of Derek.??? Anyway, the 1st shift was boring (dessert server). But the 2nd was fun! (ToGo!) Me, Josh Horton, & Katie Grapenut were it, & we only got 2 cars, so Josh & I dragged armchairs out there & we all just talked. Josh is really sweet. We were let off early, so we went down, & Travis Crucible was w/ Ellen. Sexy! I hung out w/ them & Travis is really sweet. He looks like someone & I can't figure out who. But we had fun.

  After, Laura came over & we went to drive around for a while. When we came back, Avery, Shelby, Preston, John, & Jimmy were home. We had fun!!!! Preston & Avery & Laura & I went to the playground w/ beers. I only had like 7 sips. Pres at one point looked @ me & goes "Whoa!" Avery said, "What?" and Pres, "I am like buzzing! I just looked at Courtney and she went like this!" He held up his hand and moved real fast. Then Pres, Avery, & Jessie went to get more beer from Avery's car. Pres promised me he wouldn't drive. When they came back, they had seen Phillip Mower. Avery was threatening to beat him up & Jessie got mad & ran away.

  It was like 2:30 & I thought Avery had been outside a while, & so I went to check on him. He was sitting on our steps & he looked like he was crying. He told me his whole story like we were best friends. ♥ He was going to go get Pres's car & look for her & I was like Avery, please don't. He swore to me he was okay though. But luckily she came back then. I went inside & was sitting bet. John's legs stroking his stomach and & legs. I was going to put Avery & Jessie in my room, but Shelby & Preston were *sprawled all over my bed.?? Cute! So A & J were on my parents floor. So I went down to sleep. John was like, in between my legs is fine. I was like fine for all of 2 minutes, then we folded out the bed & went to sleep. Shelby promised to make (someone) be nice to me. Hehe. Good weekend!*

♥ *Me*

I'm having a hard time after these longer entries. I want to narrate between each one, make my excuses, and make my apologies for the way I behaved when I was a teenager. I'm embarrassed that I put John through that without any thought of follow-through. But then the adult version of me goes to bed and thinks about telling the kid version to move on, that she can almost guarantee John didn't think twice about it with (much) negativity. Forgive yourself and move on. But then the anxiety says no.

April 30, 2000

Man I don't write nearly enough. This week really sucked. The four-day weekend was fun. I got to know Shelby well enough to ask him to prom. But Monday night, Jeff Anderson threatened Jimmy, & then on Thursday, after he'd seen my sign asking Shelbs, Jeff walked up to him & said "I'll see you at prom, bitch." So Shelby doesn't want to go. I don't have a fucking date to my senior prom. FUCK!!!

Thursday I also lost my bracelet & so I was crying all day. I basically haven't stopped crying since then. This sucks so hard. I can't shake this. I wish I hadn't hung that damn sign—just asked him, like Russ. And I basically ruined whatever friendship we were starting. Now he won't look at me in the halls & he has trouble talking to me on the phone. Man I hate this. I hate my class. I HATE Jeff Anderson.

Tonight something hit our window. A fist or a ball. Aud saw it, bird freaked, dogs freaked, I heard it then freaked. And now I am alone with my depressed thoughts and no Jim, no Pres, no Shelby, no parents. Just Aud asleep & the dogs locked in cages. Bloody fucking reassuring. I want my mother. Or Jimmy. Or Shelby to come over / call

& say he'll go. The latter would make me happiest. I might actually be able to stop crying.

♥ Me

It's such a familiar scene, even twenty-five years later. I've learned how to manage the panic attacks with breathing (thanks to singing and POT), and when it's uncontrollable (mostly at night), I go to sleep and start fresh in the morning. That's why I'm a morning person now when I was a huge sleeper-in-ner as a teenager. Nothing has gone wrong yet. It's a good time to be happy. We set the tone for our day, you guys.

May 7, 2000

Tonight (last) was prom & I had a really great time, regardless of Shelby. Michael was really well behaved. Andrew was damn sexy. He was really cute—like staring @ me & listening close when I talked to him. Anyway @ Palomino I got seafood linguini & we saw Brynt Brightman (& Cavell). The bus was fun.

At the dance, I got huge hugs from Josh & Joey & even Harrison. At one point I asked Joey if he had seen Kelly & he asked why it was so important for me to find her & I was like b/c she & Jess Zachary are in the same dress. He said "Don't worry, you look much better than her." And he was saying how much he liked my dress. I talked to Meredith, his date, for a long time. She's sweet.

We gambled, we danced... I danced 2xs with Michael, and a little of the song I Will Remember w/ Juan. Brent Holiday was KILLING me, he was so cute—dancing. Jennifer's was fun. We swam until 3. We watched movies. I was so cold & sleeping in a chair. Daniel's adorable, Brian was hot, & Andrew Kellogg is dead sexy.

♥ Me

May 15, 2000

Saturday night, Shelbs, Pres, & Jimmy went skinny-dipping. Aud & I joined them & Shelbs was *getting in and out, no cares. Pres was like almost backed up against me—he has THE cutest butt. Round and cute. We talked for a while & Shelbs was real flirty w/ Audrey. But last night we talked online & he called me babe & baby & said that I couldn't tell Jim & Pres that I'd worn him out b/c they'd be "jei-los." He's so darling!*

So tonight Juan came over in PJs to return my bio. His hair was all fluffy & he looked sleepy. CUTE! He and Jimmy played foos ball. Then came Shelbs. I think Drew may like me. He's cute, but he's too much of a soph.?? Anyway.

♥ *Me*

PS. I SAID HERE PRESSY & HANDED PRES HIS YRBK & EUGENE GRABBED FOR IT & PRES GOES THIS IS PRESSY'S NOT EUGEY'S! CUTE! NICE ASS!

And there was the first time I noticed someone being into me that I didn't necessarily feel as strongly about. The separation of different levels of love didn't register as early as I wish they had. I just loved so strongly and so fiercely, it didn't matter who was on the other side of the emotion. I remember if Drew became too sophomore for me, I got a little mean. What I've had to learn as an adult is to treat people nicely regardless of the level of emotion I have for them. Just because they're bugging me doesn't mean I don't love them. I just need a break, as I'm sure 99 percent of the people in my life need from me 97 percent of the time.

May 17, 2000

Tonight I was supposed to go out w/ Sarah & Dante & David & Katie & Kams & Katie but I got lost so I went to the playground cuz I saw Justin. Lauren & Ryan & some other people were there—they had found a 3.5' snake. Gross. Some more guys came up & Ben Wild threw a fb at its head. I was about to cry. Justin wrote in my yearbook that I was the best Shekinah partner ever. ♥

♥ *Me*

May 29, 2000

> *I am gradumatated. As of yesterday at 2 PM. It is now 7 AM. After grad, I went to Laura's BBQ. Tully is really sweet. We just chilled & we didn't want to leave each other. Annie & Tyler were there & others. After was the all night party. We bowled. I won $50 for best girl score & sheets & a mask... cool. I bowled w/ Juan... he was being so sweet. Derek stared at me. Katy & I chilled. Came home at 6:00 AM...been awake almost 24 hours. How much longer can I make it? I love Juan. Brian Venmo is adorable.*
>
> ♥ *Me*

I can say it sounded like I was proud of myself even if no one else cared that I walked the stage. I had to work hard to save my high school career, but I did it. Do I regret dropping out of college? Still no.

June 2, 2000

> *All I can say is I am now officially a die hard (very hard) NSYNC fan. Concert was tonight. Sigh & a half! No, triple sigh! Lord almighty above are they sexy. Justin esp...but JC and Lance...Lord. Justin wants to be black I think. The curls being as long as they were and the glasses always turned me off... but tonight those curls were in dreds & he wore a bandana for a good portion of the time...and he was rapping (the noises) and dancing by himself & he was so SEXY!*
>
> *There were 2 hot guys by us... I'd guess about 12, but cute! This was a great concert. BSB was better overall, length-wise neway. But NSYNC can dance! HOT! Man, Bye Bye Bye killed me! Sigh! Again & again. Is this illegible? I love NSYNC! BSB who? OK... I can love them both. And I DO! LORD!*
>
> ♥ *Me!*
>
> *PS My throat hurts!*

June 3, 2000

Tonight was Josh's party. FUN! It started off being boring. We sat around for 3.5 hours reading sexual astrology. But then we went on a walk & my perfect straight hair got crinkled. We played Twister in the rain. Josh & I were the last up & his butt was in my face so I fell back laughing so hard. Went inside, got some of his PJs. Watched Blues Bros and gave Jacob a back rub / chillies. All 2 hrs! Then most went home leaving me Josh Jenny & Jacob. Jacob is HOT! Built! Josh called me babe & gave me another backbreaking hug. I even (?) caught him staring... as well as definitely Jacob—when we locked eyes, one of us would always look away. Jacob gave me a back rub 2! FUN!

♥ *Me*

June 4, 2000

I went to Josh's again. I like cried at the Breakfast Club. J was making fun of me. He hit me in the face w/ a pillow. Watched Faculty. I was cold & he kept saying he could make me warmer but he never did. Sigh. He said Rod Stewart was date music—sang his fave song for me. No clue as to what he feels. Cried at Tearin' Up My Heart & Just Wanna Be W/ You. Sigh.

♥ *Me*

Oy, was this man an endless source of frustration for me. Talk about hot and cold. He was a huge flirt and gave me what I needed from that friendship, especially a scent memory linked to Hugo Boss cologne. It makes me laugh that I cried to NSYNC songs on the way home. Those were not tearjerkers. But it's about the lyrics, eh? "Speak through the music"—that has become one of my taglines as an adult. When I can't find what to say, I listen.

June 7, 2000

Shelb's b-day. Last night he stuck my $80 in his boxers & I was like you don't think I'll go after it? So he put it up his ass. Gave him the chillies. He said I could lay beside him. I should have. Laura & I sang & sang forever. Tonight I talked to Jacob—he asked for my phone #! Yea! Josh IMed me first & called me babe. Ugh. I need to have a party tomorrow night.

♥ Me

June 9, 2000

Well I didn't have a party but plenty of people came over. Lisa, Pres, Shebs, Ayla, Kelly Banion, & Corinne. It was one of the best and the worst nights of my life. Lisa got drunk & told me & Audrey that she liked Jimmy better than Preston the other day. After putting 2 & 2 together, I figured that the girl Jimmy liked that he'd never tell anyone was Lisa. Later, Lisa told Preston...or rather Pres walked in on her asking Jimmy to kiss her.

Pres playfully slapped her ass & she flipped out. She locked herself in the bathroom. Then Preston flipped out. 1:00 in the morning he was outside screaming at the top of his lungs, "I hate my fucking life, fuck everybody!" and screaming & crying. It was breaking my heart. Lisa tried to calm him down, Jimmy did, Shelby did...then Lisa & P talked & Jim & P talked in the backyard and then something made P mad again & he ran out the gate.

Shelby went after him & I heard the trash can turn over so I went out there. Shelby couldn't find him. Shelb went into the front & I heard a car drive off & I thought it was P. But Jimmy drove thru the neighbor's yard. Shelby tried to drive after him but I wouldn't let him in the car. But then J came back and they went out back to look for P.

Then I saw someone at the end of our street. I started walking down there & P started walking away. He was like, "Leave me alone Courtney I want to be alone." I ran up to him & was like "Please come home." He was mean a little more and then he looked at me w/ these sad Preston eyes & said, "I'm so sorry Courtney. I'm being so mean to you b/c

> I'm drunk." I like started to cry & was beggin him to come back. He promised he'd be okay and he wasn't stupid. He told me he loved me. Uh-oh! Made me feel really good.
>
> Then Kelly & I had a looong talk after everyone was inside. Shelby and Ayla drank more. Shelby got sick. Kelly & Ayla got in a fight & Kelly slapped her hard. But Ayla & Lisa stayed—everything is going to be fine between everyone. Except the fact that Lisa is blatantly lying to her boyfriend, herself, & Jimmy.
>
> ♥ Me

I love the fact that what sounds like a pretty intense night got labeled as one of the best because Preston told me he loved me. The "Uh-oh!" makes me giggle. I was in no way interested in stealing someone's man—ever! But after four years of crushing on Preston, finally hearing those three words was precious. It didn't matter that he loved me like a sister, and I was head over heels for him. That was on me. It didn't matter that he had a girlfriend, because we loved each other too—fiercely.

Love is nothing without trust, and maybe that's what's happened to me: I've lost my ability to trust. So now I feel like anytime someone says those words to me, it's because I give them something. I yearn for them, and I drop them often, but rarely do I feel the power behind them if someone says it back. Tell someone you love them every day. It needs to be said as much as it needs to be heard.

June 10, 2000

> First day of choir tour—Jim & I woke up really late & got to church @ 7:30 but luckily the bus was late. I'm glad we didn't have to stand around. The ride was fun as always. Boober & I actually talked, he even sat by me for a while. Em, Boob, John, Derek, & I sang together—Shekinah songs & others. We played Mush. Went to Mic D's for lunch. Got to the dorms went to Picadilly's for dinner. Then to orientation.
>
> We were being obnoxious cause we were playing "Who Wants to be a Pizzaire?" & we were chanting "Go Stars!" Then we had "devotional" and finally watched the game. I played w/ Josh's hair—

> soft! I hope something good happens for me... Boobs, Derek, or Josh? Derek!!! Yikes! Staring contest. And he was really sweet & open today!
>
> ♥ Me

Okay, now I'm just getting annoyed with myself. What in the world did I mean by "something good"? Would I have gotten with any guy who showed me interest? Holy cannoli.

June 11, 2000

> Every step he takes...I won't be watching but I'll be noticing! Derek's really becoming more outgoing. It's fun to notice. Even w/ me! Like today Josh & I were sitting down while singing & he turned around & mouthed to me to stand up. He's so cute. I think he likes Emily. But Josh & I hung out... we went to sing at an 11:00 service—horrible practice. Great concert. Then lunch then ~~free rest~~ French Q then rest then chapel w/ other churches then devotional then more free time.
>
> Walked around w/ Rinehart, David QT Pie, & Josh... did the question game, rubbed J's & J's backs... I ♥ Jordan! I wish Justin were here! James said he was really sad a/b not coming. My honey. I'm not having that great of a time, but manual labor is always fun!
>
> ♥ Me

June 12, 2000

> Today we went to Living Waters to work—awesome! My group worked on the trailer—sanding & breaking. Jordo & I played w/ a sledgehammer... David & I had a water war so I was freezing on the bus! I swear, if he was just one year older... damn! Same w/ Jordan. Derek & I got some major sun—but we were the only ones. Came home showered & played 5 games of volleyball. We slaughtered them 3 to 2. Then devotionals... I dreaded Josh's hair. We

just sat & told camp stories & worked on our senior will. FUN! I think Josh is so sweet!

♥ *Me*

Excuse me for another giggling sidenote. It's the second time I said dreads instead of what I meant, which was cornrows. Justin Timberlake also never had dreads—that I remember.

June 13, 2000

Living Waters again. David & Rachie & I used the pressure washer and sprayed the grass for bugs rather than working on the trailer. David got me wet again. But I wasn't that cold on the bus. Got home and almost immediately left for Centerville. Long trip, I was very uncomfy but I slept a lot. (I am so hungry right now!) At Brashier's we rehearsed then ate dinner (yum!) then changed and Debi, Ryno & I walked into the chapel where no one else. Dumb! But man we laughed hard.

Our concert went excellent. People ♥ed it. Then Rach & I got Brashier...and D. Lianne is so sweet! Court B's middle name is the same! Yea! We went to a party and ate homemade ice cream. Sang around the bonfire. Bo can play dead & Otis was awesome. Bud jumped the fire—gave David a chillies. He's ticklish! Then went to Brashier's. Lianne spoiled us. D is so cute around Brashier.

June 14, 2000

Got up at 8. Long bus ride home. Free time. Ate lunch. Went to the D-Day Museum. Totally cool but de ja vu! After we came home & changed. Concert at a black church. Went pretty decent. More devotional. Danced. Finished senior will & rewrote it w/ Gret. I don't remember much else??

June 15, 2000

Today was our "fun day." First was a dolphin IMAX movie. Then a riverboat cruise... Derek was being kind of rude? Oh well. Katelaine & I played celebrity Mush. We didn't even notice that the ship had moved. We like raced to the dock. They were leaving us but James & Debi waited. Then was boring aquarium. Kate & Bud & I had so much fun making a gay picture... I haven't laughed that hard in a while. Then home and dinner & then group worship again.

It was pouring. I got up w/ Jordan to go hug Jamie first who barely hugged me & then D who really hugged me then James & Debi who told me they ♥ed having me in choir & I had a beautiful voice. Then a short devotionals. Then Magnums & Kate & I ran thru the lightning. Carson & I were screaming like Mexicans at each other. Then we just hung out. We gave Derek the Dolphin the name Earl, Gret the Seal the name Bobo, & Darren the Duck the name Dexter (Poin). Taylor & Jimmy were fighting. Then I came in.

♥ Me

June 16, 2000

Back to Living Waters to paint the trailer. It stormed for us. Lunch. Then the trailer people hung around & did nada. Ellen & Rachel showed us how little their boobs are. Then we went swimming. Ryno & I sat on the edge of the pool b/c our suits were on the bus. We got pretty wet though so we decided to get in. Yuck! I had on a yellow shirt & a black bra. Oops! TK said, "Nice bra." Then we had to wear our bathing suits on the bus. At least we weren't cold. I fell SOUND asleep... so did Jordan & Little Magnum. Jordan had had Benadryl tho. Got home, got stuck on the bus with boys... dinner.

Kate, Krys, & I read for a looong time then went to the gym cause we couldn't swim cause of the rain. Watched the boys play pool. Walked to devotionals singing—senior wills went well I think. Esp. facial hair & boobs. Then David M escorted Krys & me...

we just hung out. Cooper & John C did the J-Z song. Then I went to shower & pack. Bed about 12:15.

June 17, 2000

    Got up at 9:30! Yea! We were going to go to Denny's but it was full. So we went strait to the FQ. Darren & Gret & Derek & I sat at a table at Café du Monde together... ate beinegts. Rach & Gret got palms read. We were going to get henna tats but the guy wasn't there so we just walked around. I got a lot of new shirts, & 2 nite lites. We were spose to meet at a fountain at 2 for lunch. Gret & I sat down on a bench where a homeless guy's duffel was... he came back for it & Gret started talking to him.

    I went w/ TK & Carson to the shirt stand and when we came back, our whole group was talking to this guy. He wanted us to sing "How Great Thou Art" but we didn't know it so we sang "Amazing Grace." He had his hat over his heart & he was kind of crying. Then we sang our Benediction & he really started crying. Then he said how good we are & Jordan gave him some money. Then we went to lunch at Mike Anderson's (seafood to die for). Then back to bus and to La Quinta. ~~We had quite an interesting~~

    We swam then came in & watched Ever After while we got ready for dinner at... C<small>RACKER</small> B<small>ARREL</small>! We had an interesting convo on the way a/b the man's sex organ. Kate & Jordan & John & I cont it at the restaurant. We had so much fun! This guy from a group in Austin came & talked to us. His name was Jonathan & he was very friendly & perky & Jordo thought he was gay. Then he & his group of boys serenaded Emily w/ You've Lost That Lovin' Feelin! C<small>UTE</small>! He was lots of fun.

    Juli & Jordan & I had a fun convo too. Peter Dingo came & told Kate & me how he was making Kristina mad. He couldn't stop laughing. Then we went back to the hotel & Jordo told me about Justin & Greta. Eek! And he talked a/b Graeber. I ♥ him! When we walked to our room, Kate looked like she *was going to cry so I gave her a hug & she put her head on my shoulder & told me how scared she was a/b going home & et changing.*

We (Kate 2 & Rach) had a fun convo. They played with each other's boobs again. Oh, & Jordan told me that Derek wants to get to know me better but on a slow basis. And he's paranoid that I'm following him to Baylor. Hehe, I found that exxxxtremely funny. He's what, one in 20 of my friends going? Haha! So we went to bed & got up & loaded & we watched Forrest Gump & stopped at Burger King & now we're watching Princess Bride. 3 more hours!

June 18, 2000

I guess I had fun. Of course it had to be our last night that was the best. I don't know, I don't feel like a senior. I feel like Derek & Boober are the 2 people I know the least in this group. I was hoping to have such a great time. I didn't much like just staying in once place. I think I expected too much. Rach's flirting got a little annoying… as did her laughing so much a/b every little thing! But I ♥ her! And I ♥ed getting closer to Jordan again. It happens every trip & then it goes away. It happened last year too! And Krys & Kate & I always have fun. No exception this year, but I wish I could feel comfy with the seniors!

♥ Me

Well, now to read this last entry, it sounded like my mood had taken a huge dive because the people were gone. "I guess I had fun"? I was in fucking New Orleans with some of my fave people on the planet at the time. Of course I had fun. I remember wildly missing Justin, who was my singing partner and super cute, which likely bummed me out a bit. But I also remember the fortune tellers and singing for the homeless man like it was yesterday. Those are good memories. Those are the ones I want to remember. And to look back and realize I didn't appreciate it as much as a kid breaks my heart. This poor, lonely girl. Learn your worth, child. Learn your value.

COURTNEY CANNON

June 20, 2000

> Something weird happened tonight. I was in EZ Mart & I saw this (cute) guy go to use the phones. When I came back out, he said something that sounded like my name which was impossible cause I didn't know him. But I turned around & said What?
> "Is your name Courtney?"
> "Yeeeahhh…"
> "I think you know my brother. Did you go to school with him? His name's Travis Hooey."
> "Never heard of him. I want to know how you know my name."
> "I don't know, it must have been some kind of God-send." (???) Then he said, "I need cigs."
> "Why don't you buy some."
> (Actually he asked me if I had any.)
> "I can't cause I'm only 14."
> (The guy looked at least my age.)
> "Do you want me to buy some for you?"
> "Yeah, but I don't have any $. And the thing is, I owe my bro $10 by tonight."
> Apparently he bought some cigs from a not-great guy and now the guy was going to kick his ass. I was like "I don't know what to tell you. But I still want to know how you knew my name."
> "I don't know, this is very weird." I was like, you're tellin' me?
> Then I went to Josh's & watched Sleepy Hollow. Same old same old but I got 2 hugs. And he told me I smelled good. Then I came home & some dude named Cartman7 something was like "Hi Courtney how are you. I said how are you? I don't have a profile so don't even bother. Come on just talk to me. Fine be that way. But I better see you at that West End thing Friday?" I couldn't figure that out. But apparently he IMs Jimmy 2??
>
> ♥ Me

I don't know how often stuff like that happens to other people, but for me, it's frequent and has gotten much more so the older I've gotten—small miracles and fun surprises. Honestly, it's gotten to the point that at forty-two, I expect everyone to just know me. Blame social media, ha! In Connecticut, it's mostly because everywhere I go, most people know my aunt already, so I automatically assume they know me as well.

Y'all, for the most part, it's true. I am a big personality. I am loud and colorful and often in-your-face. I can be super annoying. But if you take a break when I get overwhelming, you'll really benefit from knowing me.

June 24, 2000

> *Ketchup time! Cartman, btw was Douglas Newton. Yeah. Okay, Wed after study & swim me, Katie G, Kate Ri, Josh, Boobs, & Jordan went to Gil's to watch Wyatt Earp. At 12, we minus Jordo & Grapenut went to Ryno's to finish it. Greg slapped my hand. Movie finished at 2:15! Pretty fun. Thurs I babysat for the Honeycombs. Nolan was so excited to see me! Friday went to the West End w/ church. Got Simply Irresistible poster. Kate & I had pix done again.*
>
> *At 4 Emily Imed me & said to come over & we went swimming at her neighbor's. Boobs & Josh took off their suits. Em did 2 but she got hers back on b4 the boys got there. We cornered the guys. Josh has a nice body. After we just talked then Boobs went home. Derek, Gret & I went to M:I-2. Gooood movie! Gret sat down first then Derek went in & left a seat bet them so I sat in the middle so he could only sit by me?? Then we went to bowling @ Jupiter Lanes. That was a great night. Tonight Shelb & Ryan came over. Shelb asked for a head rub (both heads) & then had to go and ruin it by asking if Audrey would have sex w/ him & that he'd date her. Ick! Shelby!*
>
> ♥ *Me*

June 29, 2000

> *I'm at a little bed and breakfast at Baylor right now. Took the Spanish & math placement tests. Bad on Spanish. Saw Derek & Gret. I can't believe I'm going to be living here! Small dorm rooms. I hope I*

like my roommate. Tomorrow I get my classes. Yea! I hope everything goes great!

♥ Me

July 5, 2000

Last night the seniors minus Derek came over & cooked out then went to fireworks then to Josh's woods house. Me, Gret, & Boobs sang all the way there. We got pulled over the cop said we ran a red light, sped, & wove. Josh was pissed. They had taken off bc the alcohol had spilled. We got more fire & lit them till 3 AM. Talked till 4. In the morn, we lit the trash & two Roman candles were not lit & they shot off. We had so much fun!

♥ Me

July 10–July 11, 2000

Yesterday was the 1st day of camp. Jimmy & I were among the first there. We ran to Einstein's for bagels (cin raisin). On the bus (which was almost on time) I put on my headphones & was out for most of the ride. We got to camp & I had a little scare with my suitcase. Then Jimmy had to drag it up there & we told Rachel C that it was all Jimmy's. Then we had orientation & got introduced to our "song," "Uh, y'all come up here, uh, it's time to come to the place," by Darren 30+ times.

Then we ate sloppy Joes & chips. Then we went to the pool for a while & then to the lake. Then when we got tired of that, back to the pool. At the pool, we were trying to stand on the rope & at the lake, Kate & I were trying to get off the aqua jump & Bud started jumping, leaving me laughing so hard that when I got in the water, I couldn't breathe.

After pool, we went into ~~main hall~~ cabin to make our list. Funnily, almost everybody got 4 stars. And all but about 2 got at least 2 stars. Good times at date night. Then we went & showered & Amelia was trying to make me feel electric waves coming out of one of the faucets. Got dressed, went to eat fried chicken & mashed taters. Yum.

After dinner, we chilled until worship at 7. We sang & discussed the theme of camp. Brashier preached. Told about Lianne's mom. Mm... found out our real gathering song is Beastie Boys. Movie was at 9... John laid in my lap for a little, then I had to lay down. But I rubbed his hair all through For Love of the Game—bad slow movie. Rhett & Katie Lilac were holding hands. John fell asleep & I think Rhett did too.

After movie we went to bed. I got out of bed at like 7:50, put in my contax, went to eggs, bacon, biscuit, banana, Trix. After we cleaned our cabin. Then Kate & I tried going in the main cabin but someone was asleep in there. We stood outside it for like 7 mins waiting to see if they'd come out, but now we're sitting on the dining hall porch.

July 11–July 12, 2000

We had morning worship then ate lunch after Jamie, Joannah, & Juliana spoke about their joyful memories. (Tacos & nachos.) Then after we went & sat by the pool & I blew up my inner-tube & we watched the soccer players. That was when I first saw Tim—he had on khaki shorts & bare feet & he slapped hands with Cable & Luke. After we went out in the lake & inner-tubed it. I got more sunburned.

At about 3, we got out & came in the meeting room & Tim came & sat by me & asked how we were. Kate & I were trying to write notes but it wasn't workin with Tim there. I was finally like, "Are you Charlie?" Then I explained to him that I knew Greg & Austin for sure, but I hadn't remembered his name. He was like, No I'm Tim, who are you? And he proceeded to tell us all the people he met. I got crap for Luke & I got crap for Greg... Tim even told Greg over the walkie-talkie that there were some girls down there that thought he was hot. It was pretty funny.

Then we went & showered & came back & I read a little of Tears in Heaven, a story I wrote as a kid. We ate dinner (chicken fried steak) then we had chill time then evening worship. Little bit of time then volleyball tournament. Our team got skunked 7-0 but our other half made it to the champions and lost against Cable & Laws' team. I got pix of Laws & Bryson & Cable & maybe Luke. So after, I came to bed & at about 1, my #9 on Garth woke me up like an alarm clock.

Got up this morn, 7/12, went to brecky... quiet time, bible study w/ Nicole... she caught both Anna and me not listening twice. Oops. Hmm. Morning worship, lunch (burgers & fries, 1st time I prayed), then Kate & I went in search for Tim. We dribbled a soccer ball to the ropes course to see who would come. Greg & Nisha came for water jugs. Greg doesn't strike me as the most friendly of people. But either maybe he heard who the girls were that said he was hot or else maybe he's shy.??? Cute as hell anyway.

Anyway, so after we checked the lake, we went back into the meeting hall. Krystal, Jordan, & Jennifer immediately joined us & we played Egyptian Rat Screw until they left for horses. Tim had come in with no shirt & jeans & I was like, I want to go riding now! So I walked all the way down there & the girls were already on their horses. Tim: "Hey Courtney, what's up?" Me: "Not much!" I walked over to pet his horse & said, "Oh I want to go now!" "You shoulda signed up!" Then one of the horses in the corral started pulling up his lips at me & showing his teeth. Tim said, "He's trying to tell you something, Courtney. He's saying, "You could have been riding me right now." I was sad. I was like, "Have fun, be back soon." Then I went back w/ Kate & Jordan.

Instead of writing notes like I was supposed to, I talked. Jordan told us stories about Avery. Then Austin & Jessica came in & started playing ERS. I was like, "Are you playing ERS?" Austin: "Yeah, you know how? You want to play?" So Kate & I joined them (Jordan had left w/ K & J to shower). Every time Austin hit a pile, he looked away. It was so cute! He & I were always the ones to slap. A lot of times my hand ended up on his or vice versa. Warm, big hands! So Katie G joined us at one point. We played BS & Katie won then ERS again & I won for the third time. Then we left to shower.

 Came back for dinner of enchiladas. Jamie & Cable & I were trying to get Kate to eat them. Steven M sat across from us. Hmm. After ~~dinner worship dinner~~ worship I braided my hair... Oh Gret & I made the watermelon sign. Worship at 7:30. Hmm. John talked about how lying was worse than killing to him. Jimmy & I looked at each other. Um. After we hung around for a while & I got suckers for every1. I had to go back for Graham & Ryno & Jim though. Talent show was looong. Alex H & Ronnie were good. Elliott was too cute. But it was Boobs Justin Derek & Michael that really stole the show w/ 7 Bridges Road. Justin was too cute! Josh shaved his armpits & then put bbq sauce & pickles & other acidic stuff on them & Boobs ate it! Yuck!

 After that, Kate & I went & reorganized my suitcase. We girls stayed up until like 12:30 just talking, then we went to an empty cabin to see streaking boys, but we were in there till 1:15 & they never came so Em Mag & I went back. I couldn't fall asleep & then I heard the girls come back in from skinny dipping. They left again when a car came up. I still couldn't fall asleep. It was hard waking up on Thursday the 13th today. Cinnamon rolls for brecky. Then I re-braided my hair, cleaned the cabin. Now I'm here writing!

July 13–July 14, 2000

 After quiet time, we went to Juliana's bible study a/b family. I talked soooo much! After was morning worship & I almost started crying when Nicole talked. After was lunch (gross sandwiches) then free time. I stayed inside & wrote about 50 notes. Greg was the one to come at 3. We took showers at about

3:30 then I went into my cabin, scrunched my hair, & wrote a few more notes. Then I put on my makeup & went to the place.

Peter Dingo told me he told Cameron that he knew he was going to get me. I knew too. He was fun. Justin sat across from us and then made Jordan B sit next to him. Too cute, that boy is! But he always catches me staring at him & he thinks I'm giving him weird looks. In my note to him, I told him it's b/c I think he's sexy. So after dinner I got lots of pix w/ Justin, Mel, Luke, Cable, Derek, Ellen... a bunch. Then I had to change cause I was sweating all my makeup off.

Evening worship I almost fell asleep then after I stayed & talked to Debi forever. Then to the bb court to talk w/ Rach C, Katie L, Rhett, Jim, & Greta. Dance started at 10:15 & I have never had so much fun. I actually danced. The slow song, Peter & I danced cheek to head and then Lacy left Marshall so he came to me & the 3 of us were just swaying. Then Marshall was like, I have to dance with her, this is my love. So Peter got left out & I was dancing w/ M so close... like we were hugging. Poor Peter.

Then when the fast song came on, I danced with Rhett. It was so fun. Ryan Roller is too funny. Graham is really good. Luke P was trying to teach Elliott how to dance and GOD he was sexy. Then at one point, he was dancing around the floor & he ended up dancing against me. I took his hips but then he kept going, so that's all I did. It was sooo much fun. Then nice sleep!

This morning, I came to brecky with my hair frizzy but still crunched, my glasses on, & my heart pants & black shirt on. Then of course it had to be Tim doing the dishes w/ nothing but an apron on!!! I caught sight of him & turned to Jordan making yummy noises. Jessica saw me & was laughing at me & pointing & "I saw you!" She thought it was funny. Then while I was writing, he came w/ no shirt to take the waters away. HOT. After we went to Jamie's. Drew pictures. I shared about my first prayer experience. Then worship. Gret then Boobs then Josh then Mel talked.

At lunch, I got Rhett's card and ~~almost~~ started crying. My contact came out & I ran to the bathroom. Then I walked past him & he was like, Did you get mine? And I was like, Yeah that was why I started crying. Then I gave him a hug and said I ♥ U Rhett & he like whispered I ♥ U 2. (Ok, aqua jump & T or D.)

Sooo then Kate & I put on bathing suits and we went down to the lake. It started off as just us & Laura Medina with us talking with Hank a/b names. "Why do I want to call her Laura?" Then other people started coming & we got a game of T or D going. We dared Lacy to kiss Mark, who kept running. Haha. Then we dared Laura to kiss Peter, & Juliana was right there whooping On the mouth! with us. She kissed him, & there was movement on his side. We called him on it, & he said of course. We played a while longer and at 3:30 Kate & I went to write notes. Played ERS w/ Hank & Eric. I won a 4th game. Showered at like 5. Went to hurriedly write more notes. I skipped dinner. Finally finished them all. Swoosh. Hmm.

After dinner Kate & I went to get a drink & see if we could run into Tim. We pushed apple juice & it gave us a grape soda, but it still charged us $.80. We were all whining & calling Adams' various names. Dana hooked us up w/ $.20 & it was cool. We walked into the Band-aid Cabin & basically got thrown out. Well, Jordan said, "They just keep coming," and then TK told us to lock the door so no one would come in, so we left.

At 7:30 we went to worship. Then we went to get sno cones, saw Tim looking hot in a navy shirt & khakis. He was like, Hey girl what are you up to? I was like Waiting for you, actually. T: really, why? Me: There are 5 of us who want a picture with you. T: Right now? Me: Well, when are you getting home tonight? T: Late. How 'bout before y'all leave in the morning. Me: Will you be up? T: Yeah, I have to do breakfast. So we agreed & he left.

Then the 5 of us walked around. We were laughing very hard and at one point I was trying to swallow sno cone & laugh, I bent over so I could spit it out w/o getting it on my shirt, but failed & I snorted it out my nose. Ow! That's never happened to me before.

The string thing / communion thing started at about 10. We drew names. First I got Cora but I put her back & got Katie Grapenut. Jordan B had Rhett & w/o me even having to ask, she traded w/ me. I tried to trade w/ Jen for Justin, but she didn't. It was kind of better then the string thing but also not. Maris H got me. She gave me 2 hugs. Then I got up & was like, Funnily enough, if I could have chosen the one person to get, I would have chosen this person. I got Rhett Maximus. He has helped me so much in my walk with Christ & I feel very privileged to be able to give this to Rhett... then we hugged forever. Jordan was sick, but she said she could make it through.

After, I got a zillion hugs—Anna, Rachel, Jimmy, Michael, John, Jordan, Justin—everyone special & then some. Justin asked me why I was leaving. Jordan & John made me cry... Jordan just talked to me. After, we just stayed up. We were on the dock w/ Josh & Derek then the 3 of us went to the bb court. Katie G & John & some others were there. I played w/ John's hair & then Katie's while Josh, she, & I talked.

Then Katie & I walked around a long time, sometimes joined by various of Jenn Jordan Krys & Kate. Poor baby was torn up about Justin. We talked for hours. I let her cry & just stroked her ponytail. Then Justin came to talk to her & he was acting really stupid... she was acting mean. Then they went to talk & I went to find Kate & Jordan cause the other 2 were asleep. Then Jordan went to sleep & Kate & I wandered various places briefly. Ran into Jordan W. He said he hadn't had fun. I went to *sleep at 5:00. Barely could get up. I think I lost a freakin film roll!*

♥ *Me*

Church camp always brought forth the jokes about the bad kids. I remember giggling when we all wanted to go streaking, thinking, "OMG, it's true." But what I've come to understand is, we were all bad kids. We all struggled with peer pressure, with smoking, drinking, and sex. But the church kids—the holy rollers, as my best friend labeled us when I started working at Pizza Hut—got more flack when we did something naughty because we were supposed to be the examples.

Was that quite fair? Were some of us—I'm not including myself in this scenario simply because I was a good kid—more inclined toward wayward behavior because our parents (or the rest of the world) held us to a higher standard? Anxiety starts at a very young age, y'all. The next time your baby cries for no reason, give them a really good cuddle from Auntie Coco.

July 17, 2000

Went to church then to Texadelphia. Luke invited us to X-Men at 3, even tho it started off being only their grade, bc he wanted Rachel. Too cute. X-Men was pretty good. Sat by Justin. Then to Katie's. She & I had another great talk. Then to church. Then to Desperado's. Jason Patron is sooo cute! Josh gave $40. Then me Katie, DL, QT, Boobs, & Rett went to Katie's. Boobs, K, & I had more talks. We played hysterical games of Mush. Boobs & I actually talked while looking e/o in the eye. Great day.

♥ *Me*

July 19–July 20, 2000

Tonight after Watershed we went to Krystal's house. Watched the Haunting. Jason Patron—I am in love w/ yet another sophomore! Rhett sat in my lap & wove his fingers in mine & tried to put my hand on his penis. Then he rubbed the back of my neck like I was his. It felt really good! I kept thinking, this is Rhett, not a bf. I wanted it to be a bf so

> *much! If it weren't for Katie, the possibility could be there! Jordan B asked where I was & someone said under Rhett who I think was Jason. Jason kept looking at us too. Jealous? I love it being Rhett (he tickled my foot too) but I wish it had been Jason! ♥!*
>
> ♥ Me

I don't think I understood just how boy crazy I was until I started writing this. Seriously, there's a new name every page. I could sit and speculate about what drove that—hello, daddy issues—or I could embrace it and thank the good Lord in heaven I didn't end up with a disease or pregnant out of wedlock (and yes, that's a joke). But even when I started working in preschool, the boys were always my favorites.

My first year at Kids 'R' Kids, I got to work in the school-age program for the summer, and I connected with a kid named Christopher, which had always been my number one boy's name. He was nine at the time, and at the end of the summer, he told me he wished I was his mother. It was the most amazing compliment I had ever gotten—kids are brutally honest, and they're excellent at making you feel as terrible as they make you feel good—and I took it to heart. Thankfully, his real mother allowed me to be in his life, and I got to see him grow.

I remember telling my own mother about him once, and she said, "You have a crush on this kid," and it horrified me. "I most certainly do not," I replied, then spent weeks and months worrying about if I had a crush on a nine-year-old.

You guys, I did not have a crush on a nine-year-old. My heart is an equal-opportunity lover, and I believe that's what I've been put on this earth to do: love. I love fast, hard, and fiercely; and as an adult, I will apologize for none of that anymore. I've apologized for loving far more than I'd care to admit.

July 29, 2000

> *First day of senior trip—mostly driving. Nearly killed twice by macks swerving into our lanes. D is too cool. Josh put his hand on my leg, forgetting I was below him, & left it there & drug it up, then did it again later. Scared of river!*
>
> ♥ Me

Excuse me again, but the care I took to describe every tiny touch that any boy gave me breaks my heart. I crave physical touch like no one's business. If you haven't seen *Life as a House*, watch the scene with Kevin Kline in the hospital bed. Touch your people, guys. Humans need contact.

> Ok, Sunday was more driving to the cabins, Hidden Gap, very nice. 8 double beds, 8 of us. Learned Shang-hai. Up until 4, Boober snoring, Jaf & Wexler talking. At about 8, I had diahrrea & D gave me Emetrol that made me throw up. I was scared cause it was our 1st day rafting but it was cool. Rafting rocked. Awesome. Our guide, (me, Gret, Boobs, Josh) Greg was awesome. It rained! At camping, it still rained... most of us were pretty miserable. I slept soundly thru the nite, our chef Mike was hot.
>
> Next day, just me & Gret, our guide Eric was HOTTT! We had so much fun. I scraped my thigh on a rock, banged my elbow on G's t-grip, & have never been in so much pain ever. At the cabins, Em & Wexler & I hung out a lot. Played Shang-hai, Gret got pissed bc she lost & she quit. Me Em & Wex got in Jamie's bed & we got dog-piled. Smoked a pipe... hmm, lot of fun. At 5:10 AM, moved to the couch cause of Boober. Drove today. Lots of fun!
>
> ♥ Me

August 4, 2000

> Went to see Coyote Ugly w/ peeps. Lotta fun, but I kept choking up. Then in the car I was like bawling. Then went to Scott's. Now home talking to Jordan & crying.
>
> ♥ Me

August 13, 2000

> Last night, Jordan W felt me up with ice in my car. Talk about erotic experiences. It was only on my thighs but I about crashed the van. Then tonight we went a little further. I actually felt his hard on... shit. I can't believe that I could do that to someone. I think Josh Constantine may like me. And I like

> *Darren Sheffer now. Shit! Too much going on & I leave in 2 days!*
>
> ♥ *Me*

This was one of the entries I was looking forward to reading, and it severely let me down. My poor, innocent brain was too innocent for the sordid details. Oh, wait...

August 15, 2000

> *Leave tomorrow... got a great good-bye present from Jordan... at first it was more awkward, but then he started rubbing me again. He asked if he could go further, & I was like yeah, I wore underwear you'd like the feel of! So he fingered me for a long time. He knew just where to touch that I didn't. He kissed my breast through my bra... OH MY GOD. He kissed me, too, with a lot of tongue. Ah. Then I massaged him for a while & told him to undo his belt. When I touched the head, it jerked around. I pulled it out so I could see what I was doing. He tried to get me going fast enough to make him cum, but I couldn't so he had to. It was interesting to watch. Nice way to be introduced to all this... but not what I thought. Right now, I'm like, no biggie.*
>
> ♥ *Me*

There we go! It reminds me of reading *Forever* by Judy Blume for the first time in the junior high cafeteria with my best friends. Awkward AF. But I love myself for saying he knew where to touch that I didn't. Like, even in my own diary, I couldn't not compliment him. He was fifteen at the time, y'all, no expert despite what he might have thought.

Also, it wasn't until much later that I learned what a good kiss could be.

September 5, 2000

> *Lots of fun @ Baylor. Brian—beautiful green eyes, looks like Jay Mohr. Matt—likes Laura. James—very cute. Andy—"taught" me to 2-step at Ghrams's. Lot of fun @ the club, "freaked" with some random*

> guys. 24-year-old marine! Parents are divorcing. Very sad, distracting... I am sleeping horribly. Went home this weekend, am in love with a very show-offy Justin Woody! Jason was soooo sweet to me. Watched Cruel Intentions at Josh C's house. Darren says "guhls" like he's British.
>
> ♥ Me

I hope this is as funny for you guys as it is for me. I say funny lightly, because it's also super triggering, and I've been crying a lot. You guys, I do not remember being particularly heartbroken that my parents got divorced. As teenagers, we kids had been speculating about it for a few years, and I even think we settled on "They're waiting till I leave for college." Maybe they thought I would take it the hardest? Who knows?

What I do know is what I wrote in my journal, and the emotions are powerful, and for the first time in my life, I find myself wishing for a time machine. I would do anything—anything—to be able to comfort this girl as she lay sad in her bed at the end of every day, her heart longing for that requited love. Look around you, sweet girl. Enjoy the love in the forms it did come. But also, I understand her sadness. It's like starving and being offered morsels of beef jerky when the whole filet mignon with mashed potatoes, salad, and decadent chocolate cake sits tantalizing you with its scent. Not enough.

Did my parents divorcing intensify that somehow? Did I go as crazy as I did freshman year because of my reaction to the divorce? Was I already imitating my mother's illness? (More on that later.) Now I also say I went crazy lightly. My mother, who has actually gone crazy, may not be able to say the same thing I'm about to say, and that's that I regret nothing—except perhaps not grasping how to spend and save a little earlier in life. One thing I have to thank my father for, outside my existence, is a Dave Ramsey budgeting class.

November 7, 2000

> Wow, it's been 2 months. I adore Baylor. Matt doesn't like Laura anymore. I like Andy. I still think I'm in love with Justin Woody. When I called, he sounded so happy to hear from me. I get soo high when I'm around him! AHH! Too much has gone on, I should write every day. Please let me get decent grades and be able to stay in school and rush!
>
> ♥ Me

December 20, 2000

    I am sooo in love with Justin Woody! These feelings are so different than any others I've had, for Juan, for Chad, who I thought I was in love with (uhh??)... different from Josh, from Joey... this boy drives me nuts. I AM IN LOVE WITH HIM & IT'S KILLING ME! I really think I might be in love... every time I look at him, I feel like bursting into song or tears.
    When I saw Trey's car pull up & Justin get out to come get me, my heart felt like it was going to burst out of my chest & I couldn't breathe. I was like, yeah, calm down idiot. I was panicking. Gas pipe was fun. Trey laughed every time I heard them say something. Oh, I'm so in love, what do I do? He whispered to me tonight & I about passed out. I thought he kept exchanging looks with me. I took his hat and at one point he took it back but then he threw it back in my lap. AHHH! ♥ Then Greta wouldn't move over b/c he had said, "Scoot over so I can sit here, I don't wanna sit by Greta." I LOVE HIM! OH MY GOD HELP ME! I love Justin Woody with all my heart, body, & mind.

                                                             ♥ Me

January 1, 2001

    Tonight we went to Brian Wilson's house for a NY party. It was so much fun. I actually felt like Jason was flirting with me. He kept singling me out for snowball fights. He kept throwing smiles in my direction. So cute. But God I miss Justin. And I like Jason sooo much though. It hurt me to think I bother him when I go out with them.

                                                             ♥ Me

January 5, 2001

    Saw Justin tonight. Went to Oshman's an incredibly long way. So we could talk? I adore him. When he left he gave me this entirely long hug rocking me b & f, talking in my ear. I looooove hug-

> *ging him! So much! Why do I get crushes on people so out of my reach? Today 224.5. By musical, I WILL BE 200! Dammit, 24 lbs in a month? Doubtful, but possible. We shall see. Let me keep the looks on my two J's faces in my head... that's motivation enough for me. Oh, he also told me to study a lot so I'll be there when he comes next year.*
>
> ♥ *Me*

There I go again, putting my worth on my weight. As I am writing this, I am six pounds heavier than that college weight. That is a huge accomplishment to the adult who has fought the scale her entire life, and yet I understand that if I had just learned the tricks at twenty that I know now, my whole life could have been different. How many of my insecurities really come from being fat and having my mother tell me if I only lost a little?

It makes me angry every time I think about where my insecurities come from. I don't want to make excuses anymore. I want to overcome it. I already wrote about this, but I remember telling her any man worth his salt would love me despite my fat, and I was right. Yet I'm still single, which proves her point. But I'm working on proving mine: no one will love me until I truly love myself no matter what weight I am. (And that goes for all you beautiful souls as well. Insert your insecurity of choice.)

February 6, 2001

> *Friday night, we went to Kenneth from the Life Group's apt. I met Ben for the first time & he is adorable. Oh, & earlier, we went to D/FW to pick up Tiff's Ben & he is hilarious. At Kenneth's we had jambalaya & played a game called Therapy & then some of us played Uno Jenga. Zach cracks me up. We had a pillow fight, & Zach hits really hard. My right arm muscles really hurt the day after. Anyway, lot of fun getting to know everyone.*
>
> *Sunday night (2/5) church was weird. So different. I saw Mike Ashgrove & he told me it had totally changed his life. Saw Grant & both Daniels & "met" Leslie Stiller. It was intense. Had a discussion a/b Ben's name & mine. Monday night, went to Olive Garden & Head Over Heels with Tiff & her Ben,*

who can keep me laughing w/ no problems. Goofy guy.

♥ *Me*

I see my time at Antioch as one of the turning points in my journey with God. I remember learning what a testimony was and what made mine special. I learned—but didn't quite believe—what a prophet was. I learned that a prophecy cast when I was nineteen and that haunted me my entire life might not be the horrible sentence I thought it was then. (And now I'm making it come true in an entirely different way than I would have expected. Self-fulfilling, if you will.) And above all, I started witnessing my first miracles. (Forget that as an adult, I believe waking up after a sugar binge is a miracle in itself!)

February 11, 2001

Church this morning was good. Then to the Cowsills, met Nathan, too cute, burned his face on a fajita plate. Baked cakes, then to Zach & Tiff's for invitation party. Ben got me to go to Juarez. Too cute! At church, Luke started crying, so heartbreaking, I thought I was gonna cry. Another guy looked like he was having a seizure & others were dancing around. Weird. Takes a lot of getting used to. Bri & I had a good discussion a/b it.

♥ *Me*

February 28, 2001

Sun night, the 25th, I got to pray w/ Luke. He got his wisdom teeth out & it's hard for him to smile. He's so cute. We forgot what we were spose to pray for so when we closed our eyes, we couldn't stop smiling, it was funny. Jess & I have been on the outs for a while, but tonight was much better. I am so excited a/b Juarez. Scared too. I am sleepy now. Oh, Jess said when Derek talked to me, he blushed! Too cute!

♥ *Me*

March 12, 2001

> *Juarez was so absolutely indescribably incredible. I spent insane amounts of time getting to know possibly the sweetest guy I've ever met. Luke is an amazing person. He's gentle & funny & cute... oh, so cute. This is a baaaad situation. I can't like this guy even a little bit, much less as much as I do. I don't want to hurt Jessica. It's seeming inevitable though... I like him so much! I can't stop thinking about him.*
>
> *In Mexico, when he was praying for me w/ his hand on my shoulder, I could swear, when he took it off, he gave it a squeeze. Same w/ when we were praying at Sanborn's, he was holding my hand, & when we said Amen, I know he squeezed it. Oh my gosh, sooooooo much! Yikes. I need someone that knows him that I can talk to... I need Jess. I pray she'll find someone else... & leave Luke for me. It's selfish I know, but this one is for real.*
>
> ♥ *Me*

March 14, 2001

> *Oh this one is so for real. I'm calm & sweet around him & I think he might like me too. I walked up to Taylor's & Luke was leading his family up the stairs. He waved at me, then stopped & waited for me. He said "Hey Court-neh!" "like Eva" and "how's it going." Ohhh. Then he introduced me to his family, & I thought I kept catching him staring at me. Maybe this one is straight from God. I've prayed about it, been patient... is it finally my turn? This guy would be perfect for me. And I bloody can't stop thinking about him. Sigh, what am I gonna do?*
>
> ♥ *Me*

(*In tiny PS*): *Ben came behind me, put a hand on my shoulder, & said "this girl is so great!" and his mom said "I can tell!" Ahh! I wonder if Luke's told her about me?*

March 18, 2001

> *Hehe, I talked to Luke like 4 times on the phone yesterday. I got such a thrill from hearing his voice. Friday night out with the girls was a lot of fun, except Tiff wanted to talk about boys. I kept trying to change the subject. Jess, of all people, was the one pressing me. I think she had an idea, but she was acting like it was Ben. I came home & we talked about it, I told her the truth. She said she's fine with it, & that it's in God's hands. I know it is, but I'm so impatient, I can't help wanting to push it. But I am going to chill now. Let him come to me. And I pray that he will. God, I pray with all my heart that he will!!! Help me God! Please let this be the one you finally want for me.*
>
> ♥ *Me*

Two questions I've had for God my entire life are "When's it my turn?" and "Who is the one for me?" Two answers I have now: it's my turn when I make it my turn, and she/he is the one for me. I have come to believe I am the everybody friend. The O- of lovers. (And that's the only time you'll see me attach anything to do with negative to my name.) And it's my turn now. You know how I know? My Rangers took the pennant for the first time in seven years. Seven! Do you know what that means? It means we are winning the World Series for the first time in franchise history. You know how I know that? They blew it on my thirtieth birthday. My heart broke in two when my favorite player fumbled hugely. They owe me. It's. My. Turn.

(If for some reason it turns out I'm wrong and they're about to break my heart again, I'll make the proper apologies. But I'm leaving it here: We are winning the World Series this year. #CocoMagic is strong, and I will not be burned out again so quickly. 2023 is indeed the year of me. The phoenix has risen for the last time.)

God, writing it down makes it feel so good. Why is it so easy to lose faith as soon as you say it? My anxiety immediately makes me want to prepare to lose, but that makes me sick to my stomach, thinking of all the other heartbroken people, Rangers players notwithstanding. We will win, finally. And if I don't move on, I will write that over and over until I freaking manifest it into existence.

NOT THE F——ING GILMORE GIRLS

March 23, 2001

Wednesday night at Life Group, we were encouraging each other. Kaitlin said she liked my ability to trust—not have any walls. I kept looking at Luke, begging him to say something about me. He kept meeting my eyes, which was unnerving. He wasn't avoiding my gaze, but he wouldn't say anything. At the end of group, me, Luke, & Mark just chatted. People started leaving, & at about 10:20, Tiff, Zach, Luke, Ben, & I went outside to chat. The 1st 3 stayed on the balcony, & Ben & I went downstairs, just chatting. I told him about the Boxster, & he about wet his pants, it was so cute. Eventually the other 3 came down & we just played around. Then the Becks went back up, & Luke & Ben & I had a great time. AHH Luke is so cute. I took an entire roll of film. Eeee. I can't wait till tomorrow.

March 28, 2001

Sigh. Well, I had a great weekend. Friday night, some of us went bamboo climbing. I about threw up from the ride. But I got to see Luke. I was fine in the dark, I could climb great. Sat. Jim & Drew got here & we went straight to Luke's, then to the mall. Luke rode w/ me & we looked at toe socks. Lots of fun. Then we went to show the boys the bamboo. We climbed a path to Lover's Leap. We were throwing stones off into the river. Then we went to the bamboo. I got up fine, but I lost a soccer sandal. Back down, the branch broke & I fell about two feet onto my butt on the street. I was laughing until I saw my thumb. Luke thought the blood was a bracelet, so he didn't know what I had done until the blood dripped. Pain. Luke washed it out while Drew held my wrist. Luke drove for me.

We were gonna just do a butterfly, but Ben said I'd need stitches. So we went to the SLC. Luke & the guys waited, then when the stitches got put in, Luke got to come in. That was cool. He just watched & talked to me. Ben had come up about 15 mins after. That was sweet. So went to the HEB to get better bandages after the boys & I got changed for JD's. Ben bandaged my hand right in the HEB. Then Luke drove to JD's. We were way early, so we went to Crickets.

Luke was driving really fun, it was wild. We went down some one way streets the wrong way. Stayed at Crickets for like 20 minutes. Came back, drove wilder. Sooo fun. In JD's every time Luke wanted to say something, he had to get real close. Ahh. They picked me up for church the next day. Lunch was sooo good. Luke started off sitting by me, but Ben changed seats with him. The meeting, Luke looked like he might cry. After, I hung out w/ Ben at Kenneth's watching Survivor. Then the rally.

Monday, Luke, Jon, & I went to get passports. Missed it. Then dinner w/ Kaitlin. Then Luke came over. He was obviously very nervous. I thought he might ask me out, but it was just the opposite. He said he didn't know if it was how it was, but he felt there was something more than friends between us & he felt we should put some distance between us. People were saying things to him. Not to spend time alone together so much. Ah, I was sad. But I tried to make him feel calmer. Poor baby. Anyway, when he left, I cried so much. Tiff called & I was like, I'm sure you know Luke just came by. She was like yeah, are you okay? I'm not, but I will be. I still feel like that. Had good talks w/ both her & Kaitlin (again).

EMP the next morning, things were awkward w/ Luke, but that afternoon, we went to post office again, & things were a bit better. I finished his CD, gave him a great letter. Had Phil give it to him... and tonight at church was much better. We still locked eyes a few times, but we talked like people again, & played Big Booty great. He's such a sweetheart. Mark, Luke, & I played drums. Tiff & I sang together. Sooo fun.

There is something bet. Luke & I, I know there is. He knows it too, he even said it. "We just clicked really well." But he doesn't want it to progress.

I asked if that meant ever, & I don't know if he understood, but he said no. We'll see what God has planned.

♥ Me

April 12, 2001

Oh goodness. Goodness gracious me. Man oh man. I am dying. I think I am heartbroken. I must be manic depressive for real. For the past two weeks, I had the worst time. We went camping last week with LG. Luke was gonna leave early... he had school. We played ultimate frisbee, & it was so fun. Luke came & walked by me. I didn't have to seek him out. Oh gosh.

When he was about to leave, everything just hit me & I panicked, about my research paper & eq project, the choir concert, & Luke. I completely lost it when Kaitlin pulled me aside. We ended up at the bathroom cause K had a bug in her pants. I was standing in the parking lot crying & someone pulled up & honked. Not in the mood and embarrassed, I backed out of the way. Luke apologized for scaring me, & w/o smiling, I said I wasn't scared. I think I must have sounded mean, & I'm sure I scared him.

Anyway, Tiff B & Jess got out of the back & Luke went to drive off after he said bye softly. Tiff came & put a hand on me & I started crying again. Luke had to turn around. I know he saw me crying & I'm sure he knew why.

Long story short, I was in a bad mood for a while, but I ended up staying. I didn't easily stop crying, esp. when we started talking about the things God had been doing for us lately & I couldn't think of anything. Zach said some really sweet things though, & I started to feel better.

Eventually over the week, things began getting much better. God really worked in my life this week. Just little things, but that's what counts. When I asked Him to give me dreams about the Clements, he did. Sometimes in an over-abundance like the car crash... oh God, please keep them safe! My baby. Last night at church, Luke sat by me, even though he had a spot by Ben & it meant he wasn't completely in the circle. The best part, the one that made me wonder for TONIGHT was: we were supposed to pray for the person on our right. I was on Luke's, and excited a/b hearing what he'd say. Then he crawled over to Zach & whispered something, & Zach goes "Do you want to?" & Luke nodded. So Z goes, "Yeah, if you want to, lay hands on the person, unless they don't want you touching them."

To keep myself from exploding from excitement, I grinned at Taylor. She goes, "Don't touch me." Oh, God, please help me. I couldn't concentrate on praying b/c of Luke... oh GOD!! At one point, Z prayed for the whole group, & I had each hand on one each of T's & L's legs... and I was lightly squeezing Luke's at points that were important for us. And he was doing the same thing on my arm. His grip got tighter, which gave me more courage to really tighten mine. I think we were feeding off each other, oh man, oh man... this is tough. When I asked for his hand so I could pop my back, we ended up holding hands for a long time.

The physical contact, any contact... I can't get over this, oh, God, please hear my prayer. What if I fall in love with him? What if I am falling in love with him? What if I have fallen in love with him? I just pray for a resolution before summer so I don't feel like this w/o seeing him for 3 months. What am I going to do?

♥ Me

April 26, 2001

One week. Oh God, one week. What am I gonna do? My mom doesn't want me to come live there, & she won't let me have the van. AHH! I would like to stay in Waco, in my apt if possible. The Blossoms'll be here, & Kaitlin & Mark & the CLEMENTS! There's a chance I'll see him this summer! AH! Oh, dear.

At church Wed, John was saying something mean about women, & Luke's mouth dropped open & he stepped in front of me as if to protect me. It was the cutest thing. Then he turned around w/ his back to John, still between us. "Not all women," he said. Sweetie. He was so sweet when I told him about my heart.

Oh. It was a lot of fun going to the outlet mall with Ben & Mark & Jess. Then What Women Want. Oh, at church the end of the year thing hit me, & I was crying all through worship. Luke looked like he couldn't look at me, like maybe it hurt him? But Zach kept smiling at me, & I got notes from him, Tiff, & Bri. Oh, Bri & I after chapel met the band, Destination Known. Sooo fun.

After work tonight, Ben had called & I told him to have Luke call me, & he was like, in a different voice, "Yeah, this is—this is—this is—just kidding, this is Luke," like he couldn't think of anything funny fast enough. Hehe. I love him! Goodnight! God give me dreams about Luke, & wake me up well tomorrow so I can see him. Keep us both safe. I love you, Amen.

♥ Me

May 4, 2001

It's actually Cinco de Mayo. Ah, Luke. Sunday at DP, I was crying almost nonstop after someone said something about home & summer & I could see Luke turn to look at me. I looked at him out of the corner of my eye, trying not to smile. He laughed and said, "You still don't know, huh?" Then I was crying. Tiff K & Taylor prayed for me, I got 2 hugs from Mike, then back to the front.

When I went back, I first went to my seat, but Luke was at the front being prayed for, so I went to kneel on the floor. Then he did. He started crying as hard as I'd ever seen a guy cry. It was absolutely heartbreaking. I was crying harder, like sobbing, thinking what am I gonna do without him this summer? I couldn't stand seeing him cry like that.

Then I went back to my seat & Jess gave me a long hug, & I started sobbing again. Then Kaitlin came down & as soon as I saw her I started again. Long hug. Then J, T, & me went over to Luke, who was so red-eyed. (Ben gave me a hug on the way out.) J was asking Luke if there was anything she could pray for, & he said confusion. I want to know about what! Would it be okay to ask? Hmm. So he & I talked a bit... oh, what to do.

Then T & I went to Wal-Mart, I lost my wallet. EMP, we were encouraging people & Julie Cross said I had childlike faith or something. Then Luke brought up the Prophecy conference that when 2 or more people had the same thing, it affirmed it. Then he affirmed it. I got to hug him...& everyone else. It was a great EMP. Wed was a bit disappointing but then we went to the library to study, & Luke & I talked for a long time. Nothingness. We played Frisbee lots of fun. Thurs, 3 hours of volleyball & basketball, TONS of fun. OT exam sucked, psych went pretty well I HOPE! Please God!

♥ Me

May 5, 2001

Wow, I am actually writing the DAY something happens! Worked all day—lotta fun, Ryan is the biggest flirt. Got to deliver a pizza to Phil, who told Luke why? Luke called, or rather Ben did, for a cheap pizza. Spent 1 1/2 with Luke, changing oil, talking to Kaitlin, who, when we walked in, took a while to recognize us it seemed, and said she'd just been thinking about us why? Ahh! The floods were amazing tonight—I was almost floating in my van. Oh, dear. God, give me a prophetic dream a/b Luke's confusion tonight so I may have something to talk to him about... oh, dear God.

♥ Me

May 13, 2001

    Mother's Day. Today was kinda tough. I choked up a lot. Worship at church was great though. The (5!) Gulley guys sang. At Taco Bell, Luke seemed like he wasn't very happy... I said I didn't want his dad to pay for me again, and Luke goes, "Well, too bad." Then he told me to get in line at the end & pay for myself then. So I got out of line cause I was afraid I was gonna cry. He's never mean like that. I think he knew he hurt me, or that something was bothering me anyway, cause he was pretty sweet later.

    Oh, man. Yesterday we had a lot of fun. The Clements took me to graduation & we screamed so loud for Ben & two other people. At the reception was fun. The three younger Clements were playing grass & drinking helium. Luke was burping helium & you could see the gas come from his mouth. It was weird. Then to Luby's. Lot of fun. They're leaving soon. What am I gonna do? I'll be okay I know, but to wait 3 months... I wonder if I'll be able to see him at all?

                                        ♥ *Me*

May 23, 2001

    I feel like writing, but don't quite have the patience. Luke & I were great last night. We talked a long time w/ Mark, had a great surprise party for Luke & Kenneth. At work, Adolfo was being really flirty... saying goofy things. I am "smoking" again. I am such a hypocrite about that! But it feels as good as it does bad.

                                        ♥ *Me*

Full stop. That is the first time I feel like I might have straight lied to myself. I must have already been hard-core crazy about Adolfo—I believe I started working at the Hut in January!—but Luke must have occupied my heart so fully, I had no space to think about anyone else. I smoked with Adolfo because it gave me a reason to be outside alone with him. That is literally the only thing I could have meant by "it feels as good as it does bad." I can't imagine I even knew how to inhale yet!

May 25, 2001

> Worked till close last night. Lots of fun. Me & Adolfo & Steve & Wendy. I don't really know what to write, it was just lots of fun. Saw Helen, Adolfo's fiancé, for the first time. She's cute, which makes things worse. Ugh. Anyway. Luke's probably home now, & Mark's leaving soon too. Summer's gonna be weird w/o them, esp when Kaitlin leaves. But money's coming, & I'll get my car & my apartment and hopefully a roommate or two. Sigh. I wanted to go home & see Jordan & John & Michael & Justin. Sigh again.
>
> ♥ Me

May 27, 2001

> Okay, I want to stop thinking about Luke & Adolfo. All this alone time, it's about all there is to think about. Carrie W told me living alone, you get much closer to God. I hope that's true. I have been praying a lot, but is this the kind of praying I need to do? Is it selfish prayer? It HURTS to think about Luke. I'm like obsessed with what's gonna happen come the school year, or even the next time I see him. I wish he'd email me or call out of the blue, oh God how I pray.
>
> I was playing with my tongue ring at work & Adolfo made a face at me & goes, "I wonder what that will feel like on something." Rubbing his chin. Hehe I was like, what do you mean. Made me blush to the roots of my hair.
>
> Saturday I worked all night. Ben told me Adolfo could lose his job. Made me cry. Adrian & I walked to get cigs. I don't understand how AFII could lose his job & Ben bloody gets promoted. But. And I am also obsessed w/ the idea of marriage. I can't stop thinking about Luke saying he needed a gf before getting married. Oh, God, tell him I'm

> *available & head-over-heels for him. Tell him something please, I'm hurting for him. For some kind of male-human contact. I miss him... what amount of time to wait? Sigh.*
>
> ♥ *Me*

What amount of time indeed. Is it my turn yet? (I am asking optimistically and excitedly because I know it's my turn, and I can't wait to see what he has in store—after the Rangers win the World Series…) It's October 29, 2023, my friends. It's almost the holidays.

Break: So I came back to morning writing time on the heels of the news that my last six weeks of unemployment checks are denied. I'm waiting to fight it, but I'm also so tired of fighting them. It's like, how do I get through the next few months without the three thousand dollars I thought this was going to afford me?

Also, it's Monday night, and I get "some kind of male-human contact" tonight. We are making progress in so many areas. Why does money always have to be the point of contention?

May 31, 2001

> *Car back, apt move-in... lonely. I love Luke. He & Kdog helped me "break in" to my apt. Sweet boy put his head through bars. Ahh! Adolfo, Luke, Luke, Adolfo, sooo Luke. I'm in love with him. Is it bad to cuss so much? What am I doing wrong in prayer? Why can't I hear what you want to say to me. Give me direction, God. Help him come to me, or to say something that gives me a hint that I should go to him... please God.*
>
> ♥ *Me*

So I don't know if it's my mood (stupid money!) or if I've just learned a lot over the years, but if I were God, I would have lost my patience long before this. *When will you learn to take no for an answer, my girl?* It brings back the song "Unanswered Prayers" by Garth Brooks. Let me see if I can do it from memory: "Just remember when you're talking to the man upstairs / that just because he may not answer doesn't mean he don't care. Some of God's greatest gifts are unanswered prayers."

> *Just the other night at a hometown football game*
> *My wife and I ran into my old high school flame*
> *And as I introduced them the past came back to me*
> *And I couldn't help but think of the way things used to be.*
> *She was the one that I'd wanted for all times*
> *And each night I'd spend prayin' that God would make her mine*
> *And if he'd only grant me this wish I wished back then*
> *I'd never ask for anything again.*
> *Sometimes I thank God for unanswered prayers*
> *Remember when you're talking to the man upstairs*
> *That just because he doesn't answer doesn't mean he don't care*
> *'Cause some of God's greatest gifts are unanswered prayers.*
> *She wasn't quite the angel that I remembered in my dreams*
> *And I could tell that time had changed me in her eyes too it seems*
> *We tried to talk about the old days, there wasn't much we could recall*
> *I guess the Lord knows what he's doing after all!*
> *And as she walked away, I looked at my wife*
> *And then and there I thanked the good Lord for the gifts in my life.*
> *Sometimes I thank God for unanswered prayers*
> *Remember when you're talking to the man upstairs*
> *That just because he doesn't answer doesn't mean he don't care*
> *'Cause some of God's greatest gifts are unanswered prayers.*

I am not a patient person by nature; I'm an immediate-gratification person. But reading twenty-two-year-old journal entries begging God for the same thing—why was Luke telling me no not enough?—both infuriates me and lights my impatience. At the same time, I want to tell my teenage self to calm down, I want to tell God to hurry up. "Is twenty-two years long enough?" I yell anxiously inside my heart.

What I've learned since Luke (long since Luke, I won't lie) is, I'm not praying for a specific crush to work out. I'm praying for the people who will fill the holes in my heart. I know what I want my life to look like for me; the right people will fit effortlessly into that. Am I still hoping for that one love to be my best friend, my everything? Sure. But I'm also okay being my own best friend (I don't even mind being alone now) as long as I can reach out to friends. People are precious. The phrase "It takes a village" no longer just applies to child-rearing. Find your tribe.

June 5, 2001

> *Ugh. So Adrian likes me. He's a sweetheart & a half, but no way. When Adolfo asked me if I liked him, I said no, & he nearly sounded relieved. He immediately goes, "He's not a good person to go out with." I wanted to tell him I couldn't & wouldn't like Adrian cause I like him. That's giving me enough trouble since he's engaged. Maybe that's what I'm doing wrong. But I've had crushes on MARRIED guys before! Oh sigh.*
>
> *Adolfo sounds a little jealous of the time Adrian & I spend together... "Courtney, your husband's here." Haha. Wendy told him today that I like him. Basically anyway. Then she said he already knew. Oh he's so sweet. And flirty.*
>
> *We closed tonight just the two of us. I asked him if he was in a bad mood & he said yes & I asked him if he wanted me to go home & he said no. God please keep his job @ BPH safe... please, no matter how he messes up. Please don't make him want to quit. I'd never see him... and abMichael... Luke said he wanted to see me... maybe oh maybe?*
>
> ♥ *Me*

June 8, 2001

> Well Wendy told ~~AFII~~ Ben that I went over to AFII's house... so he got in trouble. And Helen left him. Man oh man. Hard day... he's quitting & going to San Antonio... this is hard. I want a date with him. I have to talk to him tomorrow... wonder what he'd say if I said, "Would it be weird for us to go out sometime?"
>
> ♥ Me

June 12, 2001

> Oh man. Sunday night AFII, Wendy & I closed & AFII was gonna come drink w/ us, but Helen showed up so W & I went to Adrian's. Then 3 of us went to my house, up until sunrise talking to Adrian a/b him liking me. I told him I like AF. He went to Dallas w/ me. Then tonight we closed & Adrian was obviously mad, Wendy told AF that the one main reason I didn't like Adrian was cause I like him. He's still in love with Helen... sad & so sweet. He had boxes in the back of his car. Oh, I feel sorry for him! I wish he'd come stay with me. I just want to be free from any crushes for ONCE in my life. I miss Luke too. Am I messed up for liking 2 guys so much at once? And what IS it that makes me not want to date Adrian? God help me please!
>
> ♥ Me

This was not the first time someone had a crush on me whose feelings I didn't reciprocate, though I didn't know that at the time. To me, this was an entirely new form of heartbreak: letting someone else down. I hated not wanting to date him, even past my feelings for Adolfo. It frustrated the hell out of me that it was the wrong guy. Of course this was before I understood just how strong my intuition was. It buoyed me that Adolfo didn't want me to date him, but at the time, I figured it was just because I wanted him to want to date me. Now I understand Adolfo is a good man, and his intuition is strong too, and I'm thankful I had him.

June 21, 2001

> *So it really isn't going to happen w/ Adrian. AF & Helen are 2+ again. He's happy again. I still flirt w/ him & he does me too. Tonight was fun night w/ ~~Laura~~ LG. This girl Laura & I had a lot of fun. Played Phase 10, like Shang-hai. Fun. Oh, I want to close tomorrow w/ Adolfo. God let him want me! I miss Luke God... I do, so much I want to see him. Oh, God. Let Tiff get fully better, & take care of Luke & Adolfo... & Adrian & Wendy & all my other friends. God I want someone to love who loves me back God! Jehovah jireh!*
>
> ♥ *Me*

June 29, 2001

> *Tonight was sooox100 fun. Adolfo is the biggest flirt. He & Steve talked about sex & all this fun stuff. Damn he's a flirt. Ahh! So cute too! Can't wait till Sunday. Ahh! Ahh. AHH!*
>
> ♥ *Me*

June 30, 2001

> *Adolfo called me bootylicious & said I have enough cushion for the pushin! Hehe, he's so cute! I wonder what he & Steve really said when A said he called me bootylicious. B/c yeah right. I wish.*
>
> ♥ *Me*

Please let more happen tomorrow, God!

Rangers in five, y'all. What a game that was last night! The closer it gets to the end, the more scared I'm getting, and I don't like it. I want to look forward to something for once without preparing myself for the dread. I feel like I don't even know how to have real friendships anymore. I keep saying I trust myself, trust my intention, and then someone acts outside the way I expect them to / prepare myself for, and my heart breaks. I also feel like these current little diary passages might make this confusing, so I'm curious how it will flow when it's all complete. As for now, I'm leaving it with this bit of advice after a night of panic attacks: make sure you're doing something to take care of yourself at least once a day. You're responsible for your happiness.

July 5, 2001

  Oh man. This is troublesome. Adolfo keeps saying these sexy things... they keep getting better. Yesterday when I was trying to get him to come to Adrian's, I told him I'd quit so he could hang out with me. And he said that would make him mad & I asked why & he answered under his breath & Wendy had to repeat it. Cause there'd be nobody to have fun with he said. "He doesn't have fun with me." she said. She thinks he likes me but is too afraid to say anything. Me too. When he looks at me... man, he's driving me crazy. This is ten times worse than it was with Luke. I like Luke more but Adolfo drives me insane w/ his words... and nothing is going to come of it...

              ♥ Me

July 9, 2001

  Ahh. Last night Adolfo came to Wendy's to chill for his "birth day." We made him a cake that said, "Have fun tonight sexy" & gave him two cards. He & I went to the Hut to try to look for Wendy's keys & we saw Melissa & she asked what I was doing w/ Adolfo & I told her we'd been making out all night & she went & told him that. He didn't seem too bothered by it either. He looked at me a lot. We kept catching each other's eyes. Ahh. Hehe the song "Wishin' & Hopin'" just came on. I wish I could do what it says. Sigh. Last night really was a lot of fun. I can't wait to see him.

              ♥ Me

July 13, 2001

  He came over on his real birthday too. My lucky day. Horse shit. He told me he'd call one way or the other & he didn't. I'm hopeless. There were these guys *hanging out the window of their pickup giving me huge grins & thumbs up. H*OT*. And this black guy was totally hitting on me, but it made me uncomfortable. When will I learn? I'm screwed for life huh.*

♥ *Me*

So that's the first time I've come close to changing a word or deleting it entirely. I'd like to think I was as open about adjectives back then as I am now. Using the word *black* here would be nothing but a descriptive word now, like saying *skinny* or *tall*. It likely had nothing to do with what was making me uncomfortable. Intuition always. But these days, it's sticky to mention anyone's anything without being labeled as racist or sexist or any other -ist. And I apologize to this man from twenty-two years ago if I made snap judgments based on the way he was dressed or the way he was speaking. I'm better than that now.

July 21, 2001

*A*HH! *So much has happened, I wish I'd learn to write every day. I dyed my hair & Adolfo says he didn't like it, & then I said I was hot & he said no you're not so I got pissed at him & I was snapping at him & basically being a bitch, & I apologized later cause I didn't want to leave mad & he said he hadn't noticed & that I'd been a big help. I like this pen. So he might be breaking up with Helen tonight. Just let him be happy God. If he stays with her... he loves her, so... oh man. Just let him be happy. Hehe, Austin & Robert & Josh, man, they are so much fun. Esp. Austin. Anyway. Oh God let everything go all right. If he decides to say "It doesn't matter" let that be okay. Just let him be happy, & want to come chill with us...*

♥ *Me*

It will never fail to amuse and frustrate me the amount of time I let go by without making changes. How did I keep saying I should learn to write every day, and then boom, five weeks were gone! Also, here comes the defining tragedy of my life. COVID threw another giant wrench of course, not to mention the little ones in between, but this…this one…

September 10, 2001

  God, so much has happened. I was planning on writing all tonight, but no way. Emily Mathers was murdered. Murdered. That pushed me a lot. People coming home, Emily, school, & work have been really getting to me. And God. He's "taking me out of my comfort zone." Ugh. So conflicted. The Tiff/Jess thing is horrible. Luke like ignores me. Ugh. But today we went to the Cowsills & Nathan... oh man, oh God! Trouble brewing again. We'll see what happens. What a cutie though! Man what a cutie. I am bound & determined to get him to come to LG or at least camping. AHH! Trouble!

  God, I give it all to you. It's in your hands. Please Lord let me at least see him Wed. Let him come to LG, please. Let the piano lesson go well. Let my car be fixed!! Please God let Pizza Hut work out. Let Luke get over the fact that I like him & be okay with spending alone time with me! OH GOD know my heart, please take care of me, I want so much to know you more! Help me help myself!

            ♥ Me

  OK, prayers: help me get over Luke. Please let someone randomly encourage me—a card, email, phone call, words, a prayer, something at Life Group please! Let someone show me I am loved! I know you love me & I'm so sorry I haven't learned to let that be all I need. I am love-starved. Anyway, you know my heart God. You know my heart.

            ♥ Me

September 10, 2001

  God, thank you for today—thank you for waking me up Lord. It was such a great day. I've promised to keep my crush on Nathan semi-secret. My feelings for Luke... could they be easing? Oh please God. I have to talk to him, for both our sakes... maybe

> tomorrow? Or should I write him a note? Help me God! Oh, Lord, keep my heart...
>
> ♥ Me

Okay, does that entry feel prophetic to anyone else? I wonder what I had been sensing to write "Thank you for waking me up" for the first time (that I remember) the morning before the country got bombed.

September 11, 2001

> Well, my feelings for Luke aren't going away, but it's becoming easier to bear. How can I like 3 guys so much all at once???!!! America was attacked today. 4 planes went down, World Trade Center was destroyed. It's so unreal. Protect Heather & Dana please God! Be w/ the families of the victims, & God... please wake me up tomorrow. I get to go to the Cowsills... let me see Nathan please, at least, and at most (for now) let him want to help make a snack and come to LG. Justin too please!
>
> ♥ Me

September 12, 2001

> Neither Nathan or Justin came, but I at least got to see Nathan. He doesn't date. Hmm. Such a good day—Life Group rocked, Ultimate Frisbee after rocked, & Luke is adorable. Hehe. Jess is making it so obvious—more so than I ever did I think. Lord, I give it all to you—I love him God, whether in that way or not I don't know—is it about winning? Cause I don't want any of us to get hurt, least of all Luke. Protect him tonight God—keep him safe, as Jess, Tiff x 2, Zach, Kaitlin, Jason, Kenneth, Ben, the Cowsills, Amanda, Bri... all my friends God & Jimmy & his friends too... and my mom. You know my heart God, it's all yours. Everything. You are the Lord of my life. I give it all to you.
>
> ♥ Me

September 16, 2001

> *Jess & I just had the best talk a/b Nathan & Luke. Oh, Lord. What should I do? Should I talk to Luke? Today was so fun... just me, J, Luke, Ben, & Nathan for lunch, then frisbee, Nathan sat real close to me on the tramp, then Scrabble & Scategories. It's so unnerving to catch the boys watching me. I want to know what they're thinking! Ohh! I wish I could read minds. Sigh. Like I say every night, God, my heart is yours. You know me. I love you. Guard us all tonight God, all of us.*
>
> ♥ *Me*

September 19, 2001

> *My mom has* ♥ *heart failure. Please protect her God, keep her healthy! Piano lesson tomorrow—let me see Nathan please & God let him come to LG! Anyway. Bless everyone God... let Nathan, Jimmy, & Drew come camping?*
>
> ♥ *Me*

The nonchalance with which I threw out these big announcements—that America was attacked and Mom had heart failure—cracks me up. I have never been accused of beating around the bush, that's for sure. But now...I do not remember my mother having heart failure.

September 21, 2001

> *Wed Natalie came to LG & we hung out—went to Grant's & Doug's, then she home, me to her house for lunch (chicken w/ fruit, yum!) Nathan is the cutest, please let him come camping!! Ah! Closed as waitress at PH. Was there until 3:30—Adolfo & I were madly flirting—I told him about Josh & he asked if he would have had a condom, would I have lost my virginity, & I was like 25% chance. Came close to saying "I thought if this was Adolfo, I wouldn't be a virgin anymore." He's so much fun... anyway, keep everyone safe for me please God, & let me AND*

> *Amanda go to Dallas tomorrow. Please let Nathan come camping. You know my heart Lord.*
>
> ♥ *Me*

I'm amused that I wrote about Adolfo's reaction to me messing around with one of our delivery drivers, but I hadn't found the event itself significant enough to record. I do, strangely enough, remember two very interesting things: he was the first person to introduce the term *dry humping* to me, and he was the first (and only) Prince Albert I've ever seen. Or felt.

I can't say it was an unpleasant experience.

October 1, 2001

> *Camping was so awesome. I can't really explain why 'cause nothing super-special happened with Luke... except for him teaching me guitar and during Winks, we locked eyes for the longest time, & he raised his eyebrow & he's so cute. At DP, Jess & Taylor & I were comparing hair smells & then Luke leaned over & goes, "What about me, what do I smell like?" And I just said, "Luke." It was his pillow smell. Oh, Jesus. So tonight Tiffany told me she liked him. For real. HOW DID THIS HAPPEN? And WHY Jesus? Oh, Lord, why? What better way to hurt me? Oh God, cast out any evil... let me be happy for either of them if it works out for them with Luke. Oh Lord help me. I am lost. Lost. I don't know what to do.*
>
> ♥ *Me*

That is the part about having a crush that I miss, the tiny things that make it so amazing—meeting your partner's gaze and feeling that heat when you realize they're not looking away. Love is powerful. It's powerful to feel seen. See people. Love people. Understand you, too, are worth being seen.

October 2, 2001

> *Protect Tiff tonight & through Sunday Lord. Bring her back safe, keep all her ♥ed ones safe... Jesus let something w/ Luke & Nathan go well— whether it be Nathan comes to LG or one or BOTH boys*

> come to Dallas—Jesus hear my prayer. Give me the strength and the RIGHT WORDS to talk to Luke. Oh, Jesus, you know my heart, I love him Lord. Keep him protected as well God... please, I don't know what I'd do without him. And for everyone I'm always praying for... Jim & Mom & AOTA. Keep them safe Lord.
>
> ♥ Me

It had been over a year at this point—over a year that I prayed for the right words to say to this man. Now that I have them to say, I can't be sure they're reaching him. So, Luke, if you're reading this, you were—and are—very loved. They are the easiest words ever to say now.

October 3, 2001

> Thank you so much for today Jesus—my time with Nathan was precious. I hung out w/ him instead of going to LG & then he came & played Frisbee w/ us. Chris & Shaky are cool. Nathan and I get along great. Never an awkward moment. He bought me a drink & I thought he said "Let me walk you out" when I was leaving but who knows. Great night. Hope we can do something fun this weekend.
>
> ♥ Me
>
> PS: Please let Grant come

October 6, 2001

> Psalm 38:9 "You know what I long for, Lord, you hear my every sigh." Oh, Jesus, how true this is! Oh, Lord. I saw Nathan tonight at Starbucks. Amanda & I went when I got off work. He's so...adorable. He's precious Lord. What is this thing that I like two guys soooo much? How can I have professed to have loved Luke...when I can feel this strongly about Nathan? Am I fickle? Doomed to love every guy I'm friends with until the day I die as an old maid? Please Lord tell me that's not for me... tell me you have someone to spend the rest of my life with. And please

Lord make tomorrow a great day—with Nathan AND GRANT please!!! You know my heart, keep everyone safe, I love you.

♥ *Me*

October 7, 2001

Well, I just ditched Dwelling Place to come meet my WBC friends at Common Grounds & no one's here. I sincerely hope people come 'cause I probably need prayer tonight. Strike that. I always need prayer. Something's plaguing me Jesus. I hope I'm not going into the depressed side.

I was watching Ben at DP & Luke's sweet face popped into my mind. I started to cry. I want to cry tonight. Lord I need to cry. Cleanse myself. You can help me if & when I trust you, right? Jesus give me a sign. Speak to me Lord, get up in my face like you are with Tiff. I know you exist, & I just want a miracle or a thousand. I want something to happen significant with either Luke or Nathan. And dear Jesus, nothing bad. I'd rather it stay like it is than something bad happen.

Luke & I got along great today. Playing piano & just talking easily. Went to Starbucks, hung with Laura & Amanda & Mark. Can't wait to move in w/ them. God give me great dreams tonight. You know what I mean, prophetic.

You know my ♥, please protect everyone

♥ *Me*

One of my favorite things to read is the backtracking in my prayers: "Nothing bad, God, please." Like I would ever pray for something bad to happen (now I trust myself, of course). I remember when Trump got COVID, everyone on my Facebook told me I was probably hoping he would get it the whole time, and I said, "Well, yes, but only so he could empathize. I didn't think he'd die thanks to being the president." And I sure was right about that. I still wonder just how horrible he felt that he hid from the public.

October 11, 2001

> *Oh, God. Didn't see Nathan at his house, so of course he didn't come to LG, & neither did Luke, so I was sulking. I haven't been walking like a Christian these past few days: lying & planning to drink & just not seeking you. Give me great dreams tonight, Lord. Please. Like Emily, I long to hear you Lord. Please Jesus. Please.*
>
> ♥ *Me*
>
> *Heal my mom, heal my leg, and let me have a great weekend. Let me hang out with Justin on Saturday. Oh God. Please open up a spot in Starbucks, so when I go in... and please don't let Nathan be scared of me.*

Back in September, there was a one-off prayer: "Let me and Amanda go to Dallas tomorrow." That combined with the above "Heal my mom" leads me to believe this was during her first major breakdown. I'll add details later (y'all have to hear this story), but I wish I could know for sure the timing. If I put myself in the same shoes I'm wearing today, reading these entries takes on an extra layer of pleading: "Please don't let someone else abandon me. Please let these people I love do something to prove that I'm not alone." I needed validation in a bad way as a kid, and I'll be honest, it hasn't gotten much better as an adult. But I know how to validate myself now, and I'm thankful for Snapchat filters and TikTok.

This next one is both so cute and so sad, I can't take it. (For visualization purposes, I was sitting on the countertop at Pizza Hut, my legs swinging freely.) "Just let someone touch me back" was always radiating from my brain, a constant prayer, a need that got harder and harder to bear the older I got. At nineteen, I was so happy for any tidbit from the men I loved, but now it's any person I love. Dogs help too.

October 16, 2001

> *Just wanted to thank you for when I asked to play with Adolfo's hair, he came & stood between my legs & then put his arms up, just like I wanted. You trying to show me you WILL answer my prayers? God, please answer a few of these: Nathan Justin & Bri*

to LG, Nathan to Dallas, off early on Sunday... you know the rest. I love you.

♥ Me

October 18, 2001

    LG was so fun. Nathan & Justin both didn't come, but Amanda & I went on a scavenger hunt w/ Luke & Jason. We brought 3 people back. Then we had other races, like eating donuts really fast & bobbing for apples & sack races. Lots of fun. Luke's such a great guy. When I couldn't do the donut, he was just like: "It's okay Courtney." He's so sweet. Then Frisbee.
    Nathan did really well to avoid me. When Luke got there, I was backing up & he was right behind me & he goes, "Hey," & I just go "Hey, you!" I was really happy to see him. Sigh. Me & Mickey had such a great talk about Ben, Nathan, Natalie, and God stuff. Then last night I had great dreams about Nathan & Luke. I love you God, thank you for everything yesterday. I pray that I get to hear you.

♥ Me

October 20, 2001

    Jess & Luke are taking their relationship to the next level. I'm so jealous but really happy. I love you Lord, gonna pray.

♥ Me

October 23, 2001

    20 years old, thank you God. Thank you for today, for my party, for my friends Lord. Oh God. How can I not be happy? I guess I need individual stuff—just cards from J & T, & God I wish Luke, but... I would be so thrilled if Nathan just said happy b-day. Please Lord, let him come tomorrow. I don't know why I'm not satisfied. Dear Jesus, please help

> me feel more accepted. Please help me know your heart.
>
> ♥ Me

I got excited reading about my birthday that year, as I remember it being really fun—the Life Group threw me a surprise party!—and then I read that I still wasn't happy, that I was having feelings of not belonging, even with those people whom I look back at now and think of as my best friends. That kind of anxiety only blooms from trauma. I never believed I was good enough to be worth staying for.

October 29, 2001

> Long weekend. Kaitlin finally got to meet Nathan & of course she likes him. How could she not? But how could she not sense I liked him? Oh, Jesus, why can't things be simple for once? Why can't I really find you, Lord? Why can't you satisfy me yet? Lord, help me be happy to be single—or God let me get a bf. Please Lord. And keep us all safe, now & for a long time.
>
> ♥ Me

November 8, 2001

> Lord, let Brandon come... & let my & Luke's relationship continue to grow stronger. I thank you so much for the changes that have already come about. Wed, Zach & John broke Jess's kitchen table, & I was trying so hard not to laugh, but Luke & I were looking at each other over J's head, & he was turning red, & when she walked away, he came closer & whispered behind his hand, "That was the funniest thing I've ever seen." We lost it. Then we started talking about the car thing & lost it again. Then in the car on the way to Frisbee, we started laughing again. Natalie was there!! WE stayed up till 7:00, talking, movies, IHOP. I told her I like Nathan. Sigh. I PRAY LORD that she'll be able to move in with us! God, how fun! Please Lord!!

Keep us all safe!!

♥ Me

November 13, 2001

Lord, God, let Natalie... all of the above! Phil Stahl is too cute. He taught me some guitar chords & he was so sweet and patient, and boy can he play & sing! He's awesome, & I had no idea! I saw him at PH tonight—cutie. Sigh. Lord, please let Nathan come tomorrow night & let us go see Shallow Hal. Fun! Keep everyone safe, & Jesus, bless Adolfo & Jimmy tonight. Show them your love, & save them God.

♥ Me

November 17, 2001

Jesus, Jesus—oh God please let Brandon come to the concert... oh, God, how fun. And let the people around us be willing to trade seats... oh Jesus! Please God! Let this week be great... and this weekend. Jesus, let money pour in from nowhere. God!
Ps 38:9, Lord!!!

♥ Me

I remember Brandon and I reconnected briefly when I was in Waco—late-night AIM conversations in which we talked about regrets of never having kissed or done more than held hands (I was fourteen, mind you). I'm glad to see he made an appearance in my journal, even a small one. He was such a big part of my life.

November 25, 2001

God, I hate when I have so much to say & no patience to write. Nathan doesn't like Kaitlin Lord, & he's even a bit annoyed by her. Oh thank you Jesus. Lord thank you for this week. I can't even write a/b it. Jesus, calm me down. Help me remember w/o having to write it Now! Nathan laughing so hard: salt in K's tea, her telling me the r & t were too close then saying not to drink the tea, me asking why, cause it was too close to the r? And him losing it—classic. And Thurs & Sun were so fun—& partying w/ my bro's friends... Taylor Sebastian's hair—him leaning into me & saying it felt great... oh Lord thank you for this week! The concert was incredible & I got to meet the band! Lord God THANK YOU!

NATHAN DOESN'T LIKE KAITLIN!

Oh, please, Jesus... you know the rest. What is wrong with me??

♥ *Me*

Well, okay, there's the concert where I met the band. It must be the one, because I don't remember meeting any other rock bands, which in my estimation means the breakdown came that night, and yet I didn't write about that. Is my timeline so skewed?

November 27, 2001

Natalie thinx Nathan is a mega jerk. Please, Lord, enlighten one of us. Open my blind eyes. Lord, Jesus, I know you can heal Demi. Please do. I can't bear to watch Jimmy hurt like he's going to. Please heal her Lord. And Jesus, help me with rent. I know I am spending frugally & saying "oh I don't care..." but what if I'm not welcome into the apt. anymore? Help me please.

Please Jesus don't let this wonderful week be ruined tomorrow.

♥ *Me*

November 30, 2001

Wow, 1 month till 2002! Wow! Well, Wed & tonight were so great. Wed, I started crying & couldn't stop cause every1 was being encouraged. THANK YOU LORD for Luke's finally saying something to me. And then Frisbee—tossed it around w/ Chris, Nathan gave me a smile & a waved, then PH w/ J & Luke. Tonight we got all dressed up & Luke said, "Wow Courtney" to me! Yeah, thank you Jesus! And et will be ok w/ rent,

> thank you again Lord. Please help me think of ways to get $!!! 715$ in two days... eek. You're the ultimate provider Lord!
>
> ♥ Me

December 5, 2001

> What a week. Demi, my mom's breakdown (she's in a hospital) & Jimmy's bday today. Plus Lauren broke up with him—poor baby, help him! Tonight was fun. LG party, then Frisbee, me Nathan Chris Shaky & Kaitlin. Played keep away, Nathan's so cute. Chris said I could be "one of the guys" next week & slapped my hand & held on to it. Please Jesus protect everyone—my bro & mom esp. Let Ben get some sleep, let Kaitlin retain info & do well in finals, & let Nathan be healthy, no more headaches!
> Psalm 38:9
> Lord, please help me!
>
> ♥ Me

Well, there you go, more nonchalance from the queen of beating around the bush. Demi, our sweet chunkin muffin dachshund, had to be put down after slipping a disc in her back. It was devastating, but more so for my brother, which made it all that much harder for me. My mother did indeed end up in the hospital for the first time, and it still feels weird to just insert details here. Let's start with me meeting the band, because there it was in some color and white.

We had dinner at a restaurant in a beautiful hotel in Dallas called the Mansion. Members of the band, including two quite famous musicians who have died since, were present, and in my memory, it was his whole band minus the lead. I have two very clear images in my mind and no idea how to link them up: the first is ordering an Angus burger and being hugely disappointed with it, and the second is of my mother slumped against me like a child, all but sleeping in the restaurant. I was mortified and kept pushing her to get off me. In my mind, she looked like she was on drugs. She could have been, for all I know.

I don't know if my mother followed the band on tour for months before this or after she got out of the hospital (the first time). I mentioned partying with my brother, which meant she wasn't at the house. But that fateful night, we were all at the house, and I believe even Amanda and Josh were present for this. She was reading the message boards on a Neil Sparkle fan site, where it had been posted he was planning on proposing to his girlfriend at one of the shows. My mother believed they were talking about her, that Neil Sparkle was planning on proposing to her. It's hard to relay the story now, as it's much better coming from her when she's healthy. But on the heels of her recent breakdown, I don't ever want to hear her talk about Neil Sparkle again.

Anyway, mind-blown over this, all I remember Jimmy and myself knowing to do is call for help. Her best friend was a nurse and lived right down the street. I remember Jimmy having to chase Mom down the street at one in the morning, then carrying her to Brenda's house. I don't know much about what happened after that, except she ended up with a severe diagnosis of borderline schizophrenia to add to her manic-depressive bipolar I. She refuses to remember that particular detail despite claiming she remembers everything.

Here's my issue: You remember everything, and you can take ownership of nothing? You're just supposed to get a free pass for being an asshole human because the chemicals in your brain are unbalanced? No, thanks. Learn how to manage your chemicals. Or you will push away any person trying to help you.

December 8, 2001

> Party at Brandon Culver's. Lisa gave me a huge, long hug & she was so drunk but so cute. Stacy Whitman is the sweetest. She & Jimmy kissed. Russ & Shelby almost fought, but Taylor & I mediated. Russ even apologized for his actions later, with a huge hug. Andrew Thomas gave me a hug! Stacy came bounding up to me in the hall, very drunk and saying, "Please tell me you remember me, I love you!" I couldn't place her face. Hehe.
>
> Okay, now can I tell you about Taylor Sebastian... holy cow that boy is fine. Razor fine. Sigh. Didn't think about Nathan once. Josh was so sweet about Mom. Very serious & so cute. And I think John Bell said he had a crush on me in 3rd grade. James South gave me a hug. Weird. He looks strange now. Fun fun night. I love my brother. Lyndsay puked like mad.
>
> ♥ Me

January 7, 2002

Wow, five years. This has been THE weirdest month—so good & so bad. I'm writing a story to help me remember. I miss my boys so much. I wish my brother would call me. Everytime I sing, "Caution, wet floor," I want to cry. I miss Taylor, & Russell, & Shelby & Josh sooo much. Dear Lord help me make it just a couple of months & LOSE WEIGHT! And help me figure out Nathan. Why he was irritating me so last night.

♥ ME

January 9, 2002

Okay... Nathan? That DREAM! All about NYE & kissing Shelbs & Russ... help me! Is it wrong to daydream like that? I can't help wishing. Oh, Lord, help me. I hope Adolfo will come Fri night. Not to mention Nathan. Lord please help me with a house or apartment!! Maybe Nat will move in too... please Lord help me! And please forgive me as you always have. I don't want to stop but I know it's a sin... geez. THANK YOU GOD FOR THE RENT HELP! I love you so much... please keep my family & friends protected, EVERYONE! Russell... oh Lord. Once again back to my sweet Russell. And will she ever learn.

♥ Me

January 22, 2002

Lord Jesus, what is it with Nathan? OK, Saturday Luke & I went shopping for Jess. He got her this beautiful sapphire necklace w/ 3 pt. diamonds. Aww. At Hallmark he was reading a card & I couldn't read it cause I'd know too much. It said, "I'm scared... & something about falling in love I think. Sweet boy! Such a great day.

Then Sunday, the Cowsills. NATHAN! Jesus help me. I kept watching for signs he was a jerk, but everything he did was just too cute! I made several Freudian slips: trying to read the last phase in

Liverpool, I said, "Two sets of threes & a run of SEX." Nathan found that very amusing. He started getting grumpy but I could get him to smile & roll his eyes & be sweeter.

Second slip I did twice. I was asking Nathan a/b the scores & I go, "How far behind you am me" or something funny. Such a cutie. Skipped Dwelling w/ Luke to play w/ Nathan... help me oh Lord... keep every1 safe, let Russ know he's loved, take care of my mom, & let me be able to go down there soon. Please continue to bless me w/ money even though I have to take off for World Mandate. I don't have to but I want to. And please God let Michael & Justin go to Juarez.

♥ Me

January 25, 2002

Tonight was the start of World Mandate. It was really great... the worship was awesome... esp. "Our God is an Awesome God." It wasn't especially moving, & like always I was feeling like a hypocrite, like I was putting on a show. But after—wait, Jim Yoats spoke & it was amazing! After, I talked to Doug a/b his blue glasses. He just immediately opened up... said they were baptizing his eyes, that he'd been dealing w/ lust, vanity, & pride lately. He said he felt like a moron in them. He said Baylor girls were bad. It was funny.

Got to talk to Daniel Shelton too... such a cutie & GOD does he smell good. Then Ben—he looked like he'd been crying, his eyes were all red, so I asked if he was tired & he said no, then if he had a headache, said no. "Just a little out of it" he said. I watched him for a while, getting up the nerve to ask him if I could pray for him... then decided I couldn't.

But then he went to leave & then he didn't, so I got the nerve & asked. He said, "Yeah!" and then stopped. I was like, you wanna tell me? And he was like, "I just can't think of anything!" His eyes had filled w/ tears again. I told him to tell me if he *thought of anything & he said he really appreciated it. He's so sweet. Ahh. I wished Nathan was there several times. I prayed for Russ & Shelbs & Mom & Jim... please God "rain down on them." I do love you & I'm sorry for being a hypocrite*

♥ *Me*

World Mandate was a huge concert dedicated to God, as I remember. We sang a lot and heard a lot of speakers. It was pretty amazing, and I'm super sad I still felt like a hypocrite. I wonder when my poor heart started to believe in myself.

February 24, 2002

Wow, it's been over 5 years and it's finally almost filled up. I have a new journal & I really want to start using it. But I have to fill this one up first. Whan an amazing thought—I actually kept up with a journal. And reading back through some of the earliest entries—look how much I've changed. Count how many guys I've liked...or professed to be in love with. Right now I am so blessedly "love" free. But there are the few crushes. Nathan, Brent, & Alex being the main ones. And I still have such a heart for Adolfo.

At Life Group the other week, we were talking about qualities we search for in a friend that we can always find in you, Jesus. Jessica was talking & she said "One of my best friends, actually my best friend, always speaks what's on her mind. She always tells me how it is." I hope & pray she meant me. She had to, right? It was so cool to hear—it made my heart swell up, & I don't even know if she meant me.

I haven't the slightest idea of how to fill this up—10 pages seems like an awful lot. (At the beginning of the book, 10 pages was a year and a half!) So. I really want to use my other journal. You've been a great friend though.

What else to say? Pizza Hut has started working me a lot—it's great. I got a 300$ check. Juarez in a week!! Ahh! What's more unbelievable is that last

Juarez was a year ago! Oh my gosh! I can remember it like it was yesterday.

Okay, now Robert's speaking on gifts of the Holy Spirit: the expression of God's love & power working thru a person to help, change, or edify another. So we're going to take notes cause I do want gifts of the Holy Spirit, I'm just scared. So! Kelly Cooker is my secret pal! That's gonna be fun! I'm kind of nervous, but so beyond excited. I love our small team. What am I saying, I love our big team too. THANK YOU GOD that Tiffany's coming to Mexico! I don't know why it feels so important. Maybe I just want her to know what she's missing.

But oh God, I'm believing in you for money! Please God—prophesy is a gift of the spirit that I would LOVE to have. Tongues I'm scared about. Falling on the floor—but prophesy would be awesome. I am jumping around a lot, but I keep thinking different things. Jesus, I want to be able to hug Nathan. I want him to come to Life Group! Why do I get these feelings for guys that I can't do anything about? AHHH! I love all my boys—Nathan, Adolfo, Drew, Russell, Shelby, Luke, Ben, GOD! I love having people pray for me. But my heart's not always in it. What can I do? I'm gonna draw to take up space.

That really sucks. I wish I could draw. I'm writing really slanted. Can I read this later? My tummy hurts. Robert is talking about prophecies, & I had missed the question, & then I thought a/b the first encouraging prophesy I'd gotten. In Juarez last year, I didn't know what a prophesy was, & I asked Luke & he said, "Here's a prophesy for you: Jesus loves you. And I know that for a fact!" That was awesome! My hand's starting to hurt!

February 25, 2002

Last night was so awesome. At first I wasn't going to go up to the front, but then I was like, God wants me to do what I don't feel like doing! So I went up to the place where I'd be prayed for words of prophesy. I was praying for myself to get prophesy as well as for someone to come pray for me. A girl I didn't even know came up and said God was showing her a sunse rise or something. It was cool. Then Amanda prayed for me & Erin Sandman came up, & then Ben Taylor & Jess—they talked to me for a long time, it was awesome. I was honest a/b not being ready to commit my life fully to God. Ben was so sweet & supportive & they all prayed awesome prayers for me. The whole night was just really encouraging. Amanda said she's seen a leaky faucet & one day the faucet was gonna explode (over dry soil) me, & a beautiful flower would spring up (me!) It was awesome. So thank you Jesus!

♥ Me

March 10, 2002

Wow my handwriting can be messy! Oh, Juarez was fantabulous! So amazing! I've got my new crushes, but I'm giving them to my God instead of crying over them. Clark Hampton is amazing, Nick Travis is amazing—what can I say, I love my boys! I love my God too! Ohh, but I need help forgiving Jessica. There're so many ways she's hurt me, & I don't even think she realizes it. I need help focusing on You. I want to hear your voice! I want to feel your love! I want to step out in faith that you love me & can heal me! I want your help in creative ways... and I want to stop completely wanting guys! It's gotten a lot better, but I've got a long way to go. I want gifts of your Holy Spirit!

♥ Me

March 28, 2002

Work is getting to be so much fun. Rudy asked me to be a manager. I'm so confused a/b it. Adolfo has faith in me. He was teasing me mercilessly tonight, & I was like "Adolfo hates me" to Ben. And he said, "No he doesn't, he's very fond of you 'cause you'll do anything for him. He knows you'll bend

> *over backwards for him." And Adolfo goes, "And like it!" I burst out laughing & blushed way red.*
>
> *Then while he was washing dishes, he said, "What do you think I said earlier when you said 'Rudy told me to stay'? Did you think I said 'why are you still here?'" When I said yes, he said, "I said 'whoa nice hair!'" That's seriously like the first compliment he's given me that I didn't have to pry for him! Oh, & he told Veronique she'd like living with me 'cause I was a really fun person. I love him! Oh, Jesus. Sigh. Can I ever win?*
>
> ♥ *Me*

I have actual butterflies remembering these exchanges with Adolfo, whom I grew up to consider my best friend for a long time. He taught me how to be friends with a man.

March 29, 2002

> *Adolfo & I talked about serious sex stuff tonight—what makes a porno good, messing around w/ Jordan & Josh... it was fun but way embarrassing. I really enjoy his company. What'll I do when he starts opening? Agh!*
>
> ♥ *Me*

And here's the first time I recall God showing up in my real life, not church life, in a huge way. I cried as I read it, because I spent a long time after it happened worrying about him if he was working alone. But God, maybe all the times I prayed for his protection were in place. Maybe it's all just a coincidence. But holy cannoli, Easter Sunday that year was the first time we hadn't closed the store together in weeks.

April 1, 2002

> *Well, PH was robbed last night by Helen & this guy Nick. It was AFII's first night not to close—man, God is good. If he'd been there, 80-20 says he wouldn't have walked out alive. THANK YOU JESUS! The poor boy thinks he would have been able to stop it! Oh God.*

So we were talking a/b it, & both he & Ben are very broken up. I was holding the money, & AF saw me, looked at me suspiciously, & proceeded to count it again. I said he was gonna make me cry. And he said, my own ex would steal from me, who else? He said, "I trust you Court," then counted it anyway. So I go, "Don't you trust me?" And he goes, "I don't trust anyone."

But then two seconds later he goes, "But consider yourself lucky. You are one out of four people in this world I trust. I tell Dawn every day I don't trust her. I don't even trust my own brothers." Then he let me take the deposit to the bank!

Yea! I really like him, & God, you know I'm begging you to take care of him. He's so special to me. What would I have done if we'd been there instead of Ben? Or worse, just him, & he'd been shot! Oh, God...

OH! I let him read the convos w/ Jordan & he said "he's got you all shaken up" cause I was typing badly. Then he stood up & knocked his drink over & goes, "You've got me all shaken up too!" I wonder what he meant by that?

♥ Me

April 10, 2002

This is THE coolest crush. I like him so much, but it doesn't hurt! I mean, I get jealous of Dawn sometimes, but it's just fun. I mean...like, a couple of days ago, he flipped me off for something & I gave him my pretend sad look and he goes, "I'm sorry, Court, I just couldn't resist." Then, quiet enough so I couldn't hear at first, "Would it make you feel better if it was an offer?" He wouldn't repeat it, but when I figured it out, he didn't say he was kidding or anything. Sigh. ♥

♥ Me

April 11, 2002

    V & I have gotten into the habit of going by Adolfo's house & usually he's in his uniform, but today he wasn't & MAN he looked fine! Sooo cute. Aww. My heart hurts. V & I went to Friday's & said we weren't gonna talk a/b Bo & Adolfo for 2 hours. We did it, but mentioned each boy 4xs, so once every half an hour. Not bad considering how much we wanted to!

♥ Me

April 12, 2002

    Even the smallest thing makes me deliriously happy. He never says bye to me, right? And today, I even had a customer & he whacked the counter to get my attention & waved at me. Oh, I love him! Tomorrow he closes!

♥ Me

April 13, 2002

    Adolfo started off today being jerky. He told Paula to send me & V home rather than him telling us. And V said she needed a man to help her, & he patted me on the back & said, here ya go. Oooh, I shot him a dirty look!

    I ignored him most of the night. But of course I started getting flirty, & we had good talks about trust issues & Helen & Dawn. That bitch is more threatened by V than me! Is she BLIND?! Damn. Anyway. I called him baby like 3 times & he didn't say anything. He's so cute. V thinks I should write him a letter. Sigh.

    Man Deric was flirty tonight too. Wow. I pushed him out the door so I could go outside & he goes, "That's sex. harass. & I don't have to take it." Pause. "But I liked it." He's so fun.

♥ Me

Funny, because as I was typing that, I sat here thinking, "Man, we wouldn't be able to get away with any of that behavior in today's workplace environment." I wonder if my heart stopped even for a split second when he said those first words.

April 14, 2002

> *Oh, I love my Pizza Hut boys. I walked in w/ my hair down & straight, & Jason's eyes followed me. He goes, "Look at you with your hair down, girl! You look like a rebel, like you're about to kick someone's ass!" Then Thomas goes, "She looks normal." Then I clocked in & he goes, "Damn you smell good. I thought it was the computer, but it's you!"*
>
> *Then in the back, Adolfo came back & he said, "Courtney, you actually look good!" I was hurt at the same time pleased. I go, "Are you surprised that my hair can look good?" And he said no. Then later I peeked around the corner to say something to Bo & he said "I really like your hair down, it looks good" & I squealed when I came back around & told Adolfo what he said & he goes, "I told you that too, but I said it first!" I love him. I hate not feeling like I can pray cause I'm not walking with the Lord. But I want my baby. So much.*
>
> ♥ *Me*

April 17, 2002

> *I closed the store with Rudy. He taught me everything. It was so fun & he seemed very happy with my work. So fun!*
>
> ♥ *Me*

May 30, 2002

> *Wow, it's been a long time. Catch up... we're staying in this apartment, but we still need money, so bad, please! God is so with us though. So much so. My baby transferred to Valley Mills. I miss him so much. I think he misses me too. I got a hug from*

him. ♥ Jason started hanging out with us, but he stopped too. I have a little crush on him, but he likes V. It's all good, I know I'll find someone eventually. I don't want to get married yet. I just want to be kissed & hugged & liked! I ♥ Adolfo—please, God, help me. Let him call or something.

♥ Me

PS I did write Adolfo a very long letter. He told V he was very flattered, but I was like his best friend & he didn't want to ruin it.

May 31, 2002

How do you fall in love with someone so wrong for you? Why is the world so unfair? I saw Adolfo today. He did his crinkly nose smile. He's so cute. He told me to be careful again. I wish I could walk in & tell him Jason & I are together, just to see if he seemed jealous. When he was talking about Amanda tonight, I got jealous but I could laugh for real. I love him. I hate this. Help me, Lord, help me!

♥ Me

June 3, 2002

I helped Adolfo & Dawn move last night. It was a lot of fun. He's so cute. Dawn said that at one point & I said whatever & she goes, Oh don't tell me that, I remember when you used to say that all the time. I got mad. I said I still think that. They fought a lot. She said she thinks he's falling in love with her. Ugh. Ugh. UGH.

♥ Me

June 8, 2002

> *Well, let's see. Adolfo told me he's not falling in love w/ Dawn. Dallas w/ Annie & Beth was a blast. I love Russell. And Justin Woody. Jason came over night. So fun, I love him. Amanda might like him too & he might like her. Ugh.*
>
> ♥ *Me*

So I was always second to another female—always. There was always someone sexier or hotter or with bigger boobs. And when you're a people pleaser who just wants to be loved, you let them walk all over you. I could almost guarantee Dawn got with Adolfo originally to piss me off. It was girl bullshit. But Adolfo was more important than drama, so I always rolled over. I never saw myself worth the fight. To be honest, I have no idea who Jason was. So unless I have the name in my memory wrong, I don't regret losing him to Amanda.

But as an adult, I do not only value myself much higher, but I also don't get jealous. I know the person (or people) who choose me will choose me because they want to be around me, and that's a special kind of peace.

June 10, 2002

> *Okay, I have spent so much time w/ Jase, & what do I keep thinking about? Adolfo! Big surprise. What it'd be like to kiss him, plans for his birthday, how he'd feel if Chuck & I started dating.*
>
> *Oh, I really like him. So different than Luke—so different. It's terrible. I want him so much! Life Group tomorrow—yay!*
>
> ♥ *Me*

Okay, excuse me, but who the fuck is Chuck?

June 11, 2002

> *Wow. I want to take Adolfo to karaoke & sing him Shakira: "Underneath your clothes, there's an endless story. There's the man I chose, there's my territory. And all the things I deserve for being such a good girl!" I mean, come on, how perfect can you get? I wish I could say I deserve everything for being*

such a good girl, but I've been such a bad one at the same time.

Jason called, told us he'd call back, & then didn't. Chuck didn't call at all. Oh, well. Ball's in their court now. I miss Adolfo. It's been a week since I've seen him. How long can I go? It's like a fast. And ~~how lon~~ what will he do when I come in after a while?

♥ Me

June 17, 2002

I lasted a week & a half. I showed him the pix of Annie & he said we looked alike. That was a great compliment. Then he goes umm, Courtney! Cause my shirt was so low cut. Then he said my mom looked really good too! I mean, come on! I was so happy! I love him! And Bo said "Who's that sexy girl in the middle?"

♥ Me

June 28, 2002

Ahh! I saw my baby today! He came into Baylor to pick up some olives... I turned around & almost had a heart attack. Yea! Talked to him a lot in the past few days... he & Dawn actually broke up but now they're back, but when I asked him tonight, he said they were doing shitty. I ♥ him! I heard Lukie talk a/b sex & condoms... classic! And Nathan said, "I was talking to this sweet old lady & said something a/b why the moon was orange, & she said 'No shit?'" I about died laughing. 2 classic moments from two unsuspecting boys. I talked to Luke a/b Nathan. Luke told Peter the story of me him & J. And I'm going to miss Nathan a whole helluva lot. A lot. How so? I never see him! Maybe that's why.

♥ Me

July 2, 2002

> Ahh. Life Group was encouragement tonight. Kelley Bryson said the best stuff. Jesus loves me. I love that you shine through me. You love me, & I am so underserving. I love you. Talked to Rudy a lot today. He says I need a boyfriend. I said I need Jesus. You're working again. Saw Adolfo tonight. I love talking to him, & I felt a little bit jealous when he was talking about Jennifer, but for the most part, it was just good to chat. I wish he'd come to Cali. Saw Natalie tonight! And my Jess is back! I've missed them both so much.
>
> Life's falling into place. I'm gonna tithe on Sunday. I'm trusting in you, Lord! I need something miraculous to happen! I love you. Thank you for loving me. Thank you for shining thru my friends. Preston Taylor... Kaitlin is seriously stalking Nathan! Protect him!
>
> ♥ Me

That was a random little insert of a name of a friend I went to high school with who also ended up at Baylor and Antioch. I wonder what special prayer that was. In high school, Preston ran with the same people who tortured the guy I'd asked to prom, so I had a bad image of him. But at Baylor, we became friends. I remember he smiled like the sun and hugged like a bear, so that was likely part of it.

July 4, 2002

> Last night we went to eat for Debbie Gayle's birthday. It was a lot of fun. I love Dustin Welley. He is hilarious. Debbie encouraged us all so much! It was so fun. Tonight Amanda & I went to Big D for fireworks & we saw the Bourne Identity. Jordan Granby is a cutie. Anyway. I am terribly sleepy. Very long day. Been awake 18 hours! But I love you. Thank you for being so faithful. Protect my loved ones tonight—you know who I'm talking about. Thank you for loving me.
>
> ♥ Me

July 7, 2002

> *Saw Nathan today. His hair looks like a Chia pet—so cute. Talked a/b Kaitlin. I really want to ask him for his number. God give me strength. I'll miss him so. Adolfo's bday is in 6 days.??? I'm praying! I tithed $20 today—help me be less frugal God.*
>
> ♥ *Me*

Let's rephrase that prayer: "Help me be more frugal, God." But seriously, did I not know what the word meant, or did I honestly believe I was miserly with my money because I didn't tithe enough?

And holy crap, excuse me while I disappear for four months while I'm hanging on to a brand spanking new journal I wanted to crack open. What in the world happened in those four months?

November 5, 2002

> *Wow, I have missed you. So much bloody stuff has happened. You don't even know about Jeff, Nate, & Brooke. I HATE this situation. I liked Jeff and Brooke could tell. She & I got to be good friends, but she's a malicious, vindictive, backstabbing bitch & I want nothing to do with her anymore. She doesn't trust me or her boyfriend, & he loves her so much that he'll believe anything she says. He needs to see the light, Lord, please! Ugh.*
>
> *I got fired from Pizza Hut about six weeks ago—hired at Hastings a week ago, start for real on Friday. Let you know how that goes. I need some help here. Do I want to move to California? Yes because I miss my mother & the rest of my family, yes b/c I am sick of the drama that is Waco, no b/c of Hastings, & no b/c of my brother. We'll soon see if Hastings is enough to keep me here—and if I can make new friends enough to keep me happy.*
>
> ♥ *Me*

God bless my sweet little heart, I knew it, depression. The more I notice the trends, the more angry I get at my adult self for letting this year vanish. Six weeks—I spent six weeks without a job as a twenty-year-old kid on her own. What the fuck did I think was gonna happen? Magical thinking—that was what my mother called it. I can't say it didn't work. Thank God and multiple guardian angels, I never ended up homeless or in a jail cell or hospital. But God, I'm lucky to be where I am.

The really annoying thing is, I remember being fired three times from Pizza Hut. I had an attitude problem and my tongue was pierced, neither of which flew with Rudy when he started. But I hated that he wanted me to get rid of a piercing I had had the entire time I worked there, not to mention you rarely saw it. But I was able to sweet-talk myself back into the job several times. I wonder what ended up being the final straw.

November 7, 2002

> *So Darrin Adele, Jeff's roommate from freshman year, is in a coma with mennicoggal menigitis... we spent Sat night with him, so Brooke and I spent the evening in the ER. I got a shot & a prescription, had a fever, & now have slight back pain. Brooke had a spinal tap & was cleared. Jeff's quite scared & he's sick too. I didn't get the chance to talk to him b/c of today's drama... my heart's hurting. Why can't something great happen??*
>
> ♥ *Me*

I marvel at my ability to overcome financial hardships, and then I get smacked with that particular memory: Two days after spewing venom about Brooke, I ended up taking her to the ER and putting myself through her misery. I remember her lying down on the ER floor because her headache was so bad. I had a huge suspicion that she was being overly dramatic for attention. But I didn't mind being ushered back immediately because we had been exposed to an incredibly contagious disease. I do wish I could remember if I was having hateful thoughts. I can't believe it was two days earlier that I was that angry, and I still took her to the damn hospital. I was a good friend.

Also, I'm really amused at my spelling of the disease. *Meningitis* is close, but I have no idea what that first word is.

November 10, 2002

> *Oh dear, 4 more pages, my faithful friend. How will my next diary compare? Will I be able to keep it like I did you? Oh dear. Anyway. I went back to the ER for Brooke's headache tonight—hypochon-*

driac that one. I was at PH and Adolfo was talking to me about Joey—a driver—and he blushed bright red when he pointed him out to me. Weird, since we know each other so well, but he still blushes around me. Brooke says that means he's attracted to me. She also told Jeff I said he had a big nose & I didn't. And I think he's mad at me. I am sad. I really pray for him to be TRULY happy. Can she change? He loves her, but they're so wrong for each other.

♥ Me

November 17, 2002

I think this'll be my last entry—it's gonna be long. Hastings is so much fun. Yesterday morning we had a six AM meeting & we had to take a really long test. This guy Erik, who I just clicked with, & I took it together and laughed thru the entire thing. He's a real cutie. Long hair & a beard, but he reminds me of Toby pre-Juarez. Anyway so he had an extra ticket to a Jackson Browne / Tom Petty concert last night & I got to go! WOOHOO! So fun. We met at Hastings at 3:00, were in Dallas by 4:40, and talked about movies the whole way there. Then we parked and walked around downtown, saw went to the West End & window shopped.

On our way to AA for the concert, we got stopped by a black guy selling roses. He handed me a rose and said, "I'm not going to charge you for this, lady." I was pleased, I thought it was b/c he thought I was pretty or something. But then he goes, "If you kiss this man." I must have turned burgundy. Erik did. I was like, "I barely know him!" And the guy goes, "On the cheek, of course." And asked Erik if he minded. "Not if she doesn't," he said. I would have kissed him on the mouth later on, but not at that point. So I kissed his scratchy cheek and he put his hand on my waist... real sweet-like. Then the guy charged Erik for the flower. Hehehe. We got stopped twice more, same deal. I wish it had been as easy as just kissing him, I could have gotten 3 flowers!

NOT THE F——ING GILMORE GIRLS

The concert was great... JB played one song I knew, and TP played 4 out of 4 that I was hoping to hear. IHOP afterwards. The people on both sides of us had been smoking out. Ick. Erik was really sleepy, only operating on 2 hours. We went to Bridgeport, to drop off a DVD, and finally to Waco. We had to keep stopping and jumping around, getting energy drinks. We couldn't think of anything else to talk about simply because we HAD to. I was really afraid he was gonna crash. He slept at my place cause I didn't want him driving another 20 minutes himself.

Work tonight, I felt this HORRIBLE jealousy when he started talking to another girl... and then again at the end of the night when Alisha walked him out to his car & he said, "Alisha's gonna be my girlfriend." Cause some 50-year-old gay guy had hit on him and was supposed to come back at midnight. Erik was really put off. Hehehe. Good night, good weekend—and this is where it ends. Farewell, and thank you for nearly six years. I'll miss you... but my new one will just be a continuation... forget replacements! Love you.

Courtney Elizabeth ♥

Of course I cried several times while reading that one, but the way I felt when reading this last paragraph... I love when I'm nice to my journal, because to me, it speaks of happiness with myself—or with God. Whichever. "You have a friend in me, dear girl." It's the still small voice I've longed to hear all my life. It's always been there. I've just never known how to listen.

You are not alone.

The Middle Ages

November 18, 2002

This seems sad to me—to open a beautiful new journal on a sour note. I am so excited about you—please stay together for me; I need you. Your mother grew old; 6 years took its toll on her weak spine & she split. Anyway so I am so sad tonight. Erik didn't work, & I saw Jeff for the first time in 2 weeks & he could barely look at me. He's very definitely mad at me. It hurts my heart, especially after that delicious dream. ♥ And I can't stop thinking about Erik either. I am sad tonight. And Jason was driving me crazy with his questions & stories. Help me, Lord, help me!

♥ Me

November 19, 2002

Tra la la I am so much happier tonight. Adolfo & Dawn came to see me at work. Adolfo said he forgot I worked there, & I said yeah right & he blushed red. After, I went to Jeff & Brooke's. Talked to Brooke, asked her straight out if when she got mad at me, it was because she thought I liked Jeff. She said no, & that she'd been friends w/ other girls who liked him. I told her I didn't like him anymore.

When he came home, I asked him to walk me out & he said he couldn't move. When I asked why, & Brooke walked out of the room, he put his fingers to his lips like he was smoking & told me not to tell Brooke. So I asked if he was mad at me & he said why would you think I was mad at you, & I said 'cause of what Brooke said I said. He was like what's that & I was like you know what I mean & he said no Courtney, explain to me. He was high. I'm planning on telling him straight out tomorrow, when he's more able to focus on me. But he seemed a bit more Jeff-like tonight... probably cause he was high.

Oh and get THIS: Brooke told me I wasn't the to worry about her thinking I was after her boyfriend... but Amanda. That about killed me! I didn't know whether to laugh or scream. Me after Nate... haha. I am crazy about Jeff... sure I like Nate too, but I did before Amanda did so she can kiss my ass. Not that I'd ever go for either of them unless they got single. I'm just not like that!

♥ Me

November 20, 2002

Okay, can I just say Cheston Damon is such a cutie! He makes the best eye contact I've ever seen. I hugged everyone when I left LG tonight... Joey, Cheston, Luke even. Brooke came! She actually had a good time! Yea! Maybe next time she'll bring her darling boyfriend, who, tonight was not high so he was being meanish again. He told Brooke he was pretending to be high so he could see if I told her! Agh! Will I ever win with those two? Please let him see the light!

♥ Me

Oh Tiff & I went to Hastings & she met Erik & Parnell & Sarah & saw Reagan. Liked Reagan. Let her get over Cheston so that she'll stop saying I can't like him please!

♥ me for real

November 24, 2002

Oh, my beautiful friend. Me & Erik have spent so much time together these past few days. Got three hugs from him tonight—very cool, very much him. I told him I wanted to go home with him & he said he wanted me to go but it would be weird. I don't want him to go. What am I gonna do without him? Be BORED! I really like him... Sarah said she thought we'd be "sweet" together because he's a virgin too... saving himself for marriage. Cute!

Ugh, what am I gonna do for Thanksgiving? Whatever it is, I sincerely hope I can give You the praise you deserve. Jimmy's sermon this morning hit home hard. Thank you for my wonderful job, for Erik, for Sarah, for Alisha & Parnell, for all my new friends. And bless my sweet Reagan. He's probably got a lot on his mind. Psalm 38:9, Lord, I love you!

♥ Me

November 30, 2002

Wow, it's December! How 2002 flew. Erik went out of town again today—not back till Tuesday! Two nights, 3 days without him! Ugh! Last night we were watching Pretty Woman & he was scratching my back and then put his arm around me. It's times like that I wish I had my TV in front of a couch... much more comfy for cuddling.

He slept in my bed, and every time I woke up, I wanted to hold his hand, but I didn't. I woke up screaming with leg cramps. He was very sweet. Rubbed my leg. When he left this morning, very long hug. Not so much tonight, but I don't know... we'll see how we feel when he gets back I guess. I miss him already. My house feels empty.

Hmm, so Thanksgiving was good. Went to Kellie's and had yummy food & 6 jello shots. Robert Reed wants to go out drinking one night! Hehe! Fun.

♥ Me

December 4, 2002

So Erik's cousin Nicci came in town... she's lots of fun—they both came to Life group & Erik wants to go again. Nicci & I have plans to go to a hospital or something for Christmas. That'd be so neat. So we played Hoopla at Amanda's... lots of fun. Then back to my house, Erik went home & as soon as he walked out, Nicci goes: "So what's going on between y'all two?" Hehe! I was like, "I don't know, I was about to ask you." So she told me he really likes me.

We talked about marriage... he doesn't want his mom there... Nicci says he's afraid his mom's gonna make some big deal out of it. But he is really a virgin! Maybe hasn't even really kissed a girl. Too cute. Sigh. I gotta talk to him now... How? God help me! Or him...

♥ Me

December 7, 2002

Went to Bridgeport with Erik & Nicci on Thursday. Met his mom. When she walked in, I was very aware that I was sitting a little close to him. On the drive home, we were just talking and I told him what Sarah had said. Then I finally got up the nerve to tell him a bit of what Nicci & I talked about.

I was like, "So what's going on bet. us?" basically. He said he was going to ask me the same thing. "I never take off your bracelet," he said. "And when I talk about you, I'm like, 'my girlfriend, uh, I mean my good friend...'" I was like aww! So we're dating! I have a boyfriend. Is that possible??! How did this happen! I guess everyone's right: when you stop looking, it just happens. I really like him, but it's hard for me to believe he likes me.

Life Group went to Salado last night & I was thinking about it a lot... I really wanted Erik there, esp. when watching Jess & Luke. Sooo cute by the way! At one point I was walking w/ Tiff & Jess came up and hooked arms with me & asked what was wrong and of course I started crying... big surprise. We talked for a long time & I told her some of what I was feeling: holding hands, the fact that I didn't know how someone I like could actually like me back. She says I need to talk to him & we need to establish lines of communication so neither of us gets frustrated. I actually need him to be the initiator... with everything. I think it's so I can feel he really likes me & that I'll know that if we hold hands or kiss, it's because he wanted to. Jess & Tiff both told me he's probably as scared as I am.

When Tiff took me to my car, she & I talked a lot too, and she was like, "Why is it so hard for you to believe someone likes you? You're sweet, beautiful, you're a great person to be around..." I just love her. She said I was her favorite & she loved me. So I don't know what it is. I love being around Erik. He makes me laugh & he's so sweet. But does he really like me or is this some kind of illusion? Ugh! I just want to ask him, do you really like me? I also want to tell him I want to hold his hand but I don't want to initiate... I think maybe he's used to girls initiating, Jess said that... maybe? See I didn't used to mind...like with Brandon, but I had no question that he liked me. So what do I do? How do I talk to him. Ugh! God be with us...

♥ Me

Oh, get this: his family all call him Jonathan. At his cousin Gina's house, she kept being like, "Jonathan..." and I'd start laughing 'cause he's so Erik! But Jonathan Erik Vega, what a great name huh? We've got "plans" to go to California at the end of January / beginning of February. And I don't think he's going to go home for Christmas. Is this holiday gonna rock or suck? Oh, I called Jimmy on his birthday and my mom Friday & she told me he was crying on the phone with her because he missed me so much. He said he wanted to pay my phone bill cause he couldn't stand not talking to me. How cute is THAT?! Aww. I love my life...

♥ Me for real

December 8, 2002

Sigh. This is such a good thing. Thank you Lord!! Erik came at 10:30 this morning... kinda had me scared for half an hour cause he didn't come by last night... but all good. Sunday service this morning. Jackson Gulley is such an incredible cutie! Aww!

After, back to Erik's until 3, then to Jackie's, who I think didn't recognize me. Then to Hastings, where I chilled, worked for a bit, & read until 8, then to Souper Salad. Our waiter might apply at Hastings. Um, back to the store at 9, customer service till 11. Met the gay guy who hit on Erik! Haha! Parnell told me how he told Erik he thought I liked him. Also said, "Erik, your babe is a pimp..." I think! Bell & Alisha are together. Aww!

Back to Erik's, watched him draw & listened to music & I colored. Back home at 2:30, he gave me the longest hug! Oh, so good. We talked a bit about not feeling like this was real, or not knowing maybe. And as much as he wants to get married, he's scared to cause of all the divorces in his family. Don't I understand that! Sigh.

Thank you Jesus for my... get this: BOYFRIEND! Wow! I love you, keep him safe tonight and all nights...and me as well please. And you know the rest.

With all my love & prayers—

Me ♥

December 11, 2002

So yeah. Last night I went up behind Erik & kind of tickled him, intention being to scare him. He put his arm around me & then slid his hand down and took mine, fingers twined and all. Cute! At Hastings till 2:45, got a good write-up, maybe gonna be a GSM. ALREADY! Up until 6 tonight...or this morn rather, went to Kettle at 4:00. Slept all day until 5 when Erik came over. Got dressed, went to Hastings to call Sarah & Alisha, went to a very closed Salado to walk around. Held hands again... I'm so scared... what if he doesn't want this? What if he only feels like he's doing it 'cause he feels like he's supposed to? Ugh!

We went to Pizza Hut & Adolfo was like, when I was on the cut table, I didn't get a chance to talk to you, all I heard was Salado. And I was like, do you think I looked good? And he said, Yeah you did! Why, did you think you didn't? And I said no, I know I did, I just wanted to hear you say it. Ugh. This is so hard. Will I never be happy? Why are other people's opinions so bloody important to me? Like I wish Erik had said something... And I still like Brent & Jeff... what am I going to do? I really like Erik. But does he like me? Is this who I'm supposed to be with right now? Or forever? I'm sure it pisses him off that I'm so flirty. But I'm such a physical person. Maybe he's not. Maybe he is but doesn't understand that I am.

How would God put me with someone who isn't physical? Don't you understand that I've got to get both that and encouragements and compliments from somewhere? Sigh. Please God help me... I'm so sorry I'm not happy. Strike that. I am happy. Very happy. But I am so confused... and very apprehensive about the next five days... he's got a lot of driving, and without me chattering his ear off. Bless him and his car, Lord. I love you, don't take him from me so soon after you gave him to me... and thank you for that, if he really likes me...?

♥ Me

December 13, 2002

Can I get a woo-hoo! And an ugh-ugh. I miss my boyfriend. Thank you Jesus for him! After all this time, what a blessing. Me, him, Alisha, & Bell went to IHOP for cocoa and fries after work last night. Then we came here for a little while, then Erik & I went to his house so I could help him stay awake.

We went to Hastings at six and sat in the car for like 45 minutes. I got the nerve finally to kind of talk to him about us. I asked if we were for real & he said again about his family and divorces. He said he didn't know what the future holds... that it could be great. We could be... how scary is that? I told him that once he started holding my hand & didn't keep doing it, it made me feel like he didn't like me. He said not to worry if he moved really slow... and that if I didn't make a move, he probably wouldn't cause he's so shy.

When Kris came over to the car, we got into Luis's car to listen to music & Erik put his arm around me & I played with his hair while he stroked my shoulder. I felt a lot better after that talk, as hard as it was. Please Jesus let him be able to bring up stuff with me... don't make it so I'm always having to do it.

I slept from 8 to 3, then to work. Jeff and Brooke came in. And Amanda & Alycia. Oh, and Adolfo & Dawn. Jackie's too cute, he moves so fast. Shay is too cool. We talked a lot. Bell, Alisha, & I went to Subway. Then to my house where they watched Count of Monte Cristo & I found songs for Erik's CD. God help me find songs that will be good & won't scare him! That is the last thing I want to do, Lord. He's going to San Antonio in the mañana. Protect him, please, Lord! He was so touchy last night... with initiation from me, but somehow I don't mind so much anymore... Protect him, God. And my mom & Jimmy. Thank you for everything in my life...

♥ Me

Reading about Erik is interesting. In my memory, our relationship was very quick, and the parts that stand out in my mind all stand out as super awkward. But this almost reads like any other innocent teenage romance. I'm sad I didn't enjoy it more while it was happening but sadder still that it hasn't happened again since then. Yet.

The other thing that bothers me is how I remember ending it. I don't. I believe I ghosted him, as well as one can when one works with someone. I remember being horribly embarrassed by him at a New Year's Eve party, and instead of talking to him, I stopped talking to him. I'm going to look him up on social media and reach out, but my goodness, I pray that he doesn't have memories of me as bad as I have of myself.

January 6, 2003

  Wow I haven't written in too long. I am so confused! I went to Bridgeport with Erik for Christmas... so much fun. His mom gave me a book called "Once Upon a Wedding." A hint? The food was great. Everything went smoothly. New Year's we went to see Jackie's band play, and come on, how cute was he? ~~Then~~ Brian & Bethany were there. Then the 4 of us went to Nettie's where I started drinking, the young ones left, Erik started drinking, we both got drunk, I passed out by 11:30 & Erik spent the night in the bathroom. Sarah & CJ came... I spent the night on Nettie's couch.
  Erik seemed very possessive of me that night & he was very silly when drunk. I felt awkward & didn't really want to be around him after that. I PMSed bad for a week. Things with us felt weird & I found myself flirting with Brian to make Erik mad. ??? What's wrong with me? I had a pretty good talk with Adolfo about it... and Sarah.
  Work has been great. But with Erik? Do I really like him or did I just really want a boyfriend? Thinking about Brent or Jeff... good God!!!! And when Nate came in the store today, my heart started going faster. Eeek, HELP me! I just want to be content! Oh Lord...

♥ Me

January 29, 2003

  So Erik & I broke up tonight. I am so sorry I haven't written... I don't think I wanted to admit what a bitch I was being. Things got so weird with Erik I could hardly look at him. Tonight he came by & said we needed to talk. I was like It's about damn time! I told him I'm too immature right now for a boyfriend. It took having a boyfriend to see that I am pretty happy being single right now. True, *if Brent asked me out or Jeff & Brooke suddenly broke up, things might change, but I need the solid friendship & physical attraction and I didn't have that with Erik.*

But Brent, oh Lord! Juarez is fast approaching. Please let me be able to go Jesus! Please! I want to be on worship so very badly! AH! Please let Cheston, Luke, & Brent go! And Reagan?? Ooh! Please Jesus! Oh Lord... my car, money, Amanda... keep my brother & mother so safe! Let them call me please!

Oh, Jesus, you know the deepest desires of my heart...even & especially those I'm not aware of... I don't have the patience right now to write it all: but one thing: I want someone who is as crazy about me as you are...someone who loves you first, but loves me completely for the person I am... and Jesus, that I can love him and be so sweetly content! Please let all about Juarez happen! Paul... Cheston!!! Brent... Lukie! I LOVE YOU ENDLESSLY and I'm sorry for being so...me!

♥ *Me*

Well, there you have it. I'm relieved to see I could own up to it, at least to myself and God. But it doesn't lessen the embarrassment as an adult, and it annoys me that I'm embarrassed about behavior that happened twenty years ago. But I could go on a loop forever, being alternatively angry and guilty. It's not a fun loop. But then I don't find any loops particularly fun.

February 10, 2003

So Juarez training started—great team! Charis, our leader, is so sweet. And there's this guy ~~Clay~~ Cody who rooms with Joey Davilla!!!! and they're both going!! Oh my God! And Brandon Mars... oh, thank you Lord! Please let Luke be able to go... please God! He's apparently going to war in March! Please God keep him safe! And my dear brother! Please Jesus don't let it get that far! HELP US!!

Oh, God, I couldn't handle it! Someone from Life Group gave me $100! Oh Lord you are amazing! My heart's hurting for my boys... keep them

> safe dear Lord. Oh, God. Tonight was Nettie's going away party. Fun! Clay, her drummer, is too cute. So is Clint. Oh, Jesus, it always comes down to this: you know my heart. You know what I long for. Please let Reagan come to LG tomorrow. And Luke & Brent! But Reagan... to Juarez too! PLEASE, I want to get to know him! YOU KNOW!!
>
> ♥ Me

February 28, 2003

> My baby Luke's last night... what a stressful past couple of days. He's leaving me! We chilled with his family for a long time. I ♥ his mother. I got to see Ben & Andrew, who I still think is the cutest Clement in the world. When I left, Luke & I hugged for a long time. He told me I encouraged him just the way I was. God protect him. I love him so much! I am going to miss him desperately. Please Jesus send me a boy like Luke. Please, God, please. He's so bloody special. Keep him safe, dear Lord. I love him. And keep my brother and His out of this war!
>
> ♥ Me

Luke going off to war remains one of the saddest and most dramatic times of my life. Even then, I couldn't believe I had a friend going off to war. That was something that happened when we weren't alive. I cried when we hugged. I slept terribly while he was gone, plagued by nightmares worse than they had been when I first met him. And of course, I had no idea what it was like for him. No idea.

March 4, 2003

> I feel kind of icky. I am having the worst trouble sleeping. And my legs still hurt so badly. Juarez is in like 4 days. Please Lord, provide me with the enthusiasm to go—thank you so much for providing the funds... now please make a way to meet March rent, make April rent, & start paying bills even though I'm losing a week of work. Please just help me feel excited about this. I know you want me

to go... but make me want to. I miss Luke's presence. Bless him immensely Lord!

♥ *Me*

I'm writing so slowly right now, literally having to force myself through line by line. I don't know if it's my current trauma freezing me or the disgust of having to wade through it again as I read it. All I know is, I'm horribly angry, sad, and disappointed in myself again, and I don't know that I deserve to be. Reading these entries proves I've been hard on myself all my life, but at what age did that begin? Are we born with anxiety as human beings? Are we born thinking we aren't enough? In my case, I was born too much and got told to be quieter or less than somehow until I was most comfortable hiding in my bedroom with my dogs and coloring books. It was not a fun life for an extrovert who loved people.

March 23, 2003

So yeah it's so time I wrote my personal stuff about Juarez. I've been back over a week but haven't really found the motivation for it. It turned out to be awesome, despite my aversion to it in the beginning & the feeling of not supposed to be there all week, until Thursday.

So! Cody and I hit it off really well. He's a total sweetie. One night, we had this really long, really good conversation where he told me about Colleen, his sort of girlfriend, & about his partying life, and we just had an awesome conversation. It was lots of fun. Leading up to it: I felt like I was supposed to pray for him, but I wasn't sure how to, so I just kneeled behind him, put my hands on his back, and prayed really softly however I felt like.

Then I got up and Ashley Heather came up to me & told me I made her feel like laughing all the time. That I was always so happy and smiley. Made me feel really good cause sometimes I feel so the opposite. But Jesus loves me, so I'm shiny.

I had seen Cody get up and go behind us, so when Ashley was done, I went to him and asked him to pop my back. When he did, he asked if I had been the one who prayed for him earlier. I said yes & he said "I didn't know who it was, but as soon as you laid hands on my back, I thought 'I have to find Courtney to pray for her.'" How cool is that?

This pen is dying. So, let me see... I was sitting next to Cody on the bus & right in front of Brent, & Brent was saying it was "caliente" on the bus. I told him it was actually "calor" and caliente meant spicy-hot, and he said, "you are caliente" or "tu es caliente" or something like that and Cody said "Ai yi yi!" I must have turned bright red. My heart hurts when I think about him... more at the end!

Let's see... Matty B, man, what a cutie! My first time on the mic this year, and I was feeling pretty apprehensive, Matt came up and squeezed my shoulders and said, "You did so good!" I was happy. Hmm. So one night on the bus, I was talking about some guy and Court Winter said, "So who do you like?" And I was like, Brent, and she said she thought we'd make a cute couple. When Jess Exum told me who she thought she was gonna marry, she was like, now you tell me! And I made her guess, and she guessed Cody, then got up to look inside, came out, and guessed Brent. She actually said, "I know who it is." Very sure of herself. She'd gone inside, looked, and knew immediately. She said she had been thinking earlier that day that we'd be cute. AHH!

So this is funny. Before I told Court, me, Rachael, and Sarah were in line for lunch and I had just been telling Sarah about my heart skipping thing. Rach came, then later Brent happened to walk by when my heart skipped, and I go, "Oh, there goes my heart!" And Rach thought I meant bc of Brent! Hehe!

Then one night, Thursday I think, the night after I told Court, I went to Rachael and said, "I told Courtney who I liked and I really want to tell you but I don't want you to tell anyone." She said who would I tell? And I said Mike and she promised not to. So I asked her to guess, and right away she said, "Well, we've already established it's not Brent." I just looked at her & she goes, "Or is it?" It was cute, she got excited. So! Yeah, people think we'd be cute, which makes it hard to guard my heart, especially when I hear him talking about dating someone, about being allowed to by God now. And Café Liso… at the end! So… hmm…

Toby had been on my heart since the second training day, and I didn't know what to pray for him, so I wrote him a really long encouragement letter. I didn't see him read it, but after a while, he came up and put his arms around me and said "Thank you. Thank you so much." I love him! He told us several times in Mexico that he loved us. And then at Dwelling Place on Sunday, he said, Love you, Courtney. And on the bus on the way home, he said he was just sitting there thinking about how much he loved us. Oh, sweet boy. He's so so special. So! Wow.

Well, one morning we were in line for breakfast and Kelly and I were talking about sweating and John Boxer said, "No, girls don't sweat! And they don't toot either." I about died. I felt like saying "Boys don't say toot!" He's so cute, he's one of my favorites. Man, he gives good hugs too. At the party at Grant's, he and Matty B were about to leave so I wanted a picture, and John had both arms around me, big time hug, and then Matty B got closer. Such a cute picture, except you can major see my rolls in my tummy. I'm so pale, in my pictures in my white tee shirt, I blend in. Hot mama, I tell you! Hehe. I love my pictures. I love my team!

So Friday night, Brooke, Sarah, & I were trying to figure out what to do and I was like, I really want to see Brent! We ended up walking to Café Liso to show Toby my pictures. We were on the couch & who walks in but Brent?!! I told him he needed to see my pix too & Tobes goes, "She has a lot of good ones of you in here." Brent sat down and goes, "So why do you have so many pictures of me, hmm?" Ahh! I was like, "I don't have that many."

Toby leaned over and whispered, "He's kind of full of himself" or something like that, and I wanted

> to tell him "funny thing is, I do have a lot of him."
> I really want to tell Toby. So! Brent goes to leave, &
> he's shaking people's hands. He gets to me, and we
> were talking while he kept shaking my hand, & I
> just didn't want to let go. He's so cute! At Hastings,
> Brooke told Nick she thought we should date. She
> thinks we'd be cute! So wow, long entry. Probably
> forgetting something, but...
>
> ♥ Me

The way I describe myself in those pictures, I sound like the Pillsbury Doughboy. Y'all, it's all in the lighting. In some of them, I look pink and happy; in some, I blend in with my shirt. But the tone of this entry is so happy. There were more people who cared about me, most especially the men, good, godly men. I'm ready for mine, finally. I know I am.

March 24, 2003

> So yeah I forgot to write about the single coolest, most important thing... on Thursday night, I prayed for Cody, for Nathaniel, then went to Toby & told him he was still on my heart and although I didn't know why, I was gonna pray for him. He'd had his head on his knees, and when I sat next to him & put my hand on his back, his eyes filled with tears.
> A few seconds into my prayer, he turned & said, "Courtney, I'm sorry, I never interrupt people when they're praying for me, but I just had to tell you Jesus wants you to know he loves you & he hears you when you call out to him." We were sitting very close, so instead of looking at him, I just had my ear to him. I said thank you & he said, "Courtney, look at me." I did and my eyes filled up & he repeated himself.
> Then we talked for a while & I told him I hadn't wanted to come & that I didn't think I had a purpose on the trip this year. Toby said I did, and whether it be tonight or two months from now, God would reveal it to me. Then he said, "I really want to be baptized in the Holy Spirit." Me, "Well, why don't you get someone to pray for you?" Toby, "I will." Me, "Where's Preston?" Toby, "He's being prayed for." I looked around for someone not being prayed for. "I

bet Courtney would do it." Him, "That would work." Me, "And I'd love to do it." Him, "That would definitely work."

So I went to get Court & asked Brandon Mars to come too. He said he didn't know how to pray and I was like, none of us do. Courtney told me to get Grant, & when he came over, Toby had one of us on each side. Grant started praying & some other people came up, Brandon and Courtney left. Grant said he felt like Toby's bracelet and watch were chains, so he slipped them off, praying freedom for Toby.

Nic Lowell was next to me now, & Grant felt that we weren't supposed to be touching him, that we should just hover our hands. So we lifted them, & almost immediately, Toby fell forward, crying, & Grant hugged him & was like, "It's okay, brother." He stood him back up & we prayed a couple more minutes, then he fell backward & we laid him on the floor. He kind of curled up & hid his face. I was half laughing, half crying. I was so excited.

Brent came over & Nic & he both prayed for him. It was really neat to have been there from the beginning. God, I love him! So! After the meeting, I went downstairs & Brent asked if he could give me a word. He was like, when you pray for someone & get involved in their personal spiritual life, watch your heart, or something like that. I was like, are you talking about Toby or YOU? It was kind of weird, but... God knows what's best! Love you!

♥ *Me*

I was so freaked out by this phenomenon when I first started going to Antioch. But now the stronger my faith, the more I understand it has always been within me. I just never listened. Just let peace wash over you. There's never going to be proof enough for nonbelievers. Just pray for peace.

April 5, 2003

So! Brooke is trying to set me up with Nick Hoffman. It's pretty funny. First time she met him, she straight up told him, I think y'all should date, y'all'd be a cute couple. Next time, she told me to go away so she could talk to him. She basically asked if he liked me, if he thought I was pretty... he said I have really pretty eyes. So now she's dead set on us being together but I'm not so sure. I mean, I like him, but I don't know how I'd feel about him hanging with Jeff & Nate.??? Plus, Brent... sigh.

Dad gave me $250, I signed the lease with Brooke. I CAN'T WAIT! Oh, she called me her best friend... how much can I trust her? I love her, & she is definitely the best friend I have right now, but how real is that? How soon is she gonna turn her back on me? Help!

♥ Me

April 21, 2003

Hmm...so this Nick thing may not be good. He's such a cutie. He's kind of dating Vanessa now. He called her perfect. Yuck. It's hard not to be jealous. Kaylan & Brad are kind of hooking up. Everyone but me... I haven't seen Brent in like 3 weeks, but I kind of make myself think about him. He'd be such a good boyfriend. But I'm completely sure he likes someone else. Sigh.

So, Brian asked me the other day, "How's it hangin'?" My typical response, "I don't know, you tell me." It rolls right over Brian every time, but Matt goes, "The correct response is..." and whispered to Brian. "What was that?" I said coyly. "Nothing, I don't want to get fired for sexual harassment." "Come on." "If you really want to know, come over here & I'll tell you, but remember it's a joke." About 5 minutes later I went back to him & said, "So what was the correct response?" "The correct response is, 'It's not anymore since you walked by.'" I laughed and must have turned bright red. It made me feel so good.

And tonight I was sitting on the counter waiting for someone to walk me, and Vicki had paged that I needed to be walked. Bell came out with Dustin & I was like, "I don't know what Vicki's talking about." Bell was like, "Well you've been sitting there complaining & it's probably getting on her nerves." I was like, "I only said it once!" Nick said, "Yeah, she's just sitting there bitching." I was like, "Shut up," cause my heart hurt cause he wouldn't take me to the concert. I walked off with Dustin and Nick goes, "You heard bitching in the old way, but I meant it like the skiers say, these hills are bitchin'!" I said yeah right, and then he said he thought I'd think it was funny.

After Dustin walked me, Nick popped my back. Felt so awesome. Sigh. I think I really like him. I don't like him "dating" Vanessa, but I'm glad she can't go to the concert. Keep him safe.

♥ Me

April 27, 2003

Friday night I was over at Jess's... we went to Ninfa's with Debs, then way later, Kelley, Nathaniel, Jabar, and me went to Denny's. Much fun, Nathaniel's so cute, Jabar's way too loud. It was so fun hanging with Nathaniel.

So, Nick came up to me at work yesterday & goes, "Tell me if you think this is bullshit. Vanessa and I work with this guy Vick, right? Tell me what to think if I see them kissing." I was like Oh my God! He was kind of crying. Poor baby must've really liked her. They weren't even really together. Hmm...we shall see.

♥ Me

May 3, 2003

Last night I spent a lot of time thinking about Brent, making up scenarios and stuff. My heart hurt. I really like him. I really like Nick too. I just went over to Denny's and saw Jeff. He's so hot! So very hot. I want a boyfriend.

♥ Me

A two-month intermission comes next, and my butt hurts from sitting on this bed, so I'm stopping for the night. But a thrill just ran through me because I saw my first mention of *Gilmore Girls*, which means I did watch it live, and I've literally been dreaming of Connecticut for twenty years. It's marvelously mind-blowing that it's written in ink, because there's a part of me who only remembers bingeing *Gilmore Girls* on Netflix.

God, I'm so tired. I want to be home. Home is where the heart is, and I will make Connecticut my home, because part of me believes that's the only way I'll ever truly heal. My heart is here.

July 1, 2003

> Well, it's been a long time my friend! I had a talk with Jennifer Balloon about bipolar disease and I told her I think I'm just manic. But I spent all night curled up crying over "Songcatcher." I have a huge crush on Jason Tizzy. Of course he's got a girlfriend. They were on the rocks for a while. We've been out to eat twice and I really enjoy his company. He always seems disappointed when we don't work together.
>
> On Gilmore Girls tonight, Rory just walked up and kissed Jess. It gave me butterflies. Same reaction when they kissed in Songcatcher. I really want to be kissed! Thought about telling Nick that when he leaves on Friday. He's moving to Dallas. I wonder what he'd say? He'd probably run off screaming. My heart hurts. Ugh. My life keeps going nowhere.
>
> I went to H-town with Jeff and Brooke to see the Justified/Stripped tour. It was awesome, the whole weekend. I am going to Cali with Jimmy, Alex and Drew in a week & a half. Work sucks, more later on Jase & Nick... not to mention Justin... sooo cute! Help me, God.
>
> ♥ Me

July 27, 2003

> Hmm, long month. Brooke & I got in a huge fight & didn't talk for 2 weeks. I went to California with Jimmy, Alex, & Drew, & when I came back, she had apologized. HUGE! Cali was a blast. We did

karaoke. Al and I did the Elephant Love Medley from Moulin Rouge & Sin Wagon together, then I did Let 'Er Rip by myself. Soo fun! It was great to see Annie & Beth & all the other cousins. My little Kevin is so grown up! 15! WOW! Jocelyn is great. Lani is a blast. I miss it desperately.

I just finished reading over a lot of old notes & crying. John Chase, Rhett Maximus, Suzanne Grant... very sad. I wish one of my friends NOW would write me something. Brent told me I should stop by someday... I want a hug from him so badly. My van has another flat... 2nd one in two weeks. I need a new job. In California! Ugh! We saw Melissa from some Real World. We went to a comedy club. Never gonna do that again. I had pulled a 48-hour day, so maybe that's why it wasn't funny... or NOT!

One of the guys we saw we later saw introduce the Carson Daly bash show. Ow, my hand hurts. Al is very cool, Drew got very annoying, & Jimmy is Jimmy. I miss that week very much. But I can't leave my friends yet... Brent being primary.

♥ Me

July 30, 2003

It's the end of July! Wow! Last night I went over to Jeff's, there was a big party going on. Jeff & Daniel were the only 2 straight guys. Josh & Geoff are too cute! Oh, and Daniel. Damn, he's sexy. We went to get a pack of cigarettes and we got hell for leaving. Then I went to Daniel's & Jeff came, but then he left, & when Daniel wanted to go, he said "We'd better get back before they think we're humping." I thought that was hilarious. Brooke asked if I'd kissed him & I was like no! But I sure wanted to... hmm.

Jeff wanted to sleep with Brooke & Debra, this lesbian girl. He was hot for it. Kinda funny. Daniel's gonna teach me guitar! Yea! He's a cutie... we *wouldn't make a good couple, we're too different, but damn I wouldn't mind kissing him.*

♥ *Me*

Yay, here is proof that at one time, I did understand the difference between friends and relationships. I feel like this is wise for a twenty-two-year-old, especially one who had never been in a real relationship (Brandon aside). I firmly believe that opposites attract is hogwash. If you can't communicate with someone, you can't have any kind of relationship, and you communicate best with like-minded people. I'm not saying we can't have different things we enjoy or view sunsets differently. But you have to find the people who understand you, who you're okay just *being* with.

I'm not saying to deprive yourself of a good make-out session every so often. I didn't get enough of those.

August 2, 2003

Do you realize almost every damn entry has a new guy in it? Could I be any more fickle? I was just rereading some of these entries & I started crying when I read about Brent. I miss him a lot. I ache for one of his hugs.

Last night there was another party at Ryan Oral's house. Pretty much the same crew, but Joey & Rose came. Joey is hilarious when drunk. I could tell something was bothering Daniel so I didn't talk to him much, but at about 5 we went to Whataburger and talked about what was bothering him. He's depressed. He hates the world. He has bloody scars on his wrists. Man, I can't tell you how my heart hurt for him. Then he said he wished Brooke would stop trying to hook everyone up. I wonder if he was making a veiled reference to moi?

I went over to Jeff's & Michelle & Ryan were making out. Then I went to Daniel's. He was hung over. He looked sick. I just wanted to hug him, for real. I really am attracted to him. I almost wish I'd never met him, 'cause I don't want him thinking I'm trying to save him or something. Even though I don't know him that well, my heart hurts to think of him killing himself. He just doesn't care... or so he says. Maybe he cares more than he can admit. Oh, Jesus, help me with this one... I'm starting to ache for him.

♥ Me

September 7, 2003

It's been too long. I've gotten really bad about writing. Why do I feel so much for people? Even people I don't know. I mean, come on! Okay, so... Brooke & I got in another huge fight but we went to Deric's to play poker & she got drunk & then we were okay again.

Nate was hitting on Kaylan majorly. He got very drunk & no one would let him drive home. Daniel was the only one there who could drive a stick. But he tried handing Nate the keys so I went & told Deric, and it turned into this huge thing. D & I followed them home, & when we got out I told Daniel I was sorry for being a bitch, but I cared about both of them. He just kind of smiled. I wonder if he believed me, & if he even cared? Sigh.

Seth, a friend of D-Shaft's, is toooo cute. Comes into Hastings a lot. The night turned out incredibly fun. Hmm. Uh...Jennifer Balloon, Kaylan, & I have been spending a lot of time together. And Megaan is a doll. Justin Woody got hired at Hastings. HOT! Justin Glamour's still the cutest thing ever. Jenn's brother Jerry came down this weekend—HOT as well.

We had a party on Friday night. At about 8, before anyone but Kaylan had come over, someone knocked on my door really loud, scaring the hell out of us. I opened the door & no one was there, but I could see car lights on the other side of the complex. I shut the door then reopened it & heard a really deep voice say "Courtney." I was like What! Kaylan & I were laughing & kept shutting the door. I went into my room to change & then bang bang again. Kaylan about died when she opened the door again & Jeff jumped out at her. Hehe! He came by to "mess with me" without Brooke! Oh, man! He is too cute. I haven't been over there in a while.

Haven't seen Daniel in over 2 weeks. He'd gone out of town. But last night I had the most delicious dream about him. When I woke up, I could remember every detail & told myself to write it down but I didn't & now of course I can't remember. But I liked it. I kind of miss him. I was very attracted to Jenn's brother, but so was Kaylan. She wants to long-distance date him, and she barely even talked to him. But he's mega hot. So I guess that's about it.

Oh, Life Group sucks. I don't want to go anymore, but I want to meet new people, and I want to feel closer to God. How hypocritical can I be? For real. I don't press in but I want to feel His love... I can't have it both ways, can I? Help me God, help me feel the way I do in Mexico. Like Mexico's closer to heaven. Thank you for letting me draw breath every day. My life, as much as it may hurt & be confusing & suck sometimes, is infinitely precious. Please let something wonderful happen...

♥ Me

September 14, 2003

What a weekend! Jerry came back into town, & me, Jenn, Jerry, & Kevin went to Austin last night. We walked around Sixth for like 2 hours but then Jenn felt sick. We'd gone to Johnny Carino's & I think that did it. Jerry's really cute. Jenn kept calling him Jeremiah. CUTE! Kaylan was acting kind of pissy, & Jenn's & my feelings were hurt. Jerry got a little flirty. Maybe I shouldn't have spent the weekend with him, but it's a little late now, huh? When Kaylan was talking about how hot he was & wanting a long distance relationship if he was interested, I wonder if she was staking claim to him? That's not really fair though.

We had a good time. Went to Ihop today & Jerry paid for all of us. He's so damn cute. He has one more year in the marines, the last 6 months on *a boat. Wanna hear something sad? He might come back for Christmas, & I am thinking of forgoing California so I can see him again. Geez! I barely know him! I wish Jenn would tell me something.*

So guess who's back in Waco? Yeah, Nathan Cowsill. I walked into Starbucks the other day and about died, he looks so good! Oh, my heart hurts. I saw Bruce Almighty with Jess today & couldn't help tearing up. Then I watched Life or Something Like It. I want someone to love me, kiss me, hold me... please? PLEASE!

Why are there people in the world who don't believe in God that are in love? Why do I have to be content with just God before I have someone love me? Why? Why do I get to spend one weekend with this cute funny guy who lives in fucking North Carolina? Why can't he stay here? Why did he have to come back for another weekend? I could have lived without getting to know him better... but thank you, God, for the little things... the weekend was really fun. Oh, make me content. Sometimes I almost wish I'd never known you, that I was clueless as to the things you can do... then it might not hurt so much when you don't do them...

♥ *Me*

Do y'all see a pattern yet? My poor, tortured, tangled heart, as the Chicks would say. I already mentioned unanswered prayers, but I'll touch on them again: just because you don't like the answer doesn't mean it wasn't answered. But I suppose it's okay to be hurt and angry about it, especially when what you wish for is all but magic.

What I mean by that is, it would be silly to be angry at God for not making me a millionaire from literally sitting on my couch all day. But being angry at God (or myself) for losing friendships or losing opportunities for relationships? That seems right, because I hold myself accountable. I whine about people not staying in touch, but the phone (or Internet or whatever) goes both ways. If I don't make the effort, why should they? I'm worth loving. I'm worth having in your life. Let me show you how. So when I don't get it reciprocated, I wonder what I did wrong, and I get sad and angry with God. And then I get distracted from writing because I go check my phone to see if there are any messages I need to answer.

Spoiler alert: there aren't, so I send some of my own. "Thinking of you." "Miss you." "Love you." "Be okay." "Be happy." I hope you feel it.

September 18, 2003

> God help me! I'm sorry I'm so pathetic. When I watched the OC, I wanted to scream & cry! I want a guy who loves me like Ryan loves Marissa. Ah, who am I kidding? I want Ryan! Nathan came into Hastings today & I walked around with him for a while. He's so cute. It's his sweet smiley eyes. I wonder if he'd ever want to hang out one on one? I really like him. Joey also came in & I went to lunch with him & Tizz. Lots of fun—love both of them. Arm hurts, you know my heart, God!
>
> ♥ Me

September 20, 2003

> Okay, yesterday was so much fun! I worked from about 8:30 to 2:30, 'cause I was helping Joey do a scan. Then I went to get my haircut, & it's so cute, I love it! Then I went back to Hastings & went to Chili's with Missy which was fun—we talked about boys. Then back to Hastings & Joey & I went to Sprint to get a new phone. One of the people who helped me, Justin, was so cute!
>
> Then we went to Starbucks so I could see Nathan. Agh! Came home, showered, looked cute, went to La Quinta & hung out with Brooke, Ryan, & Rafael, one of my new roomies. Summer, his wife, works at Denny's. They have the cutest baby, Andre Jordan, who I'm gonna call AJ. I will save so much money!
>
> Um, so then at eleven I went to Justin Woody's for a party. Jordan hugged me & almost immediately left. I felt really weird, until we all went inside & started drinking. We played "Links" or "Fuck Your Neighbor," and "Hockey." Blake, Justin's roommate, so so freaking hot. I mean. He seemed moody but most of the time I think he was faking. So, I had a lot of beers. I got flirty.

> *There was this girl, Jenny, Justin's ex... so cute! She & I clicked, & it was fun. Um, at about 5:30 Blake turned out the lights in the living room 'cause Missy & another girl, Kristen, whom Blake, Jenny, & Missy kept calling "Man Hands," were asleep on the couches. I was like "I can't see" and reached my hand back and Blake took it & twined his fingers with mine for a second. It felt great. THEN Jordan pulled me into Justin's room and stuck his tongue in my mouth. He was like, "When, when?" and I said, "I don't think tonight, sweetie." I wanted to go home. Then he asked about tonight & I told him I have to close.*
>
> *I asked Jenny & Jordan to walk me down, & I hugged Justin goodbye and he told me thanks for coming over. How fun is it that I get to hang out with him again? Jordan had his arm around Jenny's waist & holding my hand. One of the other guys, Cotter, was walking with us too. I hugged Jordan goodbye and then Jenny like three times. She made me promise to call Jordan's phone when I got home. I did, then went to bed. Couldn't stop thinking about Blake taking my hand... Missy made out with him! I want to!*
>
> ♥ *Me*

I believe that in a different life, we would have had a threesome that night. It would have been a whole different adventure.

September 24, 2003

> *So Blake started work at Hastings. He's so cute! I gave Tizz a hard time last night, about several things. Justin closed, & he said he and Blake would be at "the" party. I HOPE! If my world was perfect, Blake, Justin, Nathan, Jordan, Joey, Tizz, Justin Glamour, & Jerry, Missy, Jenny, would all be at the party, & I want to kiss the former ~~seven~~ eight. Ooh, the images... hmm, we'll see. Is it wrong to pray for something that bad? Slutty! I would be content with*

just Blake, Nathan, or Jerry. Sigh. My tummy hurts. Maybe I have food poison. Goodnight.

♥ Me

October 5, 2003

Last night was Brooke & "my" birthday party. She started off the night being a bitch—fighting with Ryan because he invited 3 people. And she finished the night being a bitch—throwing everyone out at 2:45, b/c we were supposedly spose to be out at 3. She had Rose about to throw down 'cause she called her a bitch & Joey left w/o saying goodbye. Missy wanted to kick her ass too. So did Jen.

I got so drunk. We played drinking games. Even Daniel was being nice & he started smiling & he was like, "You're right, I needed to get drunk." Connelly's rather cute. Blake...damn. I went to their house for an hour when Brooke kicked us out. Blake made me drink another jello shot. Then I sat on their couch, trying to get sober, & ended up hugging the toilet. Everclear's fucking nasty. Justin however is so hot. I just love to hug him. Even Tizz & Leah came. Missed Justin Glamour, but I knew he wouldn't come.

Brooke spent 3 hours at the beginning passed out on the ground because she had 9 jello shots in like 20 minutes. She threw up on herself. Nathan threw up all over. It was really fun for the most part, but Brooke's fucking mental! Will is hot too!!!! I mean! So is Doug. Man, Will, Doug, both Justins, Tizz, why does everyone have a girlfriend? Of course there are Blake, Nathan, Connelly... hmm.

♥ Me

Now I wonder if I was possibly still slightly intoxicated when I wrote that, because I have no idea who, like, four of those names are. But I'm also disgusted by my nonchalance writing about people throwing up, especially myself. Let me preface this next statement by saying puke is a phobia for me. So when I say I remember almost every time I've had to deal with it, I mean it. And I remember an old man throwing up on the floor of the ER when I took Brooke to get her spinal tap, but I don't remember her throwing up on herself at our party. The mind is strange.

October 15, 2003

> *So I got fired from Hastings today for "misappropriation of product & misuse of my associate discount." Sucks like no other, b/c I think the first one means taking product. I'm going to move to California at the end of the month. I'm going to hate leaving my friends… but I guess this is for the best. We'll have another huge party. Please help me Lord.*
>
> ♥ *Me*

Here is something that stands out vividly to me: me standing in line for a drink at work, getting paged to the music department, and not going back to pay for my drink. I 110 percent would have called that stealing, and I still will. But what they fired me for was stealing CDs, and that pissed me off because they were considered swag and had holes in the labels. So I got fired for a soda. Something that seemed so black-and-white to me back then was that thou shalt not steal, cheat, lie, yada yada. It has so many gray areas now. I hate that such a good worker got let go over something that small, but I also hate stealing. So ugh.

The drive that followed to California was also vivid. I cried hysterically for about an hour out of Waco, and then I stopped. I drove over seventeen hours straight through, only stopping for gas. I stopped at a Motel 6 in Arizona, thinking I'd crash hard but only slept for about four hours. I woke up at seven and couldn't go back to sleep, so I went on, arriving in Hollywood at four in the morning. The hills were burning, and I stopped my van, which had been painted by my friends, on the edge of the highway to watch in awe. It was horrifyingly beautiful. Looking back, it seems quite symbolic—out of the fire and into the flames. But like a phoenix from the ashes, she will rise again.

November 6, 2003

> *So I've been in Cali for a week now & I really miss my friends. Especially Joey. And I want a hug from Justin. I had a great dream about Nathan the other night. I want him to move to Cali. I want a job I'm going to like. I want some friends. I want*

a church I love. Sigh. I want to be in Texas...or at least rich enough to jump on a plane anytime.

♥ Me

December 2, 2003

So I went to an acting thing & got a call-back audition. I go in today to read a L'Oréal commercial. Oh PLEASE let something good happen! Thanksgiving was such a blast. Jimmy cracks me up, Helen is gorgeous, and their little boy Zachary is a doll. So is Alison. There were no fights although Beth was in a horrible mood. It was just really fun.

I got a job at Old Navy & it's got potential: Dan & RHYS! Rhys, pronounced Rise or Reese, is very funny, cute, & straight! I had a dream about him last night. Me & him & Audrey & another guy? Audrey wanted Rhys too, but he was way troubled. At one point we were trying to find somewhere quiet to talk & it took forever, finally we found an abandoned house with beanbag chairs all over. It was dark. Aud & the other guy were waiting outside.

So Rhys and I sat down & I was trying not to cry. He wouldn't let me touch him. He started telling me that he stole. He pulled on his sweater & said, "See, this I took from my job." I was like, "I don't care, I just wanna touch you." He was obviously upset about it. His hand was lying on the couch & I twined my fingers in his so our palms were on the couch still. Then Jackson woke me up before we could talk anymore. Good dream, way more detailed. I want to go to the beach or the dog park with him. Sigh. So wish me luck today!

♥ Me

January 16, 2004

Long time, lots of stuff! Christmas was the best, New Year's sucked, got in a huge fight with Mom, kind of worked it out, but she threatened to send me back to Texas. David was like, "No, we love you!"

Rocio & Ulises, two friends from work, have been giving me a hard time about Rhys. It took an hour and a half to get up the nerve, but after talking to Ulises, I asked Rhys out for tonight. It was fun—we went to the Grove to see LOTR again and OH MY GOD guess who was standing in line in front of me? SCOTT SPEEDMAN! Hotter in real life than I could imagine! Agh! Then we saw Mark Feurstein, from "Good Morning, Miami." Great night, lots of fun, hope we'll do it again.

♥ Me

January 26, 2004

So I've been getting a lot of hell about Rhys. We are planning to go to Long Beach next week, me, Ulises, & Rocio, & Rhys doesn't know yet. I hope he'll come. I'm going to ask him out again on Thursday, I think. Agh! People tease me a lot; I wonder if they say stuff to him? I hope he doesn't think I'm the one talking! Sigh. He's cute. But if he liked me, wouldn't he ask me out again? He said he had fun last time. Ah, who understands men?

So Mom's mad at me again. Money issues of course. I want to get my own place, but I'm scared to live anywhere in LA where the rent would be cheap. I wish me & Rocio & Ulises & Rhys could get a place. How fun would that be? My tummy hurts. I wonder if I can write without connecting letters. It's hard!

♥ Me

February 2, 2004

Rhys & I went to Red Lobster & Big Fish on Friday night. Jose asked him when we were going out again. I'd be interested to know what he said. I think he thinks I'm the one talking. I knew this was going to go bad, but who knew so soon? Agh!

I had fun Friday. He's so sarcastic, I hardly know when to believe him. When we were walking the parking lot, he said he hated to ask me, but did I have cash, & he touched my hand with his knuckle. He's very flirty & asked what I could keep secret about the store... but AGH! He's such a guy!

I want a boyfriend! I want Brandon Wonderful... but I want Rhys too. I had a dream about him last night. Sigh. I called him today when I went out with Ulises & Rocio, & my heart about broke when he said he was going to stay in. I was so disappointed. But I had fun.

♥ Me

February 25, 2004

So Rhys finally went out with the three of us. He said he didn't want to go see a movie, but just dinner. We went to City Walk for a little while, & Ulises wanted to see a movie, & I told Rhys he could say no. He said, "No, it's okay, I'm just along for the ride, don't even tell them anything." But I felt bad, so I said I didn't really want to see a movie. We were going to eat there, but Rocio wanted to go to Hometown Buffet. It was fun; Rhys looks really good in blue. He's sweet.

Yesterday, as like the past few days, people were kidding me. Jose & I were in the fitting room & Rhys came out of the dungeon & glanced over, & Jose goes, "Ooh, he's looking at you, you think he's jealous?" Then Rhys & I were in the break room & Kenny came in & goes, "Oh, you want me to leave you two alone?" I was like shut up, but Rhys just laughed. Then Kenny said, "Come on, guys, let's see some porno," and Rhys laughed & said, "Yeah, you got any Kenny?" I asked him to Annie's party, told him there'd be 3 kegs and I didn't even know if he partied, & he goes, "Well, I'll get to see you drunk, right?" HAHA! I really really really really really really times four million times hope that he'll go! Really times four zillion! Hope! Ahh! Please God!

♥ Me

February 27, 2004

  Well, what a surprise... Rhys isn't going to go. He is supposed to have breakfast with his sister at ten on Sunday, & he doesn't want to do six hours of driving. I have to be at work at 1:30 on Sunday, which would give us all of like ten hours in Santa Maria, after a lot of driving. I talked to Rhys on the phone for ten minutes with him going, I don't want to say no & let you down. I was like, don't worry about it, I don't want to make you do something you don't want to do, and plus you never said yes. And he said but it's always like this. I was like, it's okay, it's how you are. He laughed.

  Earlier, I was trying to convince him to bring clothes, & he was like, no I need to shower, and I said, I have a shower Rhys and he goes, I'm not ready to be naked in your house yet. HAHA! Then he was like, especially with a dog at my feet, & I was like yeah, he likes to be in the bathroom when people are showering, & Rhys was like yeah, no! But he said, are you committed to doing this and I was like yeah, but you're not, & he said, well I'm up for hanging out tomorrow, if you want to ditch the party & hang out here like go see a movie.

  Ahh! I was so disappointed. David, Liz, Little R, & Carolina all say I should go out with him, Ulises says go to the party. But practically, it's not a great idea. And anyway, Rhys wants to hang out! Sigh, decisions, decisions.

              ♥ Me

March 1, 2004

  Well, so Lani & Annie's best friend Nicole said the party was the worst in history... people snorting coke in the bathroom, peeing off balconies, & having sex in every closet. Lani almost called the cops. So I'm real glad I chose to go out with Rhys. It was so fun. I looked really cute. First we went to Old Navy to say goodbye to David, who gave me a hug & said "I'll miss you honey!" Awwwww! Then we went to the

Grove & got in line for the 10:40 show of the Passion. Sold out. 11:10 sold out right when we got up there. So we bought tickets for 9:55 Eurotrip. We had about an hour to kill, so we bought popcorn & just chilled around the lobby talking.

We finally went into Big Fish for about 20 minutes, then went into the Passion. We got great seats. The movie was phenomenal. I think Rhys even cried. We walked out in completely different moods. We went to the restroom, then I said, "What did you think?" and he said, "You'd be hard-pressed to find a more powerful movie than that." We barely said two words more than that on the way home.

When he dropped me off, I asked if he'd like to go out with me, Rocio, & Ulises again, & he said sure. Not maybe, sure! Ahh! I love to see him smile. He's too cute. I love spending time with him. Ahh!

♥ Me

March 27, 2004

I got to see American Idol be recorded! Clay Aiken performed, and come on, how cute is he?!! It was a lot of fun. I've been thinking a lot about Texas, and at the end of May, I think I want to move back. I talked on the phone to Texas tonight for half an hour—Megaan, Joey, & Rose. Megaan's party. Rose called me darlin' & said she missed my beautiful smile, Megaan told me she loved me & wished I was there... Rose said Joey talks about me all the time. God, I miss them. It was so nice to hear all that. Granted they were drunk, but still, I know they love & miss me. What do I do?

♥ Me

April 4, 2004

Mom & I got in yet another huge fight—rather she yelled; I didn't speak. She said I didn't contribute enough around the house—cleaning, $, whatever. I pissed her off cause I didn't have anything to say because I didn't want to make promises I won't keep.

I went to Old Navy Friday & gave my notice to Alex. Told a couple of people on Saturday—this is so hard! Rhys & I were going to go out Friday, but he got busy, so we planned on after work Saturday. I told Betty he didn't know I was leaving, & the girl turned around & told him!! I went over to talk to her in women's, & she goes, "He knows." I was like, "Knows what?" "That you're leaving. I wanted to see his reaction. He was really surprised. He said he'd have to talk to you about that." I almost started crying, & said so.

He was standing by a table folding, & he turned around & said, "So, Courtney, are you really leaving?" I couldn't look at him, but I was like, "looks like it." AHH!

I knew I wanted to talk to him, so I was real glad when he agreed to go to Santa Monica pier with me. We walked the promenade, then cruised the pier & then went down to the beach & sat and talked for a while. I was speed-talking the entire time because there was so much I wanted to say, to ask, but I couldn't get the courage. All evening he was joking about my leaving, saying things that made me think he didn't care. But then at one point, he asked if I planned on coming back to visit. Why couldn't I have been coy and said, "Why, will you miss me?" or something. My heart was aching.

On the drive home, he said "it really sucks that you're leaving." AHH! I told him there'd been some stuff I'd been wanting to tell him or ask him over the past few months, & he said like what, & I addressed the John, "Courtney loves Rhys" thing & told him it wasn't me. He said he hadn't thought it was, but he was just (like what) & I filled him in.

We made plans to watch Indiana Jones later this week, & he wants to smoke me out. I think I want to. Is it boy pressure? I'd rather go drinking with him. I want him to tell me he'll miss me, or that he doesn't want me to go, or that maybe someday something will happen. 'Cause if not, what's the point? I like him, but I'm 22, & I don't want to waste time liking someone who ONCE AGAIN only sees me as a friend. How can I get the nerve to ask him? Patty says I really need to act. HELP!

♥ Me

Oh yeah, I forgot to say Lisa & I went to the Tuesday American Idol, it was so fun. We got on tv. Jon Peter Lewis is soooo cute. I got Matthew Rogers' autograph—he's wicked cute.

Love,

me

April 7, 2004

So Mom & I made up, but I'm not going to live with her after two months. When I went into work today, I had to ask Rhys something over the walkie & he sounded grumpy. But then he came up to the front & said "Hey Courtney" & asked me if I was leaving. I said no, & he goes "No?" all excited-sounding, & he looked so happy. I told him I'd talk to him later, but I never did. GOD GIVE ME COURAGE!! Please, help me! We're planning a whole big thing Friday night & I really hope it works out! Please!

♥ Me

April 15, 2004

Jon Peter Lewis got kicked off tonight—I'm so sure it's not America's choice, this show makes me sick now. Why would America pick him as their wild card then withdraw their support? Pisses me off. I told Rhys I want to smoke with him. I just want the guts to talk to him—cause I've been yearning for Texas. My heart hurts. Lisa told me tonight she *doesn't want me to leave. What should I do? I'm so sad.*

♥ *Me*

April 19, 2004

Fuck my life. I should never have moved out here. I should have just moved to Austin. Who knew this would have given me six months of misery? Oh wait, I did!

I smoked out with Rhys a couple of nights ago, & it was mellow & chill. It was fun. We talked about the impending move, & I got up the nerve to ask him to drive out with me. He said, "I knew you were going to ask me, & I've been thinking about it. Now that you did, I'll give it some serious thought." At this point, I think my decision will be based on his answer. Jimmy told me tonight he wants to be left out of it. He's sick of hearing one thing, then 20 seconds later, another.

My heart's breaking. I can't decide what to do. Whatever my decision, there will be repercussions. Moving to Texas will entail paying rent again, tearing myself away from another group of friends, & most importantly, leaving Rhys before I tell him in my own goddamn words how I feel. Of course I'd miss my mom. But she makes me miserable 7/8s of the time. Of course staying here, I'll have to live with her or pay 700+$ for a 300 sq ft. room. And I'll be further depriving myself of my friends in Texas.

What I want more than anything is to buy Rhys & me plane or train tickets & go visit for a week, make my decision that way. If he decides to go with me, I will probably break down halfway there. If he doesn't, I don't know what I'm going to do. My heart is in pieces, & I can't stop crying. This is by far the hardest decision of my life, & I feel like neither is going to be right.

Devastation seems unavoidable in my life. Why did I have to move out here? Sure there's been some good—I'm halfway paid off to my rent office, I got to go to American Idol, I made friends... but then again, I made friends. Rocio, Ulises, Izzy, Lisa, Kenny, Betty, Becky, and, oh my gosh, Rhys.

He keeps telling me we won't stop being friends just because I move, that I can come visit, & I'm just like, do you realize how far 1500 miles is? Good intentions are nothing... look at Jessica, at Jennifer, or even Megaan & Joey. Friendships fall apart... but what I wouldn't do to mesh my two worlds—to move Joey, Megaan, Rose, & Jimmy here... God that'd be great. Perfect.

Lord help me please. I can't do this on my own.

♥ *Me*

My wavering between decisions seems incredibly uncharacteristic for me, and that's because I've learned to trust my gut. If something doesn't feel right, I don't do it, simple as that. I've also learned to voice my opinion. What I want matters.

I'm sitting here struggling to stay awake because of the amount of energy reliving this is taking. I keep having mini revelations that knock me down a notch, like how I've lived my entire life for other people. I'm forty-two years old, and the only thing I've done for myself is move to Connecticut, and even that has become wrapped up in my mother. But I'm on my own again, and I vow to make my dreams start coming true finally. It's always been on me, hasn't it?

April 28, 2004

Well, Rhys went with me to Texas. I gave final notice, talked to the manager in Austin—the hardest was when I hugged Ulises goodbye, for sure. He looked like he was going to cry, & that made me sad. The trip down was good—Rhys drove a huge majority of it. We got to La Quinta Waco, & my van died. Weird, lucky, thank God we got there in one piece.

Ryan Oral gave us half price on a room & OH MY GOD, told me Brooke's been missing for six weeks—that no one's heard from her & all this shit about getting engaged to a marine... she filed a cop report that Jeff hit her... GOD was it good to see Jeff.

>When we got in our room, we showered & Megaan, Alex, Joey, Rose, & Tiffany came over & we went to Roadhouse. I called Jeff afterwards & he came over. We got beer & hung out then Rhys, Tiff, Jeff, & I went to Arlington Farms hot tub until like 3:30. Rhys got pretty damn drunk; he ended up throwing up. Jeff was really fun to talk to, there was a very cute 19 year old named JD... lots of fun.
>
>Went to Austin next day, went to Chili's then took Rhys to the airport. Wasn't as hard as I thought it would be. But it was sad. Got a hug. Finally. Jim & I went to Sam's for a while, then to Ft. Worth, & we drove like eleven hours tonight, & now we're in Birmingham, AL, on our way to South Carolina tomorrow.
>
>♥ Me

Goodness gracious, I cannot believe how much driving I did that year, and I barely remember it. I'm floored that I essentially repeated history twenty years later. (That story in twenty years!) I'm thankful for this journal, but I would love some pictures to accompany every entry.

May 26, 2004

>Okay, so much can go down in 3 weeks! Carolina was fun—we met like 100+ relatives we never knew we had. Jimmy & crew found this phat house, but we can't move in until August 23. 3 months of nowheredom. I have a little problem with Sam in that I have a huge crush on him. He winks at me all the time & he's so goddamn cute! We've been playing beer pong at his house. Ben's a lot of fun too.
>
>My heart hurts though. I just want to be debt free & happy. I HATE having to live off Jimmy. Sam got an interview at Old Navy today. Please let him get the job! That'd be so much fun. We went to San Marcos tonight to buy hash. God I like him so much. FUCK!! When am I gonna be happy? Ever? I'm as close now as I've ever been: I ♥ my job, I ♥ my friends...

but the money thing's so rough. And then I go get sick & have to buy medicine. Oh God help me.

♥ Me

Yowch. That one hurts. Do y'all do that? Forgo things like medicine or shampoo, basic self-care items, so that you can pay for the roof over your family's head? The older I got, the worse it got, to where I would feel guilty if I had to use one of my own bandages or something. No longer, though. I will take care of myself and my dogs selflessly, so to speak.

June 3, 2004

There was a party Tuesday at Sam's & it kicked ass! Jim & Curtis kicked like 20 peoples' ass in beer pong, Alex & I talked a lot, Sam was all about his little redhead Brooke. I really like him though. I was trying to find out if she liked him. Courtney's a lot of fun. I drove Ryan Abrams and Josiah to Whataburger drunk. We went to Kerbey Lane after the party at like five & it was just a lot of fun. We were gonna go to the creek today but we didn't. Man, Sam sucks. This sucks. Can I lose weight? By end of July? Help!

♥ Me

You will never understand how embarrassed I am that I drove "drunk" more times than I can count. Please, for the love of God, understand that you are not better at driving when you're drunk. You might feel like it because you're relaxed and no one else on the road matters, but that's simply not the case. Other people matter. Please, please, call an Uber. Get a friend to be DD. *Don't drink and drive* or, for the love of *fuck*, text and drive. Your phone will do that for you, and if it doesn't, it can wait. Relax, sure. Breathe. Listen to music. Smile at the people who are annoying you. Don't be the reason someone loses their life.

June 7, 2004

Alex asked if I wanted to go to IHOP for lunch & then Jimmy asked where my money was. I just wanted to be like, "Don't ask me to go when you know I don't have money." I knew he was going to end up resenting me. And having Alex around is not helping. I feel like a horrible person around her. She's mean.

Like I said I was gonna get a flight voucher for Sam to go to Cali with us & they went into this whole "Sam's Jimmy's friend" thing & I didn't have the right to ask him to go. I was like, "He's my friend too," & Alex was like, "You've only known him a month." I was trying not to listen to her, but I guess she's right. No matter how long I know them, they will all always be Jimmy's friends. I'm going to forever feel out of place with them. And I signed a fucking year lease. What the hell. Fuck this. Seriously, what am I going to do? Anyway.

♥ Me

June 13, 2004

Well, this past week with Jimmy gone has been fun. I've hung out with Sam a lot. Party at his house Friday night, I got drunk. Real flirty. Ryan Abrams was like, "Am I dating you? You bark at me like a fucking girlfriend!" Ouch. Sorry I care!

Saturday was fun too. Brooke's pimp & hoes party. REAL drunk. Sam & I walked home at like 2 I guess. Then down to Blair's. Cherry bombs & more beer. Had Jimmy John's with Sam. Ahh I really like him. Too bad he barely sees me as a friend, much less anything more. I wish he'd hug me like he hugs Brooke or that girl Laura, who he kept calling Lively.

Lejla came & hung out. She's fun too. Got home at like 5 this morning, after Deeno came & crashed on Sam's couch. He's a little hottie now! Grandma called me at 11 this morning & asked if I'd heard from Mom. No one's heard from her or can get a hold of her. Beth's calling the police tomorrow. She quit her job. Fucking hate this shit. What the fuck is in her head? What if she kills herself? How will I *react? I'm scared. What if I end up like her? What if...*

♥ *Me*

Later in life, Sam told me that he felt closer to me when we first met than he did to Jimmy. He *was* my friend. I just tended to believe what people I cared about said to me, whether it was true or not.

July 31, 2004

I just reread most of these entries, & I'm all crying & shit. I haven't written in so long! Emily, this girl I work with, & I have been hanging out a lot, she's great. So is Lejla.

Tomorrow's the "day of dread." Last day in this apartment & I have no idea where to go. Don't wanna go to Sam's. Want to stay at Sarah's with Emily, but don't know how to ask. Oh, God, help me. How can I still pray when I don't know what I believe? God I'm such a hypocrite, & there's nothing I hate more.

Sam's kind of driving me crazy. Still cute, but he pisses me off about Old Navy. He's always saying what a bitch Angie is when she hired him with no reference, he's lazy & slow & ungrateful. Oh Lord what do I do? Wish we could move into the house tomorrow, only we CAN'T. Odd lease terms. I want to go to Cali soooo much for Luke & Jess's wedding, but what if I can't afford it? Ahhh! Oh God I want to go so much. I HAVE to go. Please. God, please. Anyway, headache.

♥ *Me*

These six-week gaps speak volumes. It's strange. That's about the amount of time my depression seems to hold me down, even as an adult. At forty-two, I've learned to talk, to reach out. I will never let it conquer me again. It makes me sad that I again thought I was being hypocritical, that I was questioning my faith, which is now so rock-solid, I can't believe I ever doubted.

This timeline does coincide with my mother doing her wildest wilding, however. I don't not see the resemblance, and like a phoenix from the ashes...

This next entry in September of 2004, I braved seeing her again, even after she broke down. I remember her guilting me into taking her to Jess and Luke's wedding—I had no idea why she wanted to go—but have zero recollection of her at the wedding, which is nice. It means I must have made my rounds despite her anchoring me. I'm sure I got in trouble for that. In *Garden State*, which we saw while I was out there, she blabbed my ear off about how the movie was about her. That was not an uncommon theme when she was sick. Movies and music, they were all about her and no one else.

September 9, 2004

> Okay, way too long—moved into our house, stayed with Amanda & her roommate Miriam for two weeks. Lots of fun. My house is amazing. Huge. Poker table's here.
>
> I went to Cali, my mom's crazy. Saw Garden State with mom. Went to the wedding, it was beautiful. Mom made me leave early because she was cold. I couldn't argue though. Jess looked gorgeous. It was really good to see Ben. And Zack. I got to take Joshie to go get chocolate, he was so excited. Everyone was so great. Luke told me he was really glad I came, that it was "an added bonus." Luke's mom was great, Andrew is still adorable, his wife Estrella is beautiful. Just a good night.
>
> I went out with Rhys Saturday night, we went back to the beach & walked around. Good to see him, fantastic to see Ulises.
>
> Okay so I was reading over things from old friends & came across a letter from Chad. I didn't write about the Homecoming dance, & I really wanted to read about it, so I'm gonna write about it now. We had so much fun—pictures at my house were kind of awkward; Chad kept his hand in a fist when he had his arm around me. Then we went to the Melting Pot for dinner with Suzanne & Philip. When the boys went to the bathroom, Suzie & I threw lettuce into the oil, splattering it onto our dresses. We were laughing hysterically through the whole dinner.
>
> The dance was in RHS Eagles' Nest. It was so great. We slow-danced twice, my head on his shoul-

der, his arms all the way around me. I liked him so much. I asked Suzie later if he had his eyes closed & she said he did. What a good night.

I love my house, my memories. I want to make more. I just walked into the living room in my cord skirt & a white button down & Sam asked why I was so dressed up, & if I had a date. Evan was like, oh my God, & Jimmy was like, "the guy better bring back up when he comes," cause Sam had said he was gonna fight him. I love my roommates.

♥ Me

October 4, 2004

Okay, well, I have a little crush on Evan. Hmm, who saw that one coming? I've been really moody lately. I don't like who I am. Why can't I be happy to be me? Why does what other people think, or more specifically, how they treat me, matter so much? Jesus! I talked to Jess for over an hour last night. Oh, God. I was writing my life story & writing about Rocking L Ranch & thinking about Brandon... oh, when will I be content? My birthday's in less than three weeks. I want to have a party, but I don't too, cause I want the weekend to be about me & I don't want people to come just for free beer. GOD!!

♥ Me

November 1, 2004

Well, my birthday weekend had very little to do with me. My dad & Beverly came down & I got a new bed & couches & stuff—very nice. We went to Alligator Grill on Fri then to Hut's on Sat noon. I tried to get the boys to go to dinner on Sat, but they were all dead. Katie from next door & I decided our party would be combination Halloween too. Didn't happen.

This weekend was funner though. I was super tired on Sat so I wasn't going to go out, but I did. Wore orange tights, denim skirt, black boots,

> & a black cut off sweatshirt. Fun. Went to Kevin & Luke's. Saw Crystal Fullerton & Abra Glisten, then Sam, Ryan, & I went to Mandy Booker's. AWESOME! Saw Adam Deviney & he KNEW my NAME! Saw & "met" James Fair SOOOOO Hot!! Saw the Feemsters, Katy Kirkley, who's dating Andrew... Nic Johnson... lots of fun!
>
> Our party Sunday, Amanda, Ryan, Miriam, Erin, came. I looked so good. Maaaan, the one person I wanted a compliment from gave it to me—I walked into the laundry room & Evan turned around & goes, "Whaaaat," & I repeated him, & he goes, "You look decadent!!!" I almost died. Thank God for that. Amanda must have told me 20 times I looked beautiful. Nice feeling.
>
> ♥ Me

I remember the costume I wore, and I remember seeing the pictures, but I have no idea what happened to them. I was in a beautiful jade green and purple Renaissance dress, my hair long and curly. Using the word *decadent* was a perfect choice, and looking back, it seems even more precious. On this Thanksgiving Day in 2023, I'm so thankful I journaled. I did experience love—many, many times—and it's nice to have this reminder.

November 12, 2004

> My roommates all just went to a party without inviting me. Earlier I went upstairs & there were 2 girls up there & no one said a word to me, not even "whaaat," or "Oh, my God." Why do I have to be the girl guys want to hang out with, but not date. Sometimes I even wonder if they want to hang out with me.
>
> Like Evan writing, "No death allowed" on a paper on his bed—at first I thought it was a joke, but then Sam said, "You sleep on Evan's bed every night," which made me realize Evan had said something.
>
> When I said I wanted to go somewhere cold for Christmas, Evan said, "You can come to Indiana with me." He was really drunk so I said it again a couple of days later, & he goes, "Come to Indiana

> with me." And I said, "All right, I will." And he was like, all right.
>
> Ahhh!!! I feel like even if I lose weight they won't love me. So what's the point of trying? And shouldn't whoever loves me love me for who I am, not what I look like? Jesus fucking Christ. I GIVE UP!

Excuse me, Coco. Was this a dream? Did I really have a somewhat serious-sounding invitation to go home for Christmas with Evan, and I went crazier? Please, please tell me we decided to not do it instead of me just assuming he was joking.

November 14, 2004

> Last night we went to a party at B-rat's & she & Sam got in a huge fight. Sam started crying in the middle of the party. God I wish he'd talk to me. He used to, when we first started hanging out. I wish he'd cuddle to me like he was with L Davis the other night. Maaan, every time I saw Evan hug another girl, I got so jealous. WHAT!
>
> I'm just so protective of my guys... why don't they like me? Would it be different if I asked them to talk to me? Told them how much I cared about them? God I want to go to Indiana with Evan soooo much. Please make it possible!
>
> ♥ Me

OMG, what made it impossible? Why didn't I go?

November 24, 2004

> Everyone's leaving for Thanksgiving, I'm not that upset to stay home although it would have been fun to see Josh or Jordan. I don't know what to write. I am so confused. I feel like awful for losing my faith—or throwing it away rather. But why can't I get what I ask for? In little ways, I do, but for the most part... AHH! My head hurts.
>
> ♥ Me

Oh, dear girl, that was why you lost your faith? Because you didn't get what you want? What a lot we had to learn. Sometimes, I thank God for unanswered prayers. But really, why didn't I go to Indiana with Evan?

November 26, 2004

> *I spent last night w/ Miriam & Amanda, Amanda's sis Katrina, Ryan's roomie Mike, Brad, & Marty, a guy from their work. Mike & Marty are cute. We played Balderdash, lots of fun. Worked all day today, my hips & knees hurt. Jimmy & Preston were in a car crash today. They're ok though.*
>
> *Man, I was watching Joan of Arcadia & just bawling—when "Give a little bit, give a little bit of your love to me" came on (Goo Goo Dolls) I just lost it. I miss believing in God. I hate being in Joan's place—confused & befuddled but I love feeling like someone's watching out for me.*
>
> *Can I get that back? Does God forgive me for that shit? Can I last in a house full of drinkers & smokers & keep my chin up about my faith, even when I am questioning it? God help me, I miss feeling loved—is that possible?*
>
> ♥ *Me*
>
> PS: I MISS EVAN!

All right, so we are getting somewhere. For someone who claimed to not believe any longer, why say, "God help me"? I wonder when it was that I started to understand God was *in* me, really understand that. I say it every time I get on the road: I have faith in my God, myself, and my car. I don't pretend to be God. But I understand my magic comes from within, and I believe that's powered by the Holy Spirit.

December 15, 2004

> *Well, Jimmy's 21st was fun. Party here Friday night, I got supremely wasted. Downtown Saturday, talked to Dustin a lot, lots of fun—he's cute when he's drunk. I thought Jim was gonna die of alcohol poisoning. Soooo…he's in Vegas right now. I'm going to*

Dallas for Christmas. Phillip & Claudia bought me a new computer! Ahh! Oh my God I had the best conversation online with Justin Woody. I let him read some of my stories & he said he'd never been more turned on in his life. I CAN'T WAIT TO SEE HIM! Or Josh Q... God I hope I can see him. Sigh. Justin was really drunk when we talked but STILL.

♥ Me

December 27, 2004

Justin, Justin, Justin! That's all I can think about! We had a couple more conversations, the most interesting being when he told me that for a year or two he'd been thinking I would kiss him & that he kind of wanted me to. He came over while I was in Dallas to watch Napoleon Dynamite. Ahh! Why didn't I do anything? Oh, because Jimmy and Audrey were there. But I did get 2 great hugs from him. I was very tense through the movie, just wanting to scratch his back or KISS HIM! GOD I wish he'd come down for NYE — that would be fun!

Dallas was good. It was nice to see Phillip and meet Claudia. Austin's still weird—he lives with his gf! UNFUCKINGFAIR! Audrey's very full of herself. Saw Josh Horton & Emily & David Magnum—lots of great people. God, Jordan wouldn't even look at me. Why do they have to be brothers?? Jesus! I like Justin soooo much. Can I handle this, or am I going to have to completely cut myself off from both Woody boys? I COULD NOT HANDLE THAT. Lord help me.

♥ Me

February 28, 2005

I haven't written in so long but I don't even know where to start. I went to Dallas again after weeks of begging Justin to come see me, & I was so excited. But conversations with him had been strained-feeling lately, so I didn't really think any-

thing would happen. But he assured me he wanted to see me & he promised he would.

But guess what—3 nights in D & I didn't see him. Never even talked to him. I tried not to think about it too much, overanalyze shit, but it hurt. It really hurt. Later, a fucking week later, he said he'd passed out at like ten on Friday. I was like, I called you at 5:30 and then again at 8:30. Awful. But I went out with Jim & got to see Shelby. ♥ *Ahh. So cute.*

So my "little crush" on Evan is slowly getting harder to bear. So much so that I've come really close to telling Jimmy several times & have even toyed with the idea of telling Evan. GOD! I got pretty drunk this past weekend. FUCKED UP. I had a dream that I told Kelly Willis I wanted to kiss a girl. It was a huge deal with her. I don't want to write it all down, but it was weird. I just want physical content so much. So so much.

Michael IMed me 2 times, saying he never saw me anymore. I wish he said he'd missed me. I've missed him. I wish someone from work would call me. They all hang out and never call me. I hurt inside all the time. Even when I'm happy. I'm so sick of it.

My mother tried to kill herself. Swallowed 100 excedrin in a hotel room then called the cops herself. I don't know how I am going to end up... sometimes I wish I could just do it, but I don't have the nerve. Anyway.

♥ *Me*

Well, that was the first time I knew that I ever said those words, even to myself, after I was a teenager and had learned what harm suicide did to those left behind. Reading that just prompted me to make a TikTok that described my mirror energy—November 24, 2023, if you want to help make the video go viral. But if you don't have TikTok, here's this: I am 100 percent authentically a reflection of the energy you bring.

It's no wonder I asked myself for years if I was bipolar; the mood swings were wacky. The voices my mother experiences, I attribute them to coincidences and, more than that, signs from God. I get a thrill out of them, whereas they terrify her. Does it mean with certainty that I'm not bipolar? No, I suppose it doesn't. The difference between me and my mother is, I don't bite the hands that try to help me, or at least I don't intentionally bite. And she…she tears people to shreds like the lion coming from the meek little kitty in the mirror, a picture she has always loved.

I remember telling my brother haughtily once that I was gonna kill myself. I was about fifteen, and I can recall the look of horror he gave me even then. Then James South found his brother Neal in his car, asphyxiated from CO_2, and I cried like I had never cried before. I felt like someone had carved out my heart when I saw his body, thinking of what his little brothers and his mother must have felt like. When I wrote that I didn't have the nerve, I meant it. I could never, never do something permanent if I knew it was going to hurt even one person I loved, not to mention I'm far too optimistic. Always look at the bright side of your life. I am the rainbow phoenix. If you need help seeing the silver lining, please come find me. I'll find it for you.

Also, in ten years of journaling, that's the first mistake I made (physical content) that I didn't correct myself on, even in ink. I must have been hurting so much.

March 9, 2005

> *I talked to Justin & told him I was sorry for the way I'd spoken to him. I miss him so much. A bunch of ON people went downtown on Sat. Andrew is the cutest thing ever. All the non minors left Exodus without telling me, but I had a lot of fun with the minors, especially when Angela & Jerry showed up. Jenny & I got danced with a lot. I got felt up—yuck. Lot of fun that night. Too bad Andrew's four years younger—2 cute. His friend Mallory's really nice too. Man, Mark asked me to sell my baseball ticket to his cousin. That really hurt my feelings, & I can't really seem to get over it.? Amanda called today though. So glad. I have the hugest crush on Evan. When he's in the room, I can barely look anywhere else. Ahh!*

> ♥ *Me*

April 1, 2005

> *Bout to go to karaoke with Amanda, more on that later, right now I just want to talk about Evan.*

GOD! I'm debating about even resigning the lease because it's getting so hard to be around him. He doesn't seem like the girlfriend kind of guy, but he kind of seems like he likes me sometimes. Like the looks he gives me...playful & cute. Man, I really like him. Victoria from work says I should tell him, but I'm afraid it would make the next six months (or year & a half) very awkward. Who the hell knows? Only one way to find out, & I don't think I have the nerve. Why not? Maybe I'm afraid of Sam & Jimmy's reactions. I thought about writing him a note but I'm afraid he'd show Sam or Jim. Ick, this sucks so hard. What do I do?

♥ Me

April 12, 2005

Maaan I want to tell him! What do I do? I really freaking like him. OK, so how much fun is karaoke with Amanda. We had a blast, twice in one week. No patience to write about it, I just want to think about Evan.

♥ Me

I'm reading about karaoke with Amanda, and my brain is trying to split, because the time just doesn't match. And then I realize, I had two eras of karaoke with Amanda. Three, really, but we called the third one Mandy, so… Man, my life is weird. No wonder I can never remember anything.

April 23, 2005

Last weekend I went to Dallas with Amanda to see her sister Katrina. All 3 of us stayed at Claudia & Phillip's. I spoke to Justin several times, but he never managed to get it together. I felt so stupid. I called him one last time at midnight on Saturday & he said he was going to Cable and Jansen's but he wasn't staying long. I stupidly told him that whether I went to bed or not depended on what he was doing. I waited up for him till 3:30. Ouch. I even slept with my makeup on in case he called

& woke me up. What a child. I gotta get over this Woody boy obsession. Too bad I love them so much.

♥ *Me*

May 20, 2005

Evan's killing me. I'm freakin' crazy about him. He's had a rough few days—drinking himself into oblivion, to the point where he's blacking out. I thought he was drinking to drown out hurt inside of him, & it kills me that he doesn't talk. It kills me that I've lived with him for a year & I know so very little about him. I have this whole letter to him planned out—now whether or not I can get up the nerve to give it to him is a completely different story.

♥ *Me*

Okay, y'all wanna talk about clairaudient? I picked *The DUFF* to watch on the heels of a couple of nineties movies and thinking about the moment I did tell Evan I was into him. Right as I'm wrapping up this last entry, a scene between Toby and Bianca goes down, in which Bianca says she's into him, and Toby says she has big balls. Y'all, it's almost verbatim what Evan said to me ten years earlier. If I had been my mother, I would have freaked out and said, "Oh my gosh, this movie is about me!" But because I'm (mostly) sane, it makes me laugh, gives me butterflies, and makes me wish someone were here to experience the magic with me.

June 13, 2005

Wow, okay. I gave Evan a letter, & after I felt like I shouldn't have, but we talked about it a little & he said it was "the good friend thing to do." I asked him if I was off base with it and he said no. It makes me sad to think he's so sad. So I went to Dallas again, got shafted by Justin in sooo many ways one more time. I'm giving up with that endeavor. Fuck him.

Okay, so now on to this last weekend. Friday was Ian's 21st, so we went downtown Thurs, Fri, & Sat. Thurs I wore my purple tunic & Dan H told me he loved my shirt & that I looked hot—what a great compliment. I didn't drink much, but it was fun. We met this girl who worked at Fuel & asked her to teach us to dance. She was pretty cool. Okay, so I had to be at work at nine on Friday & I definitely went to sleep at like 5:30, but I was fine all day—it went really fast.

Came home, showered, & got ready for another night out—white lace shirt & denim skirt, hair down—felt really cute. We spent the majority of the night at Fuel & most of the crowd were people we knew—Curtis, Siah, Amanda, Sarah...Dean... so yeah, I was being pretty flirty with him—asked him to buy me a drink. I bought my first shot & took it with Brooke, every other drink I had that night someone else bought me—Dean, Curtis, Blake, Jimmy, or Sam. FUN! I danced with Dean for a heartbeat, & Lauren & I danced with Blake a bit. Hannah, the waitress from the night before, tried to teach us to dance, but yeah right, two white girls? But it was fun.

Ok, so most of the drinks I had were like in the last 20 minutes, so I was good to drive home. Ian had to get out to throw up when we were like, a block from home. He was really really drunk. I had one beer when we got home & started feeling fairly good. So outside on the swing, I was scratching Dean's back and playing with his hair—he was really relaxed, & eventually he put his head in my lap & I just played with his hair.

My left arm was resting along the back of the swing, & he put his left hand on my arm & his right hand above his head on my other arm. His left thumb was kind of rubbing slowly on my arm. I kept swallowing really loudly. I was pretty nervous. But Curtis came back out & asked Dean if he wanted to go to IHOP... boo, for unwanted interruptions. So Dean sat up, but Curtis went back inside & he laid back down & this time put both his arms around my legs. I really wish something had happened. I really thought it was going to.

He came over again the next night, & I got nada, not a hug, not even a high five. Wonder if he got freaked out or grossed out. When can I ever win? Jeez!

Oh yeah so Thurs, Sam talked to me for like 10 minutes about how if anyone ever tried to hurt me, the guy would end up with a bullet in his brain. He said he & Jimmy would kill him, & then he looked at Evan & whispered, "He would never say it, but he feels the same way." Oh, I wanted that to be true. I told Sam that's why I hadn't told him anything about Justin, cause I was afraid if he ever came to Austin, he wouldn't be allowed in the house. Sam goes, yeah, if I ever found a reason to kill Justin Woody, I would do it." Aww.

A few minutes later, Evan, who had been washing dishes, turns around & says, "I haven't really been listening, but I caught the gist of the conversation, & I agree with Sam completely." I walked out of the kitchen pretty quickly cause I didn't know how to respond. God I like him so much. When I was with Dean, I really wanted Evan to come smoke, see what his reaction was. I wonder what they'd do to Dean if we ever did mess around.

Okaaaay so Sat night I was dead tired cause I'd gone into work at noon still drunk, but the day wasn't bad. But I wasn't planning on going downtown again. But I did. My roommates were talking about girls being crazy & stuff & they were getting hard to be around, especially Evan, so I went looking for Evan Dyno, who was supposed to be in the Drink, but there were way too many people, so I went to the Library to meet up with Amanda & Sarah.

We met some Marines, Milo, & James Eric Hendricks—yes, Jimmy Hendricks. He was sort of cute—bought me a drink & they both came to the house after. Good night, but nothing beat Friday.

So I want physical contact so badly. I want to bite the bullet & tell Evan I like him so I can start getting over him, cause it's so hard hearing him say girls are hot or he'd have sex with them... & I have *another year and two months living with him— he's bound to hook up with someone eventually & I'd really just prefer to be over him. Hopefully it will start to feel like it does when Sam says a girl's hot or even hooks up with them. It stings a bit, but in the end, I know he loves me... I just wish I knew Evan did. Sigh. What can you do?*

♥ Me

June 18, 2005

So a few nights ago Dean came back over & I sat outside with him for over half an ~~over~~ hour, just talking. He kept saying how good of guys my roommates were... it was as if he's scared of what they say. But at one point he put his arm around me & I laid my head on his shoulder. He kissed the side of my head & I turned slightly & whispered "do you want to kiss me?"

His left hand was already on my face, & as I turned my head, Evan walked outside. But someone inside got his attention again, so he closed the door, & I turned around again & he put his other hand on my face too. We were literally millimeters apart, I could feel his breath, & then freaking Evan comes back out. AHHH! Sooo frustrating. And then he bolted again. AGAIN! Like he can't handle being around my roommates & me at the same time. I wanted to tell him I'm a big girl & my roommates can't dictate my decisions. Grrrr.

Yesterday night we went downtown & Jimmy had trouble parking so we got out. Evan & I first, & we didn't know Lauren & Brandon got out too, so we walked quickly to Fuel. Ben gave us two shots, I hugged Hannah hello—then we went to Maggie Mae's & eventually back to Fuel. Evan was being really horny.

When we got home, I started crying out on the swing. Lauren came out to talk, & I talked a lot about Dean & Evan. I told her about work people... she said they must be crazy if they don't want to hang out with me. She was being really sweet but really loud & she kept saying I should tell Evan I like him, then she told ~~him~~ me not to like him anymore, that he was being stupid. It breaks my heart when he talks about other girls... as much as I like Evan though, I know nothing will ever happen, so I wanted to kiss Dean...a lot. And now I'm confused & hurt, & I don't like this at all.

♥ Me

June 22, 2005

Fucking Dean man. I just randomly walked outside & he & Justin were in the living room. Justin gave me five & Dean barely looked at me, but then he gave me 5 when he left... sort of missed, so he tried again. I gotta talk to him or this is going to be the most frustrating thing ever. Fuck boys! Man Evan was in a car accident on the way home from SA today. I don't want to ever lose him.

♥ Me

September 18, 2005

Man I haven't written in so long. I did talk to Dean, & he said he was dating someone, then he left for the whole summer. Now he's back & things aren't awkward but I still really want to kiss him. I'm not talking to Justin Woody anymore. Lyndsay Love came to visit this weekend—FUN. Justin is such an asshole—stood me up one too many times. Philip de la Rafael od'ed—sad!

My relationship w/ my roommates is falling apart. I HATE caring so much about them & getting nothing in return. Bitch Lauren has taken over & she's welcome to them. I really hate her. Exactly the epitome of why I don't hang out with girls. Whore.

Talked to my mom & she's positive I am bipolar. Surprise surprise. I don't want to get older, I want to stop it now. But I can't. I don't want to take medicine. I want to be happy & normal & have people love me. Because I am a great person & I love so deeply. I hate myself.

♥ Me

And therein lies the rub. Dear Coco, love yourself, or no one will ever be able to love you.

October 1, 2005

> I am always so sad. I've had some really good conversations with my mom over the past couple of weeks. She's helped me understand & come to terms with some of the shit that's going on inside me. She said emotions are doubled for us. It's the reason I get so unbelievably angry for little or no reason at all. I hate feeling like this. I want someone to understand & I am so glad I have my mom & so sad that she didn't have anybody.
>
> I want to be on medicine. I can't control it anymore & I can't keep taking it out on people when they don't understand. But I also can't live here anymore. I just can't continue to deal with Lindsay or Lauren. Lauren who has successfully wedged herself between me & my roommates. And pretty well between me & Jimmy too. He fell out of a tree yesterday. Ten feet on his head. Nothing broken. Pretty lucky to be alive. If he'd died, I would have killed myself.
>
> I am so sick of crying. I am so sick of going into the boys' house hoping for someone to be happy to see me or to ask how my day was & instead getting nothing. I am sick of having to search them out. Not one of them ever comes to see me. I wonder how long it would take before they noticed I was gone? If rent wasn't due today, I think it would be a very long time. And that breaks my heart.

♥ Me

November 25, 2005

I love having crushes. There's a guy @ work—our LP auditor—& I have suuuch a crush on him. He's on MySpace & he told Jenny I smiled too much & that it creeped him out & "he is a creepy person." So I told him I wouldn't smile @ him anymore, & he said I couldn't do it. So tonight was the first time I'd seen him. I was dressed in the elf outfit & had my back to him so I wouldn't smile. He goes, "So you're the coolest elf I've ever seen." "Coolest what?" "Elf." "Oh, I thought you said 'stuff.' Thanks, but I'm still not going to smile at you." Later he said I wasn't going to be able to get thru the entire night w/o smiling, & god if he wasn't right. He's too cute not to smile at.

I was running kids clothes w/ Cassie & I saw John coming out of the corner of my eye, so I turned around so I wouldn't smile. He was like, "You're smiling!" And I was like, "I am not!" I got my face straight & turned back to him. He was grinning & when I smiled, he just cracked up, & said, "See I knew you couldn't do it!" Ahhh! Then me, him, Robert, & Jim, our new manager were talking & Angela came up & tried to lay down across a folding cart & it fell over. So my trying not to smile @ John didn't matter anymore & I could just burst out laughing. Sooo then I was talking to Beth & the damn boy was a shop over & kept commenting on everything we said. Eavesdrop much? Then I was singing Walk the Line music, 'Ring of Fire,' & he was by himself in men's & I could see him smiling.

There was one point during the night when I was putting up clothes & he walked up w/in like 4 feet of me & I was like, "That's not fair, you're cheating, you can't do that!" And he goes, "Well it's not fair to say you're not going to smile! You can't do it, it's in your blood!"

Man I really think he likes me. It's been a while since I've had a crush like this. I love it, but I hate it too. Patience is just not something I am good at. I want him, even though he's like four inches shorter than me. Well, maybe not that much. ♥

♥ Me

There's another huge gap of time during which my depression must have swallowed me. To say it had been a long time since I had had a crush like that was alarming. Did time feel different to me back then, or was my love for Evan mostly tinged by darkness? I do know flirting with John was mostly all fun, maybe because his vibe was very, very clearly no.

But I always had to be loving someone. I felt lost without somebody to love. So I can kind of understand how two months felt like forever, especially around my birthday, my twenty-fourth (I wonder what I did that year) and the holidays.

November 29, 2005

> Ohh John's way too cute for words. I do think he might like me. I was eating LJS & he said it looked good, so I told him to have a piece, & I swear, he moved the first piece of chicken to get to the one I'd taken a bite of, & when I said it was bitten, he goes, "I'm all good." We swapped spit! Uh…well, he got mine in any case. And I swear it was on purpose.
>
> Sigh. So why does he leave comments on Jenny's MySpace & not on mine? Whatever, he's still mega-cute.
>
> ♥ Me

December 8, 2005

> Ok so he has left me some comments now, this one being the cutest: "Listen, I have to say something, & please know that when I say this I say it with all the love in my heart & I would never say it to anyone I didn't feel very close to, but you are f'ing crazy! And that is quite possibly why you are so cool. Please keep in mind that you are not cooler than me. And by cooler I mean crazier." How cute is that?!! He also commented on the picture of me with braids on Halloween, & that one says: "Alright, cough 'em

up! I know they're in your mouth, Courtney! It's not funny anymore! I left a bag of marbles right here on the table. And what, you expect me to believe you have laryngitis? Don't blink those glittery eyes at me!" Soo cute. Love him

♥ Me

January 21, 2006

Gah so many cute boys—all younger than me, except John, who doesn't, in fact, like me. Two Jesses from Pizza Hut, and JIM! Sooo cute. No one at ON likes him but me & Jenny. But I ♥ him! And Jesse Garcia, Spike, is sooo cute, but he's only 20—GASP! I think he's into me—he's so cute! Sigh. Amanda & I are gonna live together. Townhouse, very cute, very cheap. Think it should be good. My brother doesn't even care. Whatever.

♥ Me

June 1, 2006

For my 25th birthday I wanna sing my mom my life:

1. Natalie Merchant—Wonder
2. Leavin on a Jet Plane—PPM
3. Teach Your Children Well
4.
5.
6.
7. Somewhere Over the Rainbow
8. Let the River Run
9.
10. Home—Michael Buble (camp)
11. Calling All Angels
12. The Pretender—Jackson Browne
13. Puddle of Grace—Amy Jo J
14. Heaven—Better than Ezra
15. Breathe—Anna Nalick
16. Live & Learn—Cardigans

17. At Seventeen—Tara MacLean
18. Somebody to Love—Queen
19. Half Life—Duncan Shiek
20. I Dreamed a Dream—Les Mis
21. Let Me Fall—BJL
22. ~~Jesus Take the Wheel~~ Goodbye's
23. Time—Chantal K
24. Bring on the Men
25. Unwritten—Natasha B.

Maybes: Play Me—ND; The Luckiest—BFF; Beth Nielsen; Walking on Sunshine; Top of the World; Goodnight My Someone; Independence Day; Alone; Fallen; Stay or How; Evanescence; Honest?'s; Learn to be Lonely; Broken Road; In the Deep; The Rose

July 26, 2006

Goddammit John. Why does he have to be so cute when he doesn't like me? I think he enjoys being on the other end of the field for once.

"So I'm sorry I'm getting this to you late. I wanted to thank you for the card. I thought it was super sweet of you to think of me before you left. Imagine my surprise when I opened the envelope marked JOHN (all decorative and shit)...& opened the card & it said "Jim." Also, apparently you had more to say to Jim than to me. So thank you Courtney for getting my hopes up... Ass. I'm kidding. But pain does make me laugh."

Me, "Are you kidding? I was so careful about not switching the envelopes. Please tell me you're kidding. Okay so if I had more to say to Jim, I had better to say to you. Specific. Kinda like an inside joke. Since I no longer work w/ u, can we be real friends? I'm glad pain makes you happy. But tell me you're joking. Cause that's pretty embarrassing. I was really tired, really stressed, really excited, & really sad. Nice combo to write a card with..."

AHHH, ♥ him

November 19, 2006

  We went to karaoke Friday & there were a lot of Amanda's work friends there. There was this guy Dean who was really touchy-feely with me, like when I was ~~leavi~~ looking at the song book, he had his hand on my back, arm around my shoulder, kind of rubbing my ~~book~~ back. He was sweet & really flirty. At one point he had his arm around this girl Julie & he took my hand, twined my fingers in his. I held his hand for one second & then whispered to him, "You can't have us both." And he chose Julie.

  Dean was at the bar w/ Amanda & I went to go get a drink & some fight was brewing which seemed to be over Amanda. Roger was trying to break it up & Dean & I were sort of standing in the middle. Dean had his arm around me & I was kind of resting against him. Once Amanda left the bar, Dean & I were still standing there & she came back up to the bar & whispered to me, "Dean's hooked up with Julie." I know, I said.

  Why can't she have just let us be? Why, after 5 years of hearing me say I wanted a boyfriend &/or asking her to hook me up, wouldn't she just let us be? It might have been fun. Matt's friend Sean came out too, & he's really sweet too. I was rereading my entries about John Welch from last year & started crying. I just want a guy in my life. I'm going to Dallas for Thanksgiving & I really want to see Justin Woody. Will that help?

               ♥ Me

October 28, 2007

  God, those entries are so melodramatic; and here comes another. MySpace blogging has stopped me from writing here ~~because~~ but not about this—no one will ever know about this. A few years ago, I was crazy about Nathan Cowsill. I thought for a while that maybe I was trying to make myself like him because I never had dreams about him, and I banked a lot on dreams. Still do. But I wanted a boyfriend so bad back then, I kind of wondered whether I really liked him. But then I had a really good dream about him. Then he moved away, then I did.

It'd been five years; not to say I didn't think about him, I did. But I figured I was just building him up, that once I saw him, I wouldn't feel the same way. Sigh. Not the case. He looks so much cuter since he put on a little weight, he looks older. So cute. And so sweet: he makes the best eye contact when he talks. Even thinking about him right now is making me crazy. ♥

So when he came in this past weekend, he & two friends slept on my living room floor. So close. And on Sunday, watching him with Neomi was killing me. Seriously, there has never been anything cuter. We were trying to put her down for a nap, & we were laying in Natalie's bed (it said volumes that he didn't mind me coming to lay down with them), and Neomi was between us. She kept grabbing my hand & Nathan's & pulling them over her, like she wanted to be cuddled from both sides. I really thought she was trying to make us hold hands. Ha, little matchmaker. Poor kid probably just wants someone to love each other. But really, his head would come in closer & I'd swallow so hard; I was nervous having him that near me, even platonically. But I behaved really well. I wasn't loud or hyper.

And you know what really cinched it for me? Last night I had a dream he was laying (hovering) over me in my bed. Instead of waking up and screaming like I normally do when I think there's someone in my room, I simply said, "What are you doing in here, sweetheart?" Huh, right? Crazy until it comes to Nathan.

Really, here I am again, in that most familiar of places, but this time…this time I want him for so many reasons. I hope & pray to God that he can sell his business and move to A-TX. He needs to be near Neomi & Natalie. And I want to see him more. By

> *February, if I really work, I could lose another 30 pounds. Let us see...*
> *God help me.*
>
> *Courtney* ♥

Okay, now let me tell you a bit about reconnecting with Natalie too. Neomi was almost a year old when I met her for the first time at the mall with her mama, where she worked. Natalie went to hand me the baby, and Neomi reached for me like she had known me her whole life. I walked her up and down the mall corridor while her parents talked, and then I had to give her back to her dad. I remember Neomi shrieking and holding out her arms for me, a virtual stranger. I am blessed to be a baby and a dog whisperer. Who needs me to hold their baby so they can take a nap?

November 16, 2007

> *I have a cough so bad, my jaw hurts. Natalie wants to move into a house in February & start a daycare. I think it would be fun, but I'm nervous. I don't want more money issues. I want to get a sweet house with Nathan and Neil & have them help with the daycare so I can keep working at ELK.*
>
> ♥ *Me*

I'm sadder still that I don't have access to MySpace at the first mention of ELK Electric, where I worked in Austin for three years, or close to it. My manager from Old Navy, Angie, had recommended me; her mother was the office manager for ELK. It turned out to be wonderful; my first "desk job," I finally had a regular paycheck and benefits and bosses that took me out to lunch. Not to mention the insanely fun crawfish boil that Mike, the owner, did every year. It was huge; his house was settled on acres of land in Austin, and people from all walks of life came.

Now at this time late in 2007, I had already been there at ELK over a year, so let me rewind to my mother's fiftieth birthday, which I did not write about but I remember clearly. It was February of the same year, and we had all gone to California for her big five-oh. I remember being in the back bedroom of my grandmother's house in Camarillo, alone with my mom, and she somehow managed to tell me that I was the biggest she had ever seen me, and she was scared for my health. I do not think she was healthy at the time; as a matter of fact, I don't think I wanted to be out there at all, but I was.

They might not have been the kindest words, and there were certainly better ways to deliver them. But after that, I went to Jenny Craig for the first time and lost seventy pounds. I don't remember how long it took, but I do remember certain pictures where I look huge, even to my somewhat rose-colored lenses. I also remember some pics where I look super thin, and those must have been the goal ones. But I never got under two hundred pounds.

In the summer of the first year at ELK, I even made out with a guy in the field of the crawfish boil. We were standing next to my van, and he kept wanting to get in the back. I was like, "I'm not losing my virginity in the field of my boss's house with some random drunk guy." But looking back, it feels nice to know someone wanted me, even at my heaviest. So I proved my mother wrong several times over on the "If you'd only lose a little bit of weight…" front.

Her final barb this time, though, was that no one would want to marry me because I was too much of a bitch, not because I was fat. So at least she changed her tune.

February 10, 2008

> Well, the daycare thing didn't pan out, surprise, surprise. Natalie's living with Neil and GASP neither one likes it. I move next weekend. Yea, back into my beautiful one bedroom. $ may be tight for a while, but I'll get the swing of it.
>
> So I went to Cali last weekend for Grandma's 80th. I was a little nervous to see the Gees, cause I thought it would be hard to talk to Jocelyn & PJ, but they were all so great. They weren't gonna spend the night, but I talked them into it. We played GH3 until one, then we went to bed even though Joce wanted to stay up all night & "bond." we had to meet the rest of the family at 7 for breakfast.
>
> I lay there & lay there & heard someone go outside. When he came back in, I went out to see why he'd gone out. Kevin was having trouble sleeping. When I said I had the same problems, he said, "Racing thoughts?" It wasn't until I was back home that I remembered his family had thought he was bipolar. My heart went out to him then, cause for some reason, he's always been my sweetie—so special. Joce & I have an amazing bond too, but Kev…I

> *don't know. We stayed up till 4 just talking. I went back to bed & lay there till my crazy mom opened the bathroom door and yelled "Merry Christmas." WTF?*
>
> *Breakfast was fun, we went to Ry's restaurant. I love that kid too. When we were all leaving Jocelyn said she wanted to come home with me, and she was just hugging the shit out of me. Then Kevin & I hugged. Twice. Like, he really loves me too, and I could feel that. We have some sort of connection, & I miss them all so much. So much. I want to move to California.*

Now I wonder if I was off a year; maybe it was my grandma's eightieth that my mother called me a whale. I imagine I would have written that; it stuck like a dagger to the heart. But who knows? Maybe I had a whole weight loss blog on Myspace.

June 29, 2008

> *Tracy F, a woman who used to live down the street and I used to babysit, wrote the following:*
>
>> *Hey! Crazy how Facebook connects everyone! I'm out in LA and I looove it. Somethin about the sun always shinin just makes me happy... what are you up to these days? Great to hear from you!*

October 4, 2008

> *is excited she just filled up for $3.11...and sad that seems to be the highlight of her Saturday.*

October 29, 2008

> *is wishing there was some way to take back giving a full two weeks notice.*

November 20, 2008

> *Tiffany K wrote on my wall.*
>
>> *Hey, you should totally come visit me! Shannon told me she ran into you. She said you looked really*

good and that your hair was black So anyways I miss you and I think you should come see me.

December 7, 2008

is excited about the new store!

MACKIE S: *What store, Courtney?*

December 15, 2008

is enjoying sitting around the house.

December 21, 2008

Loves Christmas cause it means seeing old friends!

December 24, 2008

Is sad her step-sister didn't make it to Texas for Christmas.
Is feeling sick. Really sick.

AMY L: *OH NO, not on Christmas! Hope you're feeling better real soon. And by the way, have a very merry Christmas.*
ME: *Thank you... I'm not physically sick, but I got robbed at a gas station last night, so I was kind of nauseated. I'm better today. You have a merry Christmas too!!*
AMY: *How horrible! I hope you weren't hurt.*

December 25, 2008

got a new iPhone... so send me your phone numbers!
Merry Xmas Courtney! I just read your comment about getting robbed... I'm sorry, that sucks! But hey at least you got a sweet new phone for Xmas. You will love it!

June 6, 2009

Okay so much has happened since I wrote last, it's unreal. To make a lot of stuff condensed: I moved to Dallas to be a manager of Palio's Pizza where Jimmy is the GM & Preston is the owner. It's been almost 7 months, and while it's really fun, it's also super stressful. One of the girls I work with, Kaitlyn, is just about the equivalent of my soulmate. She's so amazing. So much has gone down... she and Jimmy are kind of dating or whatever. We've had months of conversations and stuff... she's reading over my oldest journal. It's funny to hear it through her because it makes me seem ridiculous and dramatic. I feel like I've grown in leaps and bounds even since some of the entries in this book. Who cares if a guy looked at me?? Why did I read so much into it?

June 23, 2009

Kaitlyn & I are moving into our new apartment tomorrow! Gosh I hope this one works out like none of the others have. Okay so Adolfo found me on MySpace. Jeez isn't that an interesting situation. We've texted a lot. About random shit too. He knows some of my fantasies. He loves Smallville & has a dachshund & it's just so wild to be talking to him again. I want to see him so badly so I can see if I still feel the same way because it's Adolfo or because we are meant to be together. I don't wanna analyze all the little things he's said to me because I want to have grown out of that. So I won't. I just hope he won't rule anything out because of what a good friend I am... I get my new bed Thursday! So excited.

♥ Me

July 19, 2009

Adolfo came to visit this week. When I told Kaitlyn he was coming, her response was, "Hmm, are you daydreaming?" I replied, "Yes, because that's the only way this would be happening." How come she just can't be supportive like I was with Jimmy? She says so many negative things about him. It really hurts sometimes.

> *Anyway, so it was really great to see him. He feels so good to hug. Funnily enough, although I tried finding tons of little ways to touch him, I didn't want him touching me. I can't imagine wanting to touch me if I was a guy.*
>
> *I made a vow to myself and all my Spark friends that I was going to get back on track today, and I was really good. No more excuses; I want to be below 200 for Audrey's wedding when the Gees come, and Adolfo and I discussed going on a cruise for my birthday, and by then I want to be below 190. Can you imagine? I haven't been under 200 in over ten years, and now it seems totally attainable.*
>
> *30 pounds in just over three months. I CAN DO IT! I just gotta keep Adolfo in mind, or if not him, then someone, cause how am I gonna ever let someone touch me if I feel as gross as I do? And I want so badly to be touched. And loved.* ♥
>
> ♥ *Me*

Yikes, it's hard to read that there was a time I was disgusted with myself. I wonder how much of that sticks around subconsciously. Like, you can say you're confident, but until you truly feel it, it's not true. And I always speak the truth, so here we go! There are men who like a big woman, even men who are thinner than you! Sister, make sure you understand why he loves big women. Make him understand taking care of your health, but love what he loves. Love those thick thighs when you dance (for the record, they make pretty funny slow motion videos!). Love yourself, 'cause if you can't, no one else ever will.

August 9, 2009

> *Well, I had 2 great weeks in which I lost 7 pounds. This week 4.5 of that came back. I was PMSing so that had something to do with it, but I've never gained 4.5 lbs in one week. WTF! So I'm reading the Time Traveler's Wife and watching Kaitlyn grow up, and for the first time ever I'm wishing I could do it all over again, starting perhaps with accepting to Baylor.*
>
> *What would have happened had I gone to Emerson? Would I have graduated? Would I have*

eaten four years of free pizza? Would I have met Luke or Adolfo or been married to a rich businessman by now? Maybe most importantly, would I have come to manage Palio's? Cause it didn't work out.

And also for the first time, I'm having to find a job. Without a degree. And I can no longer settle. $8.00 doesn't cut it. Hell, $12 doesn't cut it. I want to be content. I want to win the lottery, write my books, and make a real play at publication. I want to see Adolfo regularly. I want to date him. I want Tommy to ask me out. I want to date him. I want Kaitlyn to be happy and Jimmy to be happy. I want them to be together even if they don't work together. I want to stop stressing. I want to be okay with the fact that I'll be 30 in two years. My high school reunion is in nine months. What do I have to be proud of? Nothing.

♥ Me

November 12, 2009

Man, why do I only reach for this book when I feel super happy or super sad? If I could just keep up with it, maybe I wouldn't be so surprised every time I read it. I got a job at a daycare. I haven't talked to Adolfo in a few weeks because I'm pretty hurt he didn't say anything to me for my bday. My heart is full and excited and sad and tender because I miss my brother and I feel like Kaitlyn's mad at me for something or other.

And then there's Mike. I wonder if it's in my DNA to like every boy that plays a major role in my life. I don't want to say Mike is different, because even though he is now, so was Adolfo, and Evan, and Luke, and... so who knows? My heart hurts when he goes out with Lynne and soars when he looks at me. I can't tell Kaitlyn or my mom b/c I don't want Jimmy to know.

I babysat one of my kids the other night, and since then I'm sort of obsessed with them. I want to be them. I just want a baby and a loving hus-

band and the goddamn American dream. Is that too much to ask? I got a Wii fit & feel like I gained weight this week anyway. God. ♥ *I don't want to write about Mike, but Lord help me if I don't think about him all the time. All. The. Motherfucking. Time. Sometimes I want to dance and others, I just want to bawl.*

♥ Me

November 17, 2009

Mike & I went to see Pirate Radio on Friday. I got to sit by him for 2 hours, and all I wanted to do was touch him. Yikes. This is where it gets dangerous. I can handle a little crush; it's the physical part that gets nasty. Ugh. And still I eat like I do. Hmm. ♥ *him. So I decided I'm gonna go back to school to be a massage therapist. Depending on cost of course. A huge draw being...maybe I can practice on Mike! Eeek.*

♥ Me

I did indeed go to massage school, but like most things, I didn't finish it because I was too proud to ask for financial help. If I had finished my internship, would I have become a therapist? It's extraordinarily hard on the body, so I don't imagine I would have lasted long even if I had made it. However, the lessons I learned I'll take with me forever. I learned even more ways to make other people feel good through the power of physical touch and even, sometimes, in the absence of it. Hovering my hands over Justin and feeling the heat radiate from him in our first Reiki lesson was wild.

My dreams started getting bigger when I learned how much talent I had. I was good at massage therapy. I was born to make people feel good, and I could make money doing it. I crafted my entire business plan for school with my dream to be a personal therapist for the Texas Rangers. When I lost my job at this day care, I even went so far as to put on a cute sundress, buy myself supergood seats (we hadn't gone to the playoffs yet, so tickets were still cheap!), and talk to the bat girls about how they got hired. I ended up with the worst sunburn of my life but no job. I then met a friend for drinks after spending all day in the sun.

The next morning, I got up to take Ruby outside and passed out in the elevator. I hit my head on the bar on the way down and had no idea how long I was out. But poor baby Ruby was running in and out of the elevator doors as they closed and opened. The number of times that dog saw me lose consciousness is absurd.

November 20, 2009

> New Moon. Just as bad as I thought it would be. No. Worse. But still... TEAM EDWARD.
>
> I'm thankful I'm not too tired this morning. It feels like any other morning save for some sinus problems. Again. On another note...
>
> How do babies learn the word "mine"? I know I don't teach them that. I'm not sure I ever even say it. "Yours," sure. "His, hers," most definitely. But "mine"? Not a chance. And yet here sits Jacob, screaming "mine!" at Mallory because she still has turkey and he finished his first. And no, it's not his. He just wants to pretend it is.

November 21, 2009

> Today I'm thankful we've got awesome parents that let us babysit together cause we both wanted it so much.

November 22, 2009

> Suuuundaaaay. I am thankful I woke up pretty early. So excited for this week. Love my families; glad most of them are coming for the feast!
>
> LYN B: Ok, so do we get to see you Thurs?
> ME: Absolutely! We will be there with bells on!
>
> LYN: yippee!!!
>
> Man, what I wouldn't give to be a judge for the Iron Chef America Thanksgiving battle. Yum-o!!

November 23, 2009

> Oh, Ryan Tedder, how I love thee.
>
> Just recapped Jack passing out for Kaitlyn, complete with the lax body and rolling eyes. Didn't get any less scary in the later hour. My baby.

November 24, 2009

    Knock down the only wall and be a part of it all.

    Today (and every day!) I am thankful for music. I can't imagine life without it. That's as cheesy as it gets today, folks. ♥

November 25, 2009

    I'm thankful that all my kiddos left by 4:30. It's only 6 and I already went shopping at Old Navy and Ulta and now I am HOME. So sleepy.
    The ten-dollar bill is becoming extinct. I really wanted one and I got two fives. Boo.
    Worst part of allergies? Not being able to breathe. Second worst part? Not being able to sing. So awful. I don't realize how much I sing until I can't do it anymore.
    How do you measure a year? In daylights, in sunsets, in midnights, in cups of coffee? In inches, in miles, in laughter, in strife? In five-hundred, twenty-five-thousand, six-hundred minutes. How do you measure a year in the life? How about love?

November 26, 2009

    "Rent" at bedtime = surefire way to wake up with swollen eyes. Nice!

    Happy Turkey Day people. I'm thankful for you all!

    Just watched an old home video from fourth-ish grade... Martin Luther King Jr play? Featuring... lots of y'all (FB friends). Awesome. Lmao.

November 28, 2009

    I could hide out under there. I just made you say underwear.
    HA hahahaha... And on that note...Safety pin fell out; skirt came down in the middle of the street.

Luckily it's after three and there was no one to see it. Or my amazing parallel parking job in which I pulled so close to the guy blocking half my spot that I am probably dooming myself to be hit tomorrow. But fuck him. Spot stealer.

Omg there is a crib in the bed bath and beyond catalog that transforms to toddler bed, then to day bed, and finally to full bed. Is it bad that I don't even have a boyfriend and I want it??

November 29, 2009

The Noodle is curled next to me, it's cold outside, and I still have seven hours in my weekend. Life is good.

December 1, 2009

Want to go to massage therapy school soooo badly. Anyone have any brilliant ideas how to get $7200?

It's amazing the hugeness of the human brain: I just heard a song I haven't heard in years and could still do every last word. Bravo, human brain.

December 2, 2009

I posted a picture of my snow-covered windshield. Tre bizarre… After 27 winters in Texas (one in LA), you'd think I'd be used to it. But it's still a surprise. A pleasant one.

LOVES that all of her FB friends who are living in Dallas and Plano mentioned the freak snow. Hehe. It's spose to do it again Friday and then…60 by next week. Seriously???

ADOLFO: I just bought a movie on DVD. See if you can guess which one: (Woman) "Dont say it like that." (Child) "Then how should I say it? 'Get outta my way' or… 'GET OUTTA MY WAY!!' or… *sob* 'Get outta my way'

Me: Yes!!! I love it!!! I'd do Anything, baby. Man it's been a long time since I saw that.

December 3, 2009

Loud, long sigh They were insane today. Or maybe it's every day, and today I just...need a drink. Woo.

Just twisted the stem off an apple to see what letter my future husband's name would start with. I got G. I can barely think of any names that start with G, much less anyone I know.

December 4, 2009

Snowing in Houston and in Austin... The one winter I am not IN Austin!! Wow. Now come on up to Dallas, pretty white cold stuff!!

December 5, 2009

Haha so I read this thing the other day that said 78% of requests for Diet Coke at restaurants go unfulfilled. Today at Chili's I got a drink that tasted like regular, but I figured maybe I was THINKING it tasted regular. But the more I drink it, the more I'm sure. Lmao.

December 6, 2009

> Adolfo F: You know you introduced me 2 that movie "I'll Do Anything." Hahah. I owe my laughter to you.
> Me: Wow I don't remember that at all! God I love that movie though.
> Adolfo: You left your box of movies at my apt & said I could watch whatever. I picked that one. I always tell ppl "I want a compromise!!" lol
> Me: ohhh duh that makes sense. Man that was a long time ago, eh? I need to start quoting movies. I love that little girl. Wonder what ever happened to her?

> ADOLFO: *Me & my lil bro always play WM? (wat movie?). Different movie quotes. I think I can beat ya. HAHAHA. My ex always hated that I quote movies ALL THE TIME! That lil girl doesnt do any movies. Dropped off the radar.*

The little girl, whose name was Whittni Wright, only really ever did one other project according to IMDb. I went further and couldn't find a word more. Mystery! She was great.

December 9, 2009

> *Oh wow I just read the words "hot jelly donut" and got an instant craving. I am worse than a pregnant woman. I guess it doesn't help that I haven't eaten dinner yet. Babysitting Samantha. Why is it that when parents say "help yourself to anything," it makes it the LAST thing I can possibly think about doing?*

December 10, 2009

> *Got my dreams, got my life, got my love. Got my friends, got the sunshine above. Why am I making this hard on myself when there's so many beautiful reasons I have to be happy?*

You guys, I legit had a "Did I write that?" moment, in which I sounded like Urkel. Usually, I put slashes in song lyrics or quotes or something or at least I recognize it. I did none of that here, and when I went to look the words up, Google took its time (by that, I mean it didn't guess my lyric as I was typing it). But surely it brought up "Happy" by Natasha Bedingfield; I used to love her, so I added the song to my TikTok Jams playlist, where all my angel songs are. Good lyrics.

December 11, 2009

> *Need a music weekend. Whether it be Pete's piano bar, a karaoke contest, or simply singing to the loudspeaker at a bar, I must have it. Tomorrow night! With drinks! Who's up?*

> *I would do pretty much anything to go back to 1966 and see the Beatles in concert. Groovy.*

December 12, 2009

> *Wow, I just added the biggest reason ever to my "why eBay rocks my socks" list. Eff Christmas shopping anywhere else ever again. I am typing with my right hand but my left is numb.*

I would be willing to bet this was the year I got my brother, like, six Robert Graham shirts. I was so excited and thrilled with myself. I have no idea why my left hand was numb, though, or why that warranted announcement.

December 13, 2009

> *Watching the season finale of the Biggest Loser. Barfed a little when Antione proposed to Alexandra. No shocker there. Cheered a lot when Tracey lost the at home prize. Now wishing I had someone who needed to lose weight and who would drive me to succeed. "Slipping up" is too easy.*

Y'all, can you hear the grumpy? OMG. What a bad mood I was in! (Although if those people sucked as humans, I would still cheer if they lost. Sometimes, people need to lose.)

December 15, 2009

> *Ohhh my gluteus Maximus! My Skechers shape ups must finally be working, cause I've done nothing else to deserve this! No pain, no gain though, eh?*

> *Ha the kid at target just called me ma'am. Twice. Feel completely justified calling him kid. Twice.*

December 16, 2009

> *I only wanted to see you laughing in the purple rain!*

December 17, 2009

> *All I wanna do is play poker.*

Mom's surgery + some crazy-nuts kids + MAJOR crazy hormones = very bad mood. Don't want to be at work.

WTF?? WTF??!!!! Russell? Seriously, RUSSELL??? Out of all of them, and ESPECIALLY against Jakob... You should have gone home long ago. Poorly played, America. Poorly played. I still maintain Nathan should have been next to Jakob.

December 18, 2009

Taking the afternoon off to take my mama home. Then headed right back to Frisco to work at the restaurant. Woohoo for tips!!

Whoo, oven on a Friday night makes for a great workout and a sore back. Seriously, who will walk on it for me??

December 19, 2009

Babysitting Danny. This boy is so tired he's wired.

December 20, 2009

My eyeball is itching up a storm. And storms make my allergies worse, so I really wish my eyeball would chill.

Wow Brittany Murphy. Celebrities my age need to stop dying. Weird.

> ADOLFO F: *I switched my dog food to a diff brand. RACHEL RAY has her own brand so my dog had 2 switch. She gets the food... I get the bag. LOL!!!*
>
> ME: *Ha, here's hoping she doesn't get sick*

My dog's stomach is insane. If she got sick from Rachael Ray—yes, Adolfo spelled it wrong—food fourteen years ago, it's because she was a puppy, and I hadn't learned her weirdness yet. At fourteen and a few weeks, she happily eats both dry and canned Rachael Ray Nutrish, only chicken or turkey, thank you very much, because she's picky AF. We had a break for Ollie when we could afford it, but we love Nutrish now.

December 22, 2009

> ADOLFO F: My dog won't get sick, it's RACHEL RAY food! She might bark like her throat is horse though. Which would be AWESOME!!

December 23, 2009

> Okay storms, where you at???? Bring my cold front; this humid 70 is nasty.

> Glee reruns... Who knew they'd make me so happy??? They need to rerun the first two so Kaitlyn can see them!

December 24, 2009

> Yeah!!!! Snow in an hour???? And going must of the day???? Gorgeous!!!

> It's been an hour... Something is coming down but it ain't looking like snow. Let me tell you: 4 kids in the whole school is rather freaky.

> 73 degrees yesterday and today this. Wonderful. I love it!!!!

> Christmas Eve dinner = prime delicious steak and the best bernaise sauce ever = full tummy and sleepy eyes. Merry Christmas Eve, y'all!

December 25, 2009

> Merry Christmas while I'm sitting in my car trying to melt the ice off!!!!!!

> Chillin at the brother's playin games. Merry Christmas friends!

December 27, 2009

> How did a 3.5-day weekend go so fast? Thank God for another 3.5-day week and then another long weekend!

December 28, 2009

> Just wanna close my eyes. They hurt real bad. Too much cat hair this weekend?

>> ADOLFO F: Never seen Hangover. A buddy just got married in LV. My lil bro went but I didn't. I heard everyone had a BLAST. So now I'm there excuse 2 go back, so they said I gotta get married. LOL! Im a manager so of course Im working NYE. Wat about ya?

>> ME: You should see it. I'm going to LV at the beginning of March for a pizza convention! I dunno what's going to happen on NYE. The school closes at 3 and Palio's closes at 8. We are talking about having a private party at the restaurant.??

> I feel funny. And hungry. There's definitely hunger there.

> Reading Danielle Steele and holding a sleeping ten-month-old. I've never wanted a baby more.

December 29, 2009

> Who doesn't long for someone to hold? Who knows how to love you without being told? Somebody tell me why I'm on my own. If there's a soulmate for everyone.

> Snow in Plano twice in five days. How did I get so lucky?

December 30, 2009

> Love this: Mallory Kyle is talking at the top of her voice at nap time. I told her "shhhh" and she

immediately lowered her volume to a whisper. What kid knows how to whisper?? Lmao!

Ow. In pain I am. Three hours on top of a ladder hurts me. But the chalkboard is redone, so hallelujah.

December 31, 2009

Blue Moon New Year's Eve. Bad ass.
I'll be waiting / I'll be watching / under a blue moon / The taste of heaven only happens / once in a blue moon.

Kiss me at midnight / dance until the morning light / party into the new year. All my friends are here / and when the timing's right / kiss me at midnight. Happy New Year's Eve!

Time is going by so much faster than I / and I'm starting to regret not spending all of it with you.

Is wishing Kelly would get home so they can go out before it's actually time to toast…and wishing everyone a HAPPY AND SAFE NEW YEAR!!!!

January 1, 2010

My pretty hair and hot pink tights had very little effect tonight. Oh well. With a new year comes a new me.

I can't possibly be hungover. But I sure am dizzy. Maybe I just didn't sleep very well with my poor hacking brother next door.

Laziest day of my life. Lovenit. Princess Diaries on Mike's couch while he and Steph snooze nearby. Thinkin bout maybe going to get Jakes.

> LYN B: *Apparently we are very old—we showed up at Palio's @ 9:25… stayed till (a little after) 9:30… figured you guys were probably at the*

other Palio's... so we took our tired, hungry selves home... SORRY WE MISSED YOU GUYS. HAPPY 2010.

January 2, 2010

The Weight Loss Diaries, Day 1

I've played this game with myself for so many New Years, I can't even remember them all. I have also NOT played this game on several occasions, telling myself that NOT making the resolution will work better. Less pressure or whatnot. This year, I'm not so much making a resolution as becoming accountable to the 250 or so people I am friends with on this silly site. I am pretending that there is someone out there in cyberspace who is actually reading this. And there is definitely one or two people on here that I would definitely not want knowing about my horrible relationship with food, and pretending they are reading this is what's going to keep me honest and on track. Even if no one reads this at all.

I'm rereading a book called "The Weight Loss Diaries" by a woman named Courtney Rubin. I swear the girl could be me; and of course it helps that every time I open the cover, I see my name. I really finally just want to be done with all this stupid weight issue. I know I never will be; it's a lifelong struggle and all that, but I just want to finally reach my goal. For once and for real. I have a few goals actually.

The first one is to be healthy.

The second is to be able to wear a swimsuit come summer.

The third is to be in a relationship.

I know I can't pretend that my weight will solve that final issue, but it sure makes me wonder. I will get all dressed up and feel really pretty and still wonder if I was 50 pounds lighter, if someone would look at me differently. And then I get into the mindset, if I wouldn't want to touch me, how can I expect anyone else to want to touch me? THAT is my number one motivator right now. Sad to say.

It's 1:30 in the morning of the 2nd day of the new year and I'm so sleepy I'm not sure how much sense I'm making. I had a whole essay planned out in a way of explanation, but I've seemed to have lost that. So I'll sum it up:

I'm going to be accountable to all of you, pretend readers, and I'm going to make it stick this time. I will not post my weight in numbers, but I will inform you of major milestones. I am going to tell you what I ate for the day, what I thought about eating, how hard it was to pass up those things, and how sad I am that I had to eat the same thing for the ninetieth time in a row. I will set small goals and tell when they've been met. And it might be boring and redundant, but it's going to help me. Or here's hoping anyway.

For this first week, I am going to make it a goal to get up a little earlier than normal and do my Wii Fit for 20 minutes before work. I am also going to eat breakfast no matter how not-hungry I am. I am going to drink at least 7 bottles of water while I am at work and 3 full glasses when I come home.

And that's that. Until tonight, friends.

> KRISTI T: I would be more than happy to be one of your "pretend" readers if you'll have me! I struggle with food issues as well. And procrastination, but I'll tell you about that later! Let me know how the Wii Fit goes! I am hoping to get one soon! Good luck! You have my support and encouragement!
>
> KATHERINE H: Very brave and honest, Courtney. You'll have lots of readers wishing you well. The food thing is a tough battle and anyone who hasn't fought it doesn't have a clue. In some ways, it's worse than trying to beat alcoholism—you don't have to drink to stay alive, but you do have to eat. Good luck! We're all rooting for you, pretend or otherwise.

JENNIFER M: ♥ and (((hugs)))... You can overcome this!!

LYN B: Good luck, Court... I know that you view me as "small" and unable to comprehend, but I have struggled with food choices my whole life too—you said that you were going to state what you eat each day and what you "thought about eating"—instead, try to concentrate on how you were feeling about yourself—bored, angry, depressed, etc—and try to start with protein in the morning—tends to stay with you longer. I'm no expert, but I know there are many who love you and want to see you succeed. Just remember everything in moderation...including moderation—don't try to change things overnight... It's a journey, not a race.

Wow, such great responses in less than 12 hours. Y'all are awesome!!!!!!

January 3, 2010

The Weight Loss Diaries, Day 1 Part 2

Well, today wasn't as hard as I expected it to be. I don't know why, really. I did pretty much nothing as usual, but I did go to the mall and to see a movie. Mmm, smelling that popcorn was hard, let me tell you. But I had brought a fruit and nut mix in case I got hungry, and I also brought an aluminum bottle of water. It was a great idea and worked out really well cause I was really hungry by like a third of the way into the movie. Not to mention I was REALLY bored cause the movie was super slow. And yes...I am a bored eater. Always have been, and I've always known it.

I realized about halfway through the way that detailing all I'm eating for y'all will be really boring for you guys and tedious for me since I already track it on a new little iPhone app that a friend recommended. I was using SparkPeople, but somehow I like the new one, called Lose It! a lot better. So it gave me a little plan to follow, and I ended up about 200 calories short of my allowance for the day. That was factoring in about 50 calories lost by walking.

I had a huge salad for dinner, and it was almost all veggies, and it was sooooo yummy. Of course I had some dressing and cheese, but I counted it. And I had a glass of egg nog for dessert. I counted that too. It may not be the healthiest way to do this, but I also had plenty of fiber and protein and very little sodium all day. So I consider today a huge accomplishment.

But it's only day one. And I spent allllll daaaaaay thinking about food. About when the next time I could eat was, about how many calories I had left... I know it's supposed to get easier, and I certainly know the weekend is WAY worse than the weekday. It will also get easier when I go back to school. The more I have to distract me, the less I can think about food. So tomorrow is Sunday...one more day in my apartment to contend with before work starts up again. I gotta grocery shop a little...get some yogurts and stuff.

And I'm adding a "starting" photo. When I REALLY started this journey nearly three years ago, I was 40 pounds heavier. So although this isn't really the ACTUAL beginning, it's where I'm starting now. I have roughly another 60 pounds to go. A grand total of 100 would be so breathtakingly spectacular, I can't wrap my head around it.

Here I go again...

The Weight Loss Diaries, Day 2

Well, an interesting side effect of concentrating so hard on food: dreaming about it. Last night I dreamed about men and food, my two favorite topics. I don't remember much of it except I went into a room somewhere and when I came back out, all that was left was some apple dessert, and I don't much like apples when they're cooked. I was disappointed, haha. Anyway, so...I dream about guys a LOT obviously, but it hasn't ever included food. So.

Today was again fairly easy. I didn't have any out-of-control cravings. I admit, I slept really late, which of course cut my eating time significantly. But I keep reading all these studies that say sleep helps with muscle repair and stuff, so. I did my Wii Fit Body Test this morning, then I cleaned my house and went to take my mom something. I hit Target on the way and got 5 frozen lunches and some snacks for like $30. Super exciting.

When I got home, I worked out to Wii Biggest Loser, which I haven't done in like a month, since I gave Mike back his Wii. Boy, let me tell you, I may not have done it regularly to begin with, but my body certainly didn't like me stopping for that long. I upped the hardness to "intermediate" so my workout was 37 minutes and WAY more challenging than as a beginner. OUCH!! Seriously, I thought I might throw up. And yes, I was drinking water while doing it. Anyway, I worked up a great heart rate and sweat. I felt good, and then 30 minutes later was starving. So I had a healthy dinner. And now I am drinking milk with a little chocolate syrup, and I feel full and it's nearly ten.

I am so excited that this seems to be easier than it was before. I am enjoying measuring everything out, and thrilled that while 1 cup of pasta may not look like that much, it is more than filling enough. I do have one issue though: I LOVE SALT. I bought this salt-substitute and it tastes like chlorine. And I used Mrs. Dash on my edamame and chicken tonight, and I was sad and MISSING SALT. EEEEK.

Okay, so. I wanted to tell you guys who are reading this that it means the world to me. Kristi, I read your status updates and sometimes I feel sad for you. I would love to know you're happy. Kathy, I know you struggle with this stuff too, more than anyone else in our family. Thanks for being here. Lyn, if there's anything I've learned on this journey, it's that overweight people aren't the only ones who have bad relationships with food. I live with a tiny girl who has a huge problem with sugar. And of course, Jennifer...we've been together through this for a long time, and I hope one day we can both say we did what we came to do.

Again, thanks for reading. Tomorrow is another day, eh?

January 4, 2010

The Weight Loss Diaries, Day 3

Welp, today was good. Except I didn't exercise cause my roommate was home... and then I had popcorn with her because...well because food is social for me. It's comfort and fun and a bridge for relationships. She's got major cravings right now and of course it draws me in because...I let it. But I didn't eat too terribly much and I was pretty short for the day, so. I'll be back on track tomorrow.

I was extraordinarily proud of making breakfast before I left for work this morning. AND doing my Wii Fit. I felt good all day; I even had my own food instead of the school food. But I think it's easier on days off. I can concentrate more on when I'm eating and when I'm hungry and stuff like that. Eeek.

Okay, so that's really it for today. Bedtime for Courtney.

My heart belongs to Finn but my everything else belongs to Puck. HOOOOTTTTT!!

January 5, 2010

The Weight Loss Diaries, Day 4

So we are going to be doing this weight-loss challenge thing at work. It's going to be fun and competitive, especially due to Michelle, who says she's fierce. Bring it on, girl! I'm excited, cause if there's anything I'll compete for, it's moola. Woohoo.

I was so great today. I am really into white tuna in water for some reason. I had it for dinner tonight and I'm having the rest for lunch tomorrow, and it was so yummy even despite the smell. Hehe. This week feels really long because of the two super short weeks previous, and I am really excited to see what my numbers are on Friday morning.

My allergies are coming in because of the stupid weather change (appreciate the cold, hate the nose), and my throat's starting to hurt, which makes me want Lipton soup, which is so low in calories but sooooooo hiiiiiiigh in sodium. WANT IT. WANT SALT. HATE BEING DEPRIVED.

January 6, 2010

Great day! I indulged a little too much in some cheese at snacktime, and when I looked up the stats, I was a little shocked. But I still came up under in calories because of the workout I did when I came home. My allergies are draining me and I had no energy. So I didn't do cardio; I did strength-training and yoga and then free-step on my balance board. It said I burned 145 calories, but who knows?

I did have soup for dinner though. I drank a ton of water trying to balance out the sodium. But it was really yummy.

I'm so sleepy I am about to get in bed and watch Friends and hope I pass out soon. One more day till I find out how this hard work is paying off!! Night!

January 7, 2010

Can't wait to see Texas demolish the stupid crimson whatever. Burnt orange all the way baby. HOOK 'EM!!

Ohhhh Colt, you're killing me. TEXAS FIGHT!!!

Red. And...Colt!!! Come back!!!!!!!

Yes yes YES!!!!!!! Holy shit I can't take this. My throat is not up for the screaming. YIKES!!!!! We've got ourselves a GAME!!!!!!

By the way, anyone see that Crimson Goon picking his nose on the sidelines?? Diggin' for that win... Don't hit the brain.

Second in the nation, but first in my heart. Rock on, Texas.

January 8, 2010

I am amused that I cannot give a hoot about football all through the year, but come January when my Horns are in the championship, I go nuts with the rest of them. I didn't even sleep last night I was so amped up. Colt, here's hoping you do well in the future. NFL would be crazy not to get you.

The Weight Loss Diaries, Day 6

Sheesh. So the kiddos had Rice Krispie treats for snack this afternoon. I was thankfully prepared with a yogurt and mandarin oranges, but the smell... holy cow, it was the first time this week (yes, it's just been a WEEK!), where something that intoxicating was near me. EEEK. But I abstained. And I abstained again at around 6:45...

I was in the middle of working out with Bob when Jimmy texted to tell me to meet them at a wing place to watch the game. I hadn't eaten yet, and my first instinct was to stop the game and go have some wings. But I not only finished the workout, I also made salmon and rice and edamame and ate it before I went. I was full and not even a little tempted, even when they brought out some fries, which are easily my biggest weakness. (There has never been a time in my life where I could honestly say if I'm a sweets or a salt person... I love them both... but lately, salt is winning. Maybe cause I've tried to cut it out completely, and I can still have some sweet things?)

I'm pretty excited for my numbers tomorrow. Scared too, because if I don't see a significant number, I'm probably going to be really sad. Or maybe I'll suck it up and move along. I guess it depends on how I feel when I wake up. But right now I'm pretty sad-feeling. The Longhorns lost and I'm allergic to life, so my heart's kind of down. But I will keep going. Because of that, above everything else, is the one thing I can control in my life. And it thrills me to conquer it.

Fingers crossed.

Happpppy Birthday ELVIS!!! And Kate Rose.

January 9, 2010

The Weight Loss Diaries, Day 8

Triumph: 3.2 pounds down.

The early part of the day went fine. I had a couple of squares of applesauce bread at snack, but they were small. But then I delivered pizzas tonight, and of course we were busy enough that I didn't think to eat until eight when I was starving. So I had a small calzone. I am okay with it because I need a chance to have something truly enjoyable every once in a while, or else I will go nuts. I've always considered Fridays my "cheat day," and I am going to try to avoid that thought as much as I can, but I really loved that calzone tonight. And tomorrow I'll work out a little extra.

A big problem of mine is little fun-size candies. I love Nerds and Airheads, and a little box of Nerds is only 60 calories. I don't know what a little Airhead is, but... what's the good in that if you eat 20 of them? Nerds are actually okay, cause I eat like three at a time and they last for a loooooong time. But I am addicted to the chewiness of Airheads, haha. Grrr. Anyway.

I'm literally dying laughing. I just purchased a bag of mini Airheads yesterday, and it's already gone. I have a problem with sugar, but the texture of chewy candy? OMG, not good for this old jaw.

So I am pleased, obviously. Let's see if this week is as easy and as rewarding. Next week is going to be PMS-y, but I WILL NOT LET THAT HINDER ME!!!!!!!!! I will drink a ton of water and try to stay away from the sweets/salts. In fact, that's my promise to you guys. PLEASE SHOOT ME IF I SAY SOMETHING DIFFERENTLY next week.

January 12, 2010

How do you pack a workout, a nap, and a trip to Target all into one hour lunch break?

We are stardust. We are gooooolden.

The Weight Loss Diaries, Day 11

Wow, today was nuts-o. I started off the day with a Frappuccino because I left my coffee mug at work. Okay, I allotted it. Then I had lunch at the school (pasta and kielbasa) and I didn't ever want to stop eating it, and it's not anything amazing, I just WANTED IT. I have no clue how much I had or how many calories was in it, but I took a guess.

Okay, so. I wanted a sandwich REALLY BADLY for dinner, but Central Market was really far. So I came home and made a grilled cheese. But I also had a little 100 calorie Oreo bar and ice cream. LOW FAT, but still. Today was hiiiiiigh-calorie. I worked out a lot and I also drank four tons of water, so hopefully they'll balance out.

I want a treadmill so badly I'm debating pushing school back to July for THAT. I am going to have NO money for the next eight months, and I do not want to wait eight months for a treadmill. Sigh. I'm afraid I'm going to get bored of the Wii games. Plus, sometimes straight cardio is just better.

I am soo sooo sooooo full right now. I'm super sleepy too. I am trying to finish my water (accounting for half of the fullness) before bed though. I'm glad it's only Tuesday because I have a couple more days to burn some calories, but the kiddos at school were insane today. INSANE. It has to be Friday. Soon.

♥

January 13, 2010

Ugh these babies have been taken over by aliens. No lie. Give me my babies back!

The Weight Loss Diaries

Yellow! So this past couple of days wasn't the best. I didn't have a hard time not eating well. On the contrary, I had a hard time eating as badly as I did. I made conscious decisions to put everything in my mouth that I did, and I paid for it. I was tired and lacked energy and slept badly and felt grossly full a lot of the time. But today I am back on track and feel much better already.

It was great having Adolfo here, as always. And it's amazing that I've only been doing this hardcore for 11 days, and I already notice such a huge difference. I ate well today (anyway, better than I did yesterday) and worked out really hard just now. DANCE IS AWESOME. So I am prepared not to meet my goal (which for this week, by the way, is 207), but I still hope I do.

Adolfo and I talked about going on a cruise in October, for my birthday, and I hope to be at my final number long before then. MY ULTIMATE goal is to be 170 by July 4, which is when I'm planning on having my cousin-family reunion in Cali. Of course that date is not set in stone yet, and depending on people's schedules, might even happen early June. But I know if I continue on this path, I can make it. (I'd even be happy with 180, cause I believe girls need SOME cushion. We are supposed to be soft and holdable). After feeling so yucky these past couple days, I know I can make it. It only takes a few days to get your body used to something. And what I'm doing is healthy and correct, so...wish me well. It'll take an army. Thank God for two specific readers who are helping me a LOT!! ♥

June 29, 2010

First hydrotherapy class tonight. MUCH more intriguing than chair and yet somehow, I still don't want to go. I miss Carol and Jessica. Glad for Justin. Blah.

July 23, 2010

Show me the meaning of being lonely / Is this the feeling I need to walk with? / Tell me why I can't be there where you are! / There's something missing in my heart.

August 30, 2010

Wisssshing.

KRISTI T: Airplanes in the night sky are like shooting stars!
ME: For the one I looooove to find me todayyyyy.

August 31, 2010

No school for me. Mega headache. Don't touch me I bruise eeeeeasily.

September 5, 2010

I love Cupcake Wars.

Workin' hard for the money to get me to Austin tomorrow. Fingers crossed that I get at least $100.

Texas. Sucks.

September 6, 2010

Where'd all the good people gooo?

Texas Hill Country...yikes.

What kind of Austin restaurant closes at nine I ask you?

October 4, 2010

Yeeeeeah being jobless sucks. Electricity got cut off this morning. Feel like I'm 19 again.

October 29, 2010

Gross I just opened my vampire fangs and they have black mold on them!! Regular butterfly it is then. How boring.

Tonight I got told my smile was beautiful and I almost burst into tears. I am so unhappy here. I'm afraid to go to Cali for Thanksgiving for fear I won't be able to leave.

November 20, 2010

There's only two types of people in the world / The ones that entertain and the ones that observe.

Kinda excited about trying Polish food. Super sleepy though

Just word-vomited all over Jess and now feel really lonely. Fun night followed by sad heart equals contemplative Courtney.

November 21, 2010

Whose brilliant idea was it to give me NyQuil at 7:50 this morning? For the record: neither it nor the DayQuil seems to work. I'm still stuffy. And...a little disappointed that while I'm still sick, my voice isn't doing the crazy thing it was doing yesterday. At least that part was fun!

Hungry and bored. Sundays are only cool till about two PM and then they suck and I wanna go back to work. Less than 48 hours till ADOLFO and HARRY POTTER and then on my way to Cal-i-for-ni-a!!!

Waaaaay too amped about this week. My heart is about to burst.

Patrick G: goin going back back to cali cali!
Me: Plus Adolfo is coming to see Harry Potter. Good week for Courtney.

November 22, 2010

Tired but psyched.

Coffy coff. My jaw hurts.

November 23, 2010

You know I know how to make 'em stop and stare as I zone out / the club can't even handle me right now.

Saaaaad right now.

Kimi K: Don't be sad... austin is thinking about you. have a great Turkey Day. take care
Me: Kim!!! Thank you. You have no idea how much I miss you guys. I even had a dream about y'all a few weeks ago. Hope you and your fam have an awesome holiday too. ♥

November 24, 2010

How early do I have to get to the airport these days? I've never had a problem with security, even when I arrive with like half an hour to spare... Knock on wood.

Carol K: I'd get there early today for 2 reasons: 1) busiest travel day of the year, 2) new security measures have everybody very upset.
Me: Omg that was a piece of cake. Nothing has changed since the new 9/11 measures; I don't get the uproar. I got here at 11:05 for a 12:20 flight and was through security by 11:22. Borrrrrrring.

It's beginning to look a lot like Thanksgiving.

Traveling is such a waiting game. Need to learn to apparate. And hope I don't throw up on this shuttle whose driver thinks she is from Jamaica.

Dyyyyying slowly. Yow.

KATHERINE H: Where are you? In S. Maria?
ME: At Granmuh's. My allergies got worse I think.

November 25, 2010

Wow I love coming to Cali. I went to sleep at like 11 (one my time) and now I'm awake with neither an alarm clock or a dog licking my ear, and I feel awesome. I was nervous I wouldn't be raring to go by 9, and here it is 7:22. But I can't find my Granmuh...

KATHERINE H: I think she sleeps in the garage, hanging upside down with her wings folded. Did you check there?
MARK E: She's in the backyard with the dog...probably picking oranges.
ME: Lol y'all!! Mark, she explicitly told me she would not be picking oranges today, no matter how much I wanted juice. She turned out to be still in bed. I figured since Minnie was sitting outside MY door that Granmuh had to be somewhere else, but I beat her awake.
MARK: Katherine was closer, then, with her guess.
KATHERINE: You beat Granma?

November 26, 2010

Watching "Charlie St Cloud" with Kev and Harper. Good end to an awesome day surrounded by the best family anyone has ever known. Whoever marries us is a lucky fool. And a little crazy too.

It is colder than a polar bear's butt in the Grover beach house. This is wrong on so many levels. I went to bed with my hair wet and instead of drying overnight, it formed icicles. And I formed pneumonia. Sigh.

Watching "Sex and the City 2" and feeling a little lost. I feel like I'm starting at the end.

November 27, 2010

Yeaaa Orcutt Burger!!! I'm so excited.

Like I said: this is the worst part about coming out here. Hate. Leaving.

November 28, 2010

Loved the plane ride home. I was in like first class. I had two feet of space in front of my knees, my own tv, and a free blanket that Ruby is now happily chewing on. Now I'm watching "Sex and the City" the show from Season 1, simply because it has to be done. I hope I like it.

Suuuunday. Wish I was still in Callllliiiiii.

November 29, 2010

Can I move to California in March?

ANNETTE W: No. You will miss J-fred's birthday!
CAROL K: Why wait?

ME: Annette, it would be the end of March if it happened at all. ♥ Carol, because my lease is up then.

Need sugar. Or sleep.

Anyone know anyone who needs a roommate in the Plano area for a few months starting in January? Male or female!

November 30, 2010

LUKE C: hey Courtney! How have you been? Long time no see! You movin to Cali???

ME: Hey yourself! Been good. Not moving to Cali anytime soon. my whole family beside my Brother and a couple of aunts is there and I miss them. How are you?

Bahhhhh I will have no possessions left if I leave my dog out of her cage, but I will have no dog left if I leave her IN her cage!! What do y'all think about upgrading her to a palace-size cage and leaving some toys inside with her??

    CARINA H: I think that's a good solution
    RICH B: Crating young with lots of toys gets them used to it. If she whines don't let her out because you'll be re-inforcing that behavior. She'll get used to it, mine did. He's at 5 months and when I say "crate" he goes right into it and lays down, sometimes after his nightly outing he just goes straight there for bed.
    ME: Rich, she's very used to it, she's 11 months and was in it most of her life. I just feel bad cause she's by herself sooo much. It feels cruel. A pen would be perfect if Ruby couldn't jump six feet straight into the air. Hahahaha.
    ANNE N: I use a gate with my dog so she can be in a room...though she's started jumping over it to sleep on our couch... I'll take suggestions too.

December 1, 2010

Today is my little girl's first birthday! Wow, we made it a whole year without her chokin on something...

Put on your yarmulke / it's time to celebrate Hanukkah! So drink you gin and tonica / and have a happy happy happy happy Hanukkah!

    ERICKA C: Ahhh... Adam Sandler! His sense of humor makes him super sexy

December 2, 2010

During the girlie time of the month, the need for chocolate waaaay outweighs the want to lose weight. I've given in. To half a whole box. Second half will probably come after dinner. Lucky there's only 9 pieces in a box.

PS Choxie is the wickedest thing ever invented. Best flavors in the world. So creative. A few years ago, when the commercials came out, I thought it was fake. Not fake. And soooooo amazing.

December 3, 2010

Bout to go into a sugar coma. But. It was good.

There's a calm surrender to the rush of day / when the heat of the rolling world can be turned away.

December 4, 2010

I'm curious how posting a cartoon from your childhood turned from something fun to date us all to a supposed fight against child abuse... Is that possible?? How is posting a picture of a cartoon gonna do anything? Does someone donate a dollar for every cartoon posted???

ADOLFO F: its fun and let's everyone know u fight against it. Just awareness is all.
ME: Good point.

December 5, 2010

I keep wanting it to be Monday so I can see my babies and then I remember I have to take my test first. Yikes.

Just finished cleaning the bejeezus out of my apartment. I hate vacuuming so much that instead I opted to manually pick up every red thread or cotton ball or carpet fiber from Ruby's toys and/or carpet-mauling.

I'm tired and even though I didn't work today, I'm still ready for bed at five... WTF.

Any Dallas friends want to start a Glee Club? I miss singing in a group...

> *Changing my profile pic back to my fave cartoon simply in the hopes that someone out there really is doing something to fight child abuse... I like to think I fight it every day when I go to work and hug my kids... but this can't hurt, right?*

> *Looking over my kinesiology tests to prep for tomorrow. It's all Greek to me. How the hell did I manage to pass that class???? Fingers crossed there aren't that many kines questions tomorrow.*

> *Whoa-o I want some more / Whoa-o, what are you waiting for / Take a bite of my heart tonight.*

December 6, 2010

> *Soooo nervous. There is $200 at stake here; I have no other option than to PASS!!!!*

> CAROL K: *You will! Good luck!*

> *YEEEEEEAH flying colors baby!!!! What a relief!!!!!*

> KENDRA R: *Good job!!*
> CARINA H: *woo hoo!! AWESOME*

> CAROL K: *Knew you would! Congrats.*

> *I ♥ "Private Chefs of Beverly Hills." PS, Willow Smith, you are 10 years old. You don't have swag so quit whipping your hair.*

I responded to a comment no longer showing.

> *Lol!! Maybe if their parents could hear, they wouldn't let their CHILD sing about having SWAG!!! Kids grow up too fast as it is; no need to encourage it!*

I'm not sure I agree with myself now. I'm sad, first of all, that I was that blunt to a kid even if it was in social media land, and she had no chance of seeing it. That song annoyed the crap out of me, no doubt, but the me now wants to cheer for a ten-year-old brave enough to do that kind of thing. Singing about having swag (or falling in love or having sex or any number of things!)

at too young of an age is always going to make people uncomfortable. But I suppose if the parenting is there and those kids are aware of the difference in a performance and real life, it can't hurt. Go, girl! Though I do hope the material has gotten better over thirteen years.

December 7, 2010

> *Bellyache. Finally have had enough chocolate. I put my hands up / they're playing my song! Rice for dinner? Me thinks so.*
>
> *Message me a number 1-500 and I'll tell you how I feel about you in a post. I feel like playing games too!!*
>
> *272, I already looooove you and I've only known you a month!! I'm so glad we have the room right in front so you can visit all the time. I'm excited to keep working with you and hopefully you won't say anymore disgusting things to neighboring class teachers.*

I'm both saddened and thankful it doesn't say a name here. I love that even thirteen years ago, I was willing to stand up for myself and could still tell someone I loved them even after they gossiped about me. That's my magic, y'all. The door is never all the way closed.

> *OMGleeeee!!!! Bawling like a baby as usual. I ♥ Brittany. But they REALLY need to bring Kurt back cause I hate the Warblers lead singer and the fat girl is a completely unfunny joke and a totally wrong fit.*

Y'all, that sounds so mean, but I still feel the same way. More power to the actress herself, but Lauren Zizes—or however you spell that—was a waste of a story on that show. You could have done much better for Puck. I don't mean because she's fat. I'm fat. Guys like fat women, even guys who look like Puck. I mean because she's horrible in every other way. There's no way any of them would have put up with her. Sorry not sorry.

> *66: girl, being intimidating is never something I intended!! I'm so glad we can chat now and I get to read some of your posts. You've always*

been beautiful on the outside, and now I'm learning your spirit and heart matches! And just keep playing... You'll beat me soon!!

December 8, 2010

Okay so Adolfo and I were talking about remakes... Are we the only people who would be totally psyched to see a remake of "The Labyrinth" starring Justin Timberlake as the Goblin King and Dakota Fanning as Sarah? Cause I need it to happen now.

> JENNY W: Noo!!! Do not wish that horrible idea of a remake into existence! PERFECTION DOES NOT NEED A REMAKE!!!!!!!!!! And above all else, it pains me SO MUCH that you chose Justin Timberlake. Really? REALLY?!

> ME: Lmao PLEASE he would kill it as the Goblin King. Like I said to Adolfo, not-quite-gay but definitely not-quite-straight and a ROCK STAR!! It's gonna be remade someday, it's inevitable. I just hope they do it justice.

Instant karma's gonna get you / gonna knock you right on the head / Well we all shine on / Like the moon and the stars and the sun / Well we all shine on / Everyone come on!

Limitless undying love which shines around me like a million suns / it calls me on and on across the universe.

Everyone who wants Cliff Lee to return to Arlington, donate $1 to the Rangers' fund. Maybe that way they can beat the Yankees' $150 million offer. Jeez. Us.

I replied to a comment that was no longer visible.

> Good opinion. I would love to have Lee back, but if it costs too much (I'm hoping his heart is in the right place and he can be happy with what we

can pay him), then I can't wait to see what we pull together. Whatever the case, WE WILL ROCK THEM.

December 9, 2010

A YEAR without writing! WTF! I won't even bother writing about what has happened. Starting today, I will write at least once a week. I'm working at a different daycare now, with infants and two coteachers I love. It seems so much happier than Parker Chase. Adolfo and I talk all the time. Right now we have a bet going on whether the Rangers (who I've become obsessed with) will win back Cliff Lee. ♥ Let's see... today was good. Still stressing about money but I PASSED my MASSAGE TEST and Phillip paid for school so I am almost a licensed therapist. Awesome. Just gotta find a way to be therapist to the Rangers. ♥

♥ Me

December 10, 2010

Nothing much to say today. I've been (playfully) trying to convince Adolfo to come be a manager at Palio's, because he's really unhappy at work. I think it would solve so much for him—he'd be happy, work less, live closer to home, and be near me. I really love him and just wanna make out with him once to see if that part would hold any appeal. I've really wanted to write lately but I'm at an impasse—can't finish "Diary of a Stranger" and can't begin the track story in an adult enough way.

♥ Me

I don't know why I was never able to finish *Diary of a Stranger*, which fifteen years ago, I was sure was going to be my first published novel. I molded it after my own life but got a little fantastical with it as well. I froze when Peyton, my main character, came home from Ireland. She had the choice between two amazing men, and she couldn't make it. I couldn't make it. Now I understand why. She didn't love herself enough. Maybe I'll be able to successfully write fiction after I get all this shit out? Perhaps that's a good subtitle.

December 9, 2010

I'm feeling the need for a large shopping trip. I'm also feeling the need for money with which to do that. Or I'm going to have to rely on school food and pasta.

MISHA T: Tomorrow is chicken spaghetti
KATIE V: & it was delicious!

Victoria's Secret models are some of the hottest people on the planet. Brava, women.

If dirt were dollars / I wouldn't worry anymore.

Bummed that I won't be able to afford Christmas presents. For anyone. Y'all expect something in May. Yea!

I've always hated when people say "PREE-sen-tay-shun" but I just realized it's a word from PREE-sent, not PREH-sent. So I guess even though it sounds stuffy, it's correct. Stupid English language, make words different.
SUSAN P: I am right there with you Courtney...

December 11, 2010

Headin off to the intern clinic. Justin, we miss you!

JUSTIN: Well once I get a good commission ck I'll be in there but till then I have to pay the bills

Yowch. First massage tore up my shoulder... Not. Good. Plus I saw everything that lady had to offer. Double not good.

KENDRA R: Well that was nice of her to share that with you! Lol

Yea working at Palio's for the first time in over a month!! Come see me if you love decadent pizza.

MISHA T: *Which one?*

ME: *Legacy.*

MISHA: *Bummer. My husband is going to the little elm one right now to get me some bread!*

Raise your glass if you are wrong in all the right ways.

December 12, 2010

Can't stop watching "Sex and the City." Anyone know a dog whisperer?

ME: *In two completely different realms of statuses.*

Good morning starshine / the earth says hello!

JOCELYN G: *Great song*

Who would you want the heroine to choose: her first boyfriend, who she was crazy about and compares every guy after to, or a cocky, funny, sweet Irish guy who she can't get enough of?

Wow, Molly Ringwald was originally slated to play "Pretty Woman" and Eric Stolz turned down Marty McFly in "Back to the Future." Wouldn't those have been different?

December 12, 2010

Yesterday was good—I had 3 massages and they were all really happy. One even tipped me & rebooked with me next week. Then I got to work at Palio's for the first time in a month & it was great to see everyone again. Today I've just been chilling— Target to Secret Santa shop.

♥ *Me*

December 13, 2010

Yesterday I accidentally let a candle burn down to nothing so that it filled my apt with smoke. Now I officially have the worst. Headache. Of my life.

"I love the view from up here / warm sun and wind in my ear / We'll watch the world from above as it turns to the rhythm of love."

Wow eating lunch at 11 in the morning makes me sooooo hungry by dinner. I know I should be full but I still want more.

Anyone with an iPhone needs to get the Talking Tom app and sing it Christmas carols. So fun.
ERIN G: Is it free?
ME: Yup. And awesome.
ERIN: Will do, then.
ME: Hahaha Talking John is hilarious too. It's an amoeba choir.

December 14, 2010

Fave "Sex and the City" quote so far: Carrie, "It's like a Danielle Steele novel in here." Aiden, "Whoo, from a writer, I'm pretty sure that's an insult."

Oh, Cliff. So disappointed. Do I still lose the bet if he didn't choose the Yankees?
MATT J: Cliff knows whats up, you didn't really think that he was going to stay in arlington did you?
ME: No but I certainly didn't think he'd go to Philly. This should be an interesting season.
MATT: yeah, no one up here thought that he would either. big surprise.

I hope they never lose Cruz. I'll cry a lot.

December 15, 2010

Wow I've got a classroom full of barfing babies. More so than usual. Beware the stomach flu, I guess! Sweet immune system to the rescue!!

Sitting on the couch watching "Blue's Clues" with Jasper. Looking at Fam Jam pix and missing my family as usual.

December 16, 2010

Here's the situation / been to every nation / nobody's ever made me feel the way that you do.

No one ever misses me as much as I miss them. Wonder why. I'm pretty cool!
DAVID M: *I miss u duh! Phone goes both ways lol*
DINA G: *So not true! Miss ya!!!*

ME: *Thanks guys.* ♥ *Love you all.*

Here's to you / raise your glass to everyone / here's to them / underneath that burning sun / Do they know it's Christmas time at all?

December 17, 2010

More pain in my right leg than your entire body. Need. Massage.

Back to school for parents' night out. LOVE that it's just gonna be Ashton and 2 from the next class... I feel serious Ashton-cuddle-time coming on!!
NICOLE O: *Where are you working?*
ME: *Kids R Kids in Frisco. Legacy and Lebanon. It's. Wonderful.*

December 17, 2010

This was a pretty good week. But I found out they're demolishing Adolfo's Papa John's when the new year starts, and he's being demoted. More reason to move out here. I love my job so much—my babies are so sweet, if not super loud sometimes. I can't wait to be done with the intern clinic so I can massage for money on Saturdays cause daycare doesn't pay much but I love it.

♥ *Me*

December 18, 2010

> What's everyone's favorite Christmas movie?
> JYNNI L: Too many to pick but Christmas Vacation with Chevy Chase and of course Charlie Brown Christmas... u?
> MARK R: Bad Santa with Billy Bob Thornton
> DAVID M: A Christmas story, oh and the holiday
> MISHA T: A Christmas Story!
> CAROL K: It's a Wonderful Life.
> ME: Love Actually. And I'm sad to say, of all these listed, I've only seen two, and they're both listed by YOU, Jenny! (There must be another Jenny missing.)
> ADOLFO F: Silent Night, Deadly Night. Does that count as a Xmas movie? I feel it should. LOL

> ME: Never heard of it. Sounds fun though.

> Sometimes Dr Pepper really tastes like pepper. Coincidence?

December 19, 2010

> I'm getting to the point where I dislike weekends. I can only take so much down time.

> Day full of fudge-making, house-cleaning, dog-grooming, and poker-playing. What a Sunday!!

> My Top Words of 2010: I'm annoyed that such little words count... but if they didn't RANGERS would be #1!!! Yea!!!! For 2011, it WILL BE. Who's up for a road trip to AZ in February??

> Holy crap. Losing entire set of keys in Target with Ruby locked in the car: better or worse than losing entire wallet in Target?? Cause I've now done both.

> Tostitos with a hint of lime are wicked addictive.

NOT THE F——ING GILMORE GIRLS

> *My first foray into fudge-making was very successful. I am much impressed with myself.*

December 20, 2010

> *Longest. Poker. Game. EVER.*
>
> *There's a rose in the fisted glove / and the eagle flies with the dove / and if you can't be with the one you love, honey / love the one you're with.*
>
> *Dilemma: so tired I could fall asleep right now, but there's a full moon total eclipse on the winter solstice, which hasn't happened in 464858264847 or so years. Dare I set an alarm???*

December 21, 2010

> *Early morning: Ruby woke me up to go to the bathroom but it's only just started. A little crescent shadow over the moon. Looks pretty much like a regularly waning moon. I'm afraid there's no reddish-brown wonder for me. I'm too old to do this again in two hours. Thanks for the early wake-up call, Ruby. Next time use an alarm clock.*

I'm laughing that at twenty-nine, I felt too old. But here I sit at forty-two, planning to be camping the next time there's a lunar eclipse. In my RV. On our great American road trip.

> *Aghh the cast of "Glee" will be at Hot Topic at the Galleria from 3-6 today!! No fair! Someone go for me and molest Harry Shum for me!!!!*
>
> *"Rhythm of Love" by Plain White T's = total goodness.*

December 22, 2010

> *I am unnaturally obsessed with the song "Bottoms Up." Which is unfortunate considering my hatred of Nikki Minaj.*

December 23, 2010

>I HATE *holiday traffic. And the way people act when they're shopping/driving/being.*
>
>*I am going to go to bed earlier tonight than I do on a work night. So. Tired.*

December 24, 2010

>*Is it wrong to get back in bed after Ruby wakes me up at 8:30? Technically she let me sleep in an hour, but if I'm not gonna sleep on my mini-break, what the hell else am I gonna do?*
>
>*I don't like this feeling. I almost feel nervous. Wish I was in Cali.*
>
>JOCELYN G: *we do tooooo, Angel*
>ME: *Thanks baby girl.* ♥

December 25, 2010

>*Definitely slept till 2 today and definitely ready to go back to sleep again.*
>
>*'Twas the night before Christmas and all through the house, not a creature was stirring, not even a mouse... Merry Christmas Eve to all of you. Hoping y'all with kids young enough to still believe the magic have the most fun ever!!!*
>
>*#1 most desired thing this cold Christmas morning: my family. #2: a boy and a fireplace. When those fail, I will happily take my puppy, a warm bed, and "Harry Potter and the Deathly Hallows." Miss you, Cali gang.* ♥
>
>HARPER H: *We miss you here in Connecticut too!*
>
>ME: *Miss you too. Hope y'all are having a grrrrreat day.*
>
>*Merry Christmas to my Facebook friends: family, people in my daily life, old Lake Highlands classmates, Jimmy's old buddies... Merry Christmas, one and all.*

Said the little lamb to the shepherd boy / "Do you hear what I hear / Ringing through the sky, shepherd boy? / Do you hear what I hear? / A song, a song, high above the trees / with a voice as big as the seas!"

Christmas dinner with my dad and his friends. Love my dad. ♥

December 26, 2010

Oh after-Christmas sales, I heart you!!

Wow my allergies must really be sucking the lifeblood from me. I've slept a lot this weekend but I'm still exhausted.

Yea I'm glad I still woke up early. Today might be bizzzzeeee.

Ruby is a walnut. That's it.

December 27, 2010

Happy Golden Birthday, Michael M!!

Has anyone played "Just Dance" or any other dance games for Wii? What are the verdicts?
  MISHA T: We have just dance 2. Had a blast dancing last night.
  ME: Is it a good workout?
  MISHA: if you do it on dance mode it is. I was sweating after three songs.

I like how when a two-year-old talks and you don't understand them, they have infinite patience repeating themselves over and over when you say "what?" They never raise their voice or get frustrated at your stupidity. Yet when they start asking "why?" over and over, we don't offer them the same patience. Bad adults.

December 28, 2010

So good to babysit the Buckley boys. I missed that special Danny smile. Really wish I could make myself go to bed, but I was so cold last night, I'm kind of dreading it.

Three more days to find a roommate. Anyone know someone who needs a place to crash for two months? Plano area, awesome place, $650! I'm getting nervous!

God I'm so glad to be off work. Tuesdays are the slowest day ever. Even with Jenny there. But today was the opposite of a time warp. It was a time suck. Jeez.

December 29, 2010

I have "ah big booty, big booty, big booty, ah yeah, big booty!" stuck in my head. Although I sub "booty" for "Ruby." Anyone know that game?

KATIE V: I think I have a new song for our Ruby. Oh gosh!
ME: Lol!! It's so addictive.

CARINA H: We used to play that game all the time.

Well it's Dec 29, rent is due in three days, and I'm officially out of ideas. How to get $600, folks? Suggestions welcome.
CLARISSA M: Donate plasma. You can get like $50-$100 for that at least. Take something valuable you own to the pawn shop.
DINA G: I hear ya sister, same boat, but need $1900 for mortgage & late fees. Sucks & so ready for better financial year than the past 2!!
ANNETTE W: Move to a cheaper place? Gamble... no not that. Babysit more!
ME: Clarissa, I thought about both... I have so few things, and nothing worth any value. Annette, we aren't allowed to babysit at the new school... People still do it on the side, but

> it's "illegal." Speaking of that though, I'll text you this weekend, I want to bring J his presents. And a poker game might just be the answer.
> ANNETTE: That's one of the reasons I like Parker Chase. A lot of schools won't let the teachers babysit.
> NICOLE O: I thought u were working?
> ME: Well, they say it's to protect families and teachers from things like valuables going missing. But if there's trust on both sides, there's no problem. Nicole, I am working. But I had a roommate but he had to move out (long story) and now I have to make $1100 rent myself. I'm lucky to get that in one month of work. I posted ads on craigslist and have done everything I can think of short of picking up a homeless person, but no roommate to be found.

I don't even know what roommate situation this was. My luck with roommates is astounding.

> I want to be a Dallas Cowboys Cheerleader. And the next JK Rowling. And a girlfriend. And a mom.
> CAROL K: What happened to The Rangers therapist?
> ME: Um. And massage therapist for the Texas Rangers. Duh!

Woo-hoo, I did put it in writing thirteen years ago, the one name I keep thinking as I write this. Thirteen years later, can we go for 50 percent and get a man-friend involved too?

December 30, 2010

> Cause when the roof caved in and the truth came out, I just didn't know what to do / but when I become a star, we'll be living so large / I'll do anything for you.

COURTNEY CANNON

December 31, 2010

What's going on tonight for everyone? New decade means big party!

Jelly Bellies are crack.

Rise of the Machines

January 1, 2011

Well, that's that. A new year (a new decade? Is it 2010-2019 or 2011-2020?) is upon us. Hopefully better than the last. Happy New Year, y'all.
JENNY W: The decade change was last year. Happy New Year!

I have a cleaning energy. Too bad my dog doesn't. She's partied out [with picture of baby Ruby crashed across my lap].
So much cleaning and only halfway done. And my apartment still has a weird smell... Someone come over and tell me if I'm imagining it! PS: moving queen sized mattresses around by yourself makes for some very sore fingertips and a tight SCM.
I wish falling asleep for ten minutes always made me feel this refreshed.

The Weight Loss Diaries, January 1, 2011

Wow, that is insane. 1-1-11. Wack. Anyway. There are no New Year's resolutions this time around. I can't start and fail another year. I always say I WILL do it this time, and then something happens and I lose all resolve. For the past month, I've been eating like a madwoman. Thank God my job keeps me up, down, and all around, or I would have gained back the 65 pounds it has taken me nearly 4 years to lose.
I can't believe another March is almost upon me. March 2007 was when I started this whole journey, the month after my mom's 50th birthday. She

said she'd never seen me bigger, and that it scared her. Now I weigh less than I did in high school. But here it seems to stop. It's been especially bad these past few days, and while I blame it on the intense stress, I can't put fault entirely on that. I've stuffed myself so full sometimes, I feel like puking, and at that point I'm like, no chance will I ever eat again. And then the next day... it starts all over.

What in the WORLD in my head keeps me thinking it will be different?? Bingeing always feels bad. Praise God I'm not bulimic, but isn't this just as bad? I'm still hurting myself, even if I keep it inside. I don't know what to do anymore, and all I can say is that I'm taking it one day at a time. I keep waiting for the moment that it's going to click: this is not what you want right now. Thankfully, my co-teacher has proven to me several times already that she has the strength to say no if she doesn't want something... vanilla cupcakes, for example. And hopefully her influence will start to rub off on me.

Once I get over this massive $1100 rent payment that I have to make all by myself, I am going to buy "Just Dance" for Wii. I also can't wait to start massaging again. That always burns a few extra calories. I'm also going to buy a calendar for my bathroom wall, right above my scale. I want to find a Biggest Loser wall calendar, but I don't know if they make those. Something inspirational anyway, and I am going to start weighing in once a week again. I still do my Wii scale every morning, but I have to start being accountable to myself again. Even if I gain, at least I need to see the numbers. Anyway!

I don't know why I do this to myself... it doesn't make me feel better when I'm sad... it actually makes me feel worse. But it's an addiction. One I would gladly trade for something else... but I don't like coffee that much, I HATE smoking, and drinking puts chub on your body too... I wish I could trade food for dancing... maybe this game will help with that, cause I LOVE to dance. But I also really love food. YIKES! Let the games begin...

Happy New Year, all!

Starting weight (again)(at last scale-time): 211.8

Goal for January 8 (Elvis's birthday!): 209.8

So weird!! Mark Salling was an answer to a crossword puzzle in People magazine! It's one thing to see his picture everywhere, but this is a whole new level of craziness.

CLARISSA: I TOTALLY saw his CD at Target! I was like WHHHATTTT???

ME: Omg a CD on his own or with Glee?? You know he went to my high school?

CLARISSA: It was his solo CD!!! I saw it in the Best Seller's section. I didn't know he went to your HS! How cool!

ME: A kind of mind-melter. Lake Highlands has churned out some stars, but Mark beats them all now.

January 2, 2011

Well, I've gained like 8 pounds over the past 3 days. I'm chugging water like a mad woman today, hoping to flush my body. I made a calendar for my weight loss. I'm gonna get back on track if it kills me. I have to pay $1100 rent by myself so I have less than zero money to go grocery shopping. I need fruit and fiber for my house—school lunches will do the trick. Not the healthiest food, but it's small portions. I don't even know what else to write. I'm keeping a Weight Loss Diary on Facebook. I wanna lose 40 (including the 10 I put back on) by June & Cuz Jam. Right now I'm 216. Jeez! This month was crazy for me. I want that thing to click back into place. We'll see...

♥ Me

I'm only gonna break break your break break your heart.

"All you people can't you see, can't you see / NKOTBSB!" There's something absurd about watching middle-aged men bounce around to songs they first performed as teenagers yet... I. Can't. Stop.

Cadbury Eggs. Really?? It's too early for Valentine's day, people!! Whoever is in charge of retail, let me clue you in: people look for Cadbury Eggs around Easter. They want sweaters in winter and bathing suits in summer (spring is fair enough). You're just driving people who are trying to lose weight CRAZY!!

49 calories short of my limit today. Of course that's not factoring in exercise.

I posted a picture of Ruby lying on the treadmill: yes, the treadmill has become a dog bed. Anyone want to buy it from me? $50 O B O. I basically need someone to haul it away.

The Weight Loss Diaries, January 2, 2011

So my guess for my weigh-in was way off. As of this morning, I was 216. That's unbelievable so I am keeping my goal the same, hoping that it was a fluke on the scale. 6 more days to get to 209... we will see.

The Weight Loss Diaries, January 3, 2011

Holy crap. So I just bought a calendar for my bathroom wall. It's a Food Network calendar, and there's recipes and stuff in it. So I went back through last year's Elvis calendar to see what I weighed every day... this day last year, I was only 9 pounds heavier than I am now. EEEEEEKKK!!! What's worse... in APRIL, I was only three pounds away from being under 200!! THREE POUNDS!!! That's so many months just wasted. I wrote the weight I was last year in my new calendar in hopes that will light a fire...

Today was pretty easy eating-wise. Until I went to Target for some groceries on an empty stomach. That was fun. I managed to stay on budget, and I used a gift card from one of my families to buy Just Dance 2. I was so hungry by the time I got home that I didn't do it yet... but I will tomorrow... fish and edamame and rice for dinner... so yummy! But now it's 9:12 and I feel hungry again... hopefully cereal will do the trick. And it all starts again tomorrow.

On the bright side, my Wii said I lost 2.9 pounds since yesterday. That's exciting and kind of another good way to light a fire.

The Weight Loss Diaries, January 4, 2011

I'm so happy "The Biggest Loser" is on again so soon. I hope they continue to be back-to-back... it makes MY journey much easier. I am a little astonished that I didn't cry during the first five minutes... I usually do. It wasn't even the show itself that made me cry tonight... it was the song they played while the contestants pushed the truck: "Dare you to Move," by Switchfoot. "Dare you to move, dare you to move, dare you to lift yourself up off the floor." PERFECT. Dare me to do something and say I won't... great song for the occasion.

I spent all day being starving. I felt like I didn't stop eating. My metabolism has certainly kicked back into gear, and if I can keep it up... fingers crossed. I massaged tonight, so no dance workout. It's going to be hard to do it on nights when I massage. I might do it during lunch, but that is of course after I find a bloody apartment that doesn't cost as much as a house.

COURTNEY CANNON

The Weight Loss Diaries (and More), January 5, 2011

Well, it's getting somewhat easier and somewhat harder. As I mentioned yesterday, my metabolism is going at such a rate that I feel hungry all the time. And then I get busy, and don't eat, and then I'm STARVING by 6. Which is what happened tonight and I almost got Chick-Fil-A for dinner, but luckily I was on the phone and missed the turn I would have taken, so I just went home. HA. Made a burger and fries, but made it the good way...and measured everything out. Also danced my non-existent ASS off at Just Dance 2... BAD. ASS. GAME. I chose the "intermediate" program for the first week... which they predicted would be about three songs a day, and turned into 5 for me cause I am TERRIBLE at dancing, so I got "perfect" like once. It was so fun though... I am determined to memorize those dances. My shoulders hurt...which just goes to show what a full-bod workout dancing is. LOVE.

On a separate note, but also attributing to my intense calorie-burning today: I found the apartment of my dreams. It's at a brand new complex, and while it's a little on the pricier side, it's so gorgeous it's worth it. Plus, and get this: for $30 I get to move in and get free rent for two months. That's right. They're running a special that's $99 for admin, application, and deposit (which normally totals $375...) and that also includes March rent. But since I work in the area, they knocked it down to $30. WHAT! As if that isn't good enough, if I sign a 12-month lease on a certain floor plan (which happens to be the one I want), I get April rent free too. WHATTTTTT!!!!! The silver lining is too good to ignore the clouds... Now all I need is to be approved, which may or may not happen, but for $30, I'll take my chances. EEEEEK!!!!! So I spent the entire afternoon running at the mouth to anyone who would listen, more than usual, and had so much adrenaline, my blood never slowed down. I hope I burned some stuffs.

AND another note: I watched a 30th-anniversary special for Michael Jackson tonight. My guess it was 12-13 years old. But it was stellar. 98 Degrees and N Sync performed, as did Usher and a bunch of other people... but my attention was on Usher, and Justin Timberlake, for the 5 seconds he was on stage... I've always known they idolize him, but you should have seen their faces. They were like kids in a candy store, especially JT.

I would do anything anything ANYTHING to be able to see MJ in concert... he was amazing. I started crying when they sang "Heal the World," just thinking... this man is DEAD. UN. REAL. Every time I see anything on him... it's been over a year, and it's so weird. People in the audience were crying and screaming in ecstasy... can you imagine having that kind of impact on people?? And he's "Gone Too Soon..."

In my head, I see you all over me / In my head, you fulfill my fantasy / you'll be screaming ohhhh / in my head, it's going down.

Omg, Ruby made the worst mess in her cage. It must have been poop AND barf because it was EVERYWHERE. Was it the avocado and Nerds she snuck last night? And the idiot wonders why I don't give her people food.

January 7, 2011

I want to do a Disney cruise now that I'm grown. Who's down?
   ANNETTE W: Done it twice. Doing it with Jasper this summer. Can't wait!
   ME: Omg Annette how fun is it for an adult?? I did it when I was ten or eleven and it was, expectedly, magical. I want to go soooon.

So bodily broken, didn't want to do my dancing tonight but then thought how annoying it would be to do it tomorrow and have my Wii remind me that I skipped a day. Now I'm glad I did it but reaaaaallllly nervous about giving four back-to-back massages tomorrow. I hurt.

January 8, 2011

"It's always better when we're together."

Happy birthday to the King of Rock and Roll!! And Kate Rose. And a bunch of other people.

Do you think Natalie Portman can really dance? She's so hot.

The Weight Loss Diaries, January 9, 2011

Hey, party people! Well, I didn't hit my 209 goal, but I did lose 4.4 pounds this week! I'm at 212 even and super excited. My body hurts like a mo-fo, whether from this new dancing video or massaging or both, I don't know, but I'm sore in places I didn't even know existed. I'm gonna just keep chuggin' along... my friend Adolfo is coming in town this week, and I'm planning on a nuts-fatty dinner with him Tuesday night, but I promise to work extra hard for the rest of the week to balance it out! Not to mention, I did 4.5 hours of massage today, and in effect didn't come NEAR eating what I should have to fuel my body after THAT workout. Hopefully that will give me a good jump start. I'm a bit nervous about being home all day tomorrow. It's always harder to not eat when I'm bored. I would almost just rather sleep the whole day away. It's so much easier at work.

So I'm going to do a "journey in pictures" blog...or a pictures folder. I am gonna include high school pix to show what I looked like as a senior... since I weigh less now than I did as an 18-year-old. And then pix at my heaviest, which was in February of '07. That means in one month, it will be four YEARS of doing this... and I've got 55 pounds to show for it. Used to be 65, but this past couple months SUUUCKED.

NOT THE F——ING GILMORE GIRLS

Anyway. I'm doing this mainly because I really don't feel like I look that different. With Biggest Loser contestants, you usually can't even recognize them. So not the case with me. I mean, 65 pounds is a lot of weight! Maybe when I reach my final goal, it'll be more pronounced? But I can't find pix of my mom's 50th birthday, where she told me she'd never seen me bigger, nor my G-ma's 80th bday, which was exactly a year and 25 pounds later. Those are the two events that stand out in my mind, so I'm going to fish around for those pix, and when I get them, I'll have a little album for your viewing pleasure. Or horror, as the case may be. If I can't find them, NONE of you will know what I looked like at 265… which may be just as well. GROSS. And stunning… I will never understand how I got that big.

Okie doke, y'all…another week is upon us, and I hope it's another stellar one… please keep reading, and I'd love feedback… for those of you who don't know, I am a narcissist through and through, and I thrive on people watching me.

Bless my heart for ever thinking that loving myself as much as I did made me a narcissist. Also, I am in the exact same position right now. Now four years on this journey, I am 55 pounds down from my heaviest, which this time was 280! This time, I will reach my goal and stay there.

First snowfall of the season. Hopefully there's more to come.

Watching Legally Blonde and coming to terms with the fact that I love Reese Witherspoon more than the average bear.

November 10, 2011

Well, I lost 4.5 lbs the first week. PSYCHED! I made rent, thanks to Jimmy & Annette, who bought 10 hours of babysitting. Hmmm… I found the most beautiful new apartment & if I get approved, I get 2 months free. WHAT! Let's see—Adolfo is coming up tomorrow. Super excited of course. Get to go to Fogo or fondue, and I gotta work hard for the rest of the week to balance out. We are gonna watch movies all night and all Wednesday. Fun. AJ's dad asked if I babysat yea!! I ♥ my AJ. Anyway I guess that's really it so far.

♥ Me

Who noticed that entry read November 10, 2011, mere days after pledging to write weekly? But it alarmed me that I seemed to be talking about the same thing, so I flipped the page and realized I made a dating error. But then here I come to insert some photographic memories, thanks to my iPhone, and that is of the delightful day I adopted my sweet dog: January 14, 2010, a day written down in infamy.

I went with a friend to see the puppies, determined not to have a blonde and not to have a female. Here comes the singular blonde and singular female, climbing into my lap like she owned me. Little did I know, she did. I wanted to name her Penny Lane, but then someone on Facebook said we went to high school with a girl named that, and I was like, *nope*! So she became Ruby Rose. She was tiny as a baby, and my friend who went with me nicknamed her Tater Tot. I was convinced she was a full-blooded dachshund, but her terrier legs betrayed her later in life. She is the redheaded stepchild in a family of purebreds, but she is my everything.

There's a meme where someone is standing in front of a dog sitting on a throne in heaven, and it says, "So let me get this straight. Your entire species is dyslexic?" Or you know, something like that, but it's so accurate. Dogs provide forgiveness, second chances, and unconditional love no matter how we abuse or disappoint them. You can talk to a dog, pray to a dog, and hope to a dog. All I know is, all dogs definitely go to heaven.

This will likely not be the only time I write about my angel dog, but it was fun to remember the smile I got when she clambered into my lap. So back to business…

January 12, 2011

I am so ridiculous. I want to tell Adolfo what I got him for Christmas but I can't so I'm making him guess.

So exciting to have a day off in the middle of the week. Fun planned. Fingers crossed the school doesn't call.

> *If I said I want your body now / would you hold it against me?*

> *Jeeeeeez, please remind me never to go in a Condom Sense with a boy who is not my boyfriend.*

> *Pic of Ruby being scratched by Adolfo, looking into the camera, her eyes sparkling from the flash, "Hypnotized by the thought of popcorn and kisses."*

July 28, 2011

> *A 15-year-old girl holds hands with her 1 yr old son. People call her a slut; no one knows she was raped at 13. People call another guy fat. No one knows he has a serious disease causing him to be overweight. People call an old man ugly. No one knows he had a serious injury to his face while fighting for our country in the war. Repost if you are not okay with bullying or stereotyping in any form.*

August 25, 2011

> *Out bowling with Adolfo, my score was 333 after the third game. And 444 after the fourth. Unreal. (And yes, there are pictures.) Then I watched him play Guitar Hero.*

August 27, 2011

> *I'm thinkin Chick-Fil-A for my final carb-filled dinner.*

August 29, 2011

Weight Loss Diaries, Atkins Day 2

> *First day at work: BINGO! Never had one sugar craving (a real one, anyway. Doesn't mean I didn't think I wanted something sweet. Thank God for Extra Desserts gum). I only felt hungry once, and that was at 11:30, roughly four hours after I'd eaten breakfast. I'm a little nervous to partake in one of the Atkins*

bars because it's 3 net carbs and I am only allowed 20! But it wasn't an issue today. Weight: 214.8 (down 1.2 pounds from yesterday!)

Breakfast: Coffee with half and half and four Splendas (4 net carbs), 2 eggs, 2 Owens sausage patties, 1 laughing cow cheese wedge (1 net carb), 3 Benefiber tablets (5 net carbs... SO ANNOYING!!)

Lunch: 3oz tuna in water, half a cucumber with salt (2 net carbs), 1 boiled egg, 1oz cheddar cheese (1 net carb), a couple squirts Ranch Wishbone spray

Snack: 1oz mozzarella cheese (1 net carb)

Dinner: 6oz (!!!!!!) 93/7 ground beef made with chili powder, cumin seed, and salt (tacos without the shell... AWESOME!!!), 1oz cheddar cheese (1 net carb), 1/2 c edamame (2 net carbs).

17 net carbs...and 1300 calories. MUCH more acceptable. But not enough veggies... I'm going to get the hang of this really quickly. I'm having a Fresca for dessert right now and watching "Tough Cookies" on the Food Network so I can dream of the sweet things I can't have. A friend of mine told me about a candy store for diabetics somewhere that I forgot the name of, but in a couple of weeks I plan on checking it out. I've got to find a carb-free candy. LOL. But then again, maybe in a couple of weeks, I won't even miss it. Here's hoping.

August 30, 2011

Weight Loss Diaries, Atkins Day 3

WOW!!! That's all I can say. Day 3 began with a bang: I'd woken up once in the middle of the night having to pee from so much water. I had a hard time falling asleep both the first time and when I woke up. But I got out of bed pretty easily and weighed myself and...4 pounds down from Sunday!!!! Whoop!! Weight: 212. Breakfast and lunch and then naaaaaaaaap. Woke up not feeling great with NO appetite. Made myself eat an Atkins bar just to stay full through the night. Delicious AND nutritious at 10 g fiber, 19 g protein, and only 2 net carbs.

Yeah the cucumber was the only veggie I got today but I also only had 10 net carbs. Now I'm popping two Tylenol PM and going back to bed. Tired. Even with the vitamins and this new sugar-free diet. Hope my body gets used to it soon. LOVE this weight dropping thing. ♥

August 31, 2011

It's amazing how a friend's hard time can make me feel so out-of-sorts. I can think of nothing that should be stressing me out and yet I just want to curl up in bed and watch movies. I'm empathetic. And wish it would all be over.

Weirdest headache ever. RAIN please!

September 5, 2011

I set fire to the rain.

This weather makes me wants to go to the State Fair. Three more weeks! Wish I could afford to go every day!!!!!!!!!

Jamming Bruno Mars Radio on Pandora, finishing cleaning my apartment, and dreaming about how good white rice would taste with the pot roast I'm having for dinner.

All right, Texas, the cooler weather was nice but WE NEED RAIN!! These fires are scary.

September 6, 2011

Wow!! I could legitimately wear a jacket right now!!

Catch 22 of the day: I'm in so much pain pretty much all I wanna do is lay down, but I think laying down is what caused my pain in the first place. Preeeeeetty positive this girl needs a new mattress.

> *If you want to view paradise / simply look around and view it / Anything you want to, do it / Want to change the world / there's nothing to it*

> *It's weird that hair grows longer in certain body places than others. Wouldn't it be wicked annoying if your arm hair grew as long as your head hair? Just sayin.*

October 12, 2011

> *Nelson Cruz = Sexiest Man ALIVE*

> *CRUUUUUUZ in 111 AGAAAAAAIN!!!! WTF is THIS!!! LOVE HIM!!!!!*

October 29, 2011

> *I knew it was over last night, as hard as it was to admit it. One more year, here we come.*

(Or twelve years.)

November 1, 2011

> *Well so much for writing every day, eh? I used to use this book for writing things I didn't want other people to know, but this time I'm gonna write it like a story, and it's a story I've shared with everyone, because it's not one I want to forget.*
>
> *Saturday night was Val's party. I looked super hot & I knew it. A vixen vampire wench with red hair, I felt sexy & confident & ready to have a good time. When Nathan showed up, Val jumped on me immediately, "Tonight's the night with Nathan!" I rebuffed her because I wasn't drinking yet, and come on, he's a cute 25 year old who's two inches shorter and 50 pounds smaller. But she was insistent.*
>
> *So the more I drank, the more outgoing I got. When he took off his wig, I asked to put color in his hair, & he let me. So somehow I started playing with his hair & that turned into a massage. He was falling asleep & was obviously really into it. Eventually*

I stopped & he said, "Okay, your turn," and started giving me one. He was pretty good, and then all of a sudden he said, "I'll be right back," and disappeared for like half an hour.

This is when it starts getting blurry—the timeline gets a little skewed. We had spent some time outside with Kirsty, and we were being flirty & I even took a drag of his cigarette. Then somehow we went back inside (to listen to Bryce play guitar) and Val pulled me into her room to tell me Nathan had sent Crista a text that said, "I need Courtney's #, I'm into that." Lol.

I was buzzed enough to not get nervous. We went back into the living room & somehow it got decided that we'd watch "Anchorman." This is where I lose track completely—cause I said I didn't want to watch a movie, that I'd fall asleep, but I have no idea how I ended up back outside alone with Nate.

So he had me sit down so he can finish my massage. I ask him how long he could keep it up & he said he could go all night. We were listening to the movie & the song "Afternoon Delight" comes on & I asked what other movie it was from (I forgot to mention he's a huge movie freak, & we traded quotes). He didn't know, so I gave him a quote. "How do you like dem apples?" By this time, I was leaning backwards into him & he was squeezing my upper arms, his chin on my shoulder. He still couldn't get it from the quote, so I said "Matt Damon" & he got it.

He was sort of kissing the side of my face & I asked him if he wanted to move, so we got up & went to sit on the patio bench. I had my feet up on the table & I was shaking uncontrollably—whether from cold or hormones or a mix of both, it was intense. We started kissing easily & it was amazing—not slimy or smoky, perfect amount of tongue, a little lip sucking & biting action. He. Is. A. Phenomenal. Kisser.

Anyway, I wish there was a way to write down all that happened—it's going to fade eventually and it was so wonderful. He'd kiss my neck & my chest & the top of my boobs (I was wearing a corset). After about two hours of kissing outside, he asked if I wanted to go lay down for a while. I totally did—and if we'd had a bed and a condom, I probably would have slept with him. But both rooms were occupied (I found out later that Val wanted to kick Crista out of the bed for us!). So we stood in the hallway & made out for another hour.

 I'm getting butterflies just thinking about it. Damn it was so hot—I was running my hands up & down his spine, over his butt—& he was doing the same, & I didn't even care that he was touching my stomach. He kept saying I was a great kisser & "so sexy" but then he was also saying how soft I am (I hope he meant my skin, not my fluff) & how "comfortable" lol! So it was so awesome, and I said I didn't want him to forget it, and he said the same back to me. Then he got my number & said he wanted to do it again & fucking kissed me goodbye in front of all our friends—not a peck, a real kiss. F!!!

 I told Val & Crista all about it & they said I should invite him over for breakfast. So I did. I wonder if he'd come (his phone had died), what would have happened. Anyway, long story short, a few days later he told me he didn't want a relationship. I told him that was fine; all I wanted to do was kiss him. So we decided to be friends with benefits—and then NOTHING. I didn't hear from him for a week. I knew the instant I got okay with never seeing him again, he'd text me. And he did, last night (11-11). I asked him to hang out tonight & no answer. It's like he wants to do the initiating, but he won't. Fucking boys. Now he's got me hooked all over again & I have to go through another week hoping...

♥ Me

November 6, 2011

 I am thankful for my imagination. Wishing for an outlet...

Ohhhhhh emmmmmm geeeeeee, all new episodes of Beavis and Butthead!!!!! I'm so excited to watch this show when I'm actually old enough to appreciate it!!!!!! Don't judge. (Get it?)

This getting dark at 6 PM thing gets old before it's new.

November 20, 2011

Third night of waking up at an ungodly hour. Although this time I can't get back to sleep.

> *KATHERINE H: Kelly Clarkson looks a lot like my niece Courtney.*
> *KATHERINE: I should add that I'm watching the AMA awards, not just fantasizing about kc.*

Quite possibly the worst headache of my life.

I'm thankful for three shifts at Palio's this weekend. $70 in tips doesn't hurt either.

November 21, 2011

On this 21st night of thankfulness, I'm feeling a sense of déjà vu. Have I done 20 nights of the same stuff??

> *MEGAN G: If you'll be my bodyguard, I can be your long lost pal*

> *ME: You can call me Al*

I'm thankful for my amazing co-teachers. You ladies make it much more fun to come to work. Thank you for always being my sounding board, even and especially when it has nothing to do with work.

Ruby is not digging the thunder. And I am.

November 22, 2011

Feliz in the rotaaaaation!! Is it April 1 yet???

So far the only negative I see in being up this late on a work night is that I'm really freakin' hungry.

1 hour of sleep didn't faze me yet. Talk to me after working at Park and Preston. Come seeeeee meeeeee!

Jeez, the nap thing didn't even work. Apparently my body has stopped needing sleep.

Park and Preston in Plano, people. Please prepare participate in pizza.

Finally pictures of the new store.

KATHERINE H: Thanks! It's gorgeous. Can't wait to eat there.

Finally sleepy. And so slow at work. Probably why I'm sleepy. Not to mention this long day stuff is about to wreak havoc on my knees.

I'm thankful for money. I'm thankful for money. I'm thankful for money.

I am an adult. That's pretty scary for all the real adults out there.

November 23, 2011

Four day weekend stretching ahead of me. Joy!

Fun night at Valerie's.

November 24, 2011

I'm thankful for vanilla vodka and Valerie Cheese. Not necessarily in that order.

Happy Thanksgiving!! On my way to the brother's, then to one family LUNCH in Dallas followed by another family DINNER in Plano. I've only been through one Thanksgiving where I don't have an appetite, and that was when I had the stomach flu. Interested to see what today has in store!

> KATHERINE H: *Happy turkey day, Court. Give your mom and bro a hug for us and keep one for yourself. Maybe next year in Cali?*
> ME: *Absolutely. Hopefully every year from now on. We are all going to get rich over the next eight months.*
> RYAN U: *Just found out that Courtney, Jocelyn, Kevin, Trevor, Harper, Patrick, Anne, Kealeilani and Rozie aren't coming to thanksgiving. this is just not what i wanted. screw the turkey and ham i just want cousins to come play with me.*
> MEGAN U: *Seriously!!! So not the same*
> ME: *Love you Ry.*
> JOCELYN G: *I don't even like ham, ya know.*
>
> HARPER H: *I wish I was with you guysss. it's so much more fun with the fam.*

I posted a picture of lunch at Nanny Anne's, complete with deviled eggs, a picture of Ruby looking adorable in a purple bow captioned, "Thanksgiving festive," and pictures of Audrey, Grace, and Norah captioned, "Grace torturing Norah. And vice versa."

November 27, 2011

> *Give me everything tonight / For all we know / We might not get tomorrow / Let's do it tonight*
> ME: *Learned all over again (a couple of times this weekend!) how true these words are. My heart goes out to everyone who's lost someone too soon.*
>
> *Watching Cast Away: I know it's fictional, but could anyone walk away after six solitary years without some serious psychological damage??*

I'm live on TikTok right now, and a woman in my chat said she was having trouble waking up after fall break. I was rubbing my face and said, "Luckily, the dogs wake me up, so I've never really gotten offtrack, so to speak, even when I'm sleeping all day." And then, y'all, here comes this entry. Wow!

November 28, 2011

It's amazing how quickly your body falls out of the waking-up-early routine, even and most especially when you don't get to bed that early. And while I mean me to an extent, I really mean Ruby, who had to be CARRIED out of the bed.

25 and freeze windshields!! If I had known, I'd a left my house much earlier than 6:17. But I LOVE IT!!
ME: Freezy not freeze. DYA.
LISA P: oh man! Thx for the warning!
CRISTA L: Dislike your crazy

NATHAN: "I'm a narcissist."
Me: "Me too."
Nathan: "Yeah, if there was another one of me running around, I'd f*** him." Bahahahahahaha.

November 30, 2011

Watching American Horror Story: This show freaks me the eff out and disturbs me in countless ways but I can't stop watching it.

December 1, 2011

Happy birthday to the sweetest, funniest, cutest, most aggravating, monkey-buttiest dog in the world. You're a teenager now, Ruby. No wonder you've been so damn moody.
JUSTIN J: Happy b-day Ruby. Good day to be born.
MEGAN G: Ruby!!!! Happy birthday!!!
KATHERINE H: We love Ruby! She has fans in New England.

December 2, 2011

KISS FM was discussing an ESPN discussion: Peyton Manning for Tony Romo next year? Which is better, a old sore Manning or a... Romo?
ME: And of course that's supposed to be AN old sore Manning.

ANDREW B: *Romo is a great QB*
NICK C: *Romo is not great but he is good and he didn't have to have anything in his neck fused together. PS. hey peyton look left now look right oh thats right my bad you cant lol*

December 3, 2011

Ashton started off his dinner gesturing at the mac and cheese when he wanted more. He ended it SIGNING for more!! I'm so excited!!

Watching Sister Act: I remember watching this in theaters and everyone clapped at the end, which I hadn't heard anyone do in years. Great.

December 4, 2011

Watching Sixteen Candles—Love John Hughes films!!

Any of y'all FMJH/LHHS people remember Tiger Bull's? I got a weird craving for their chicken tenders the other day and it's stuck in my head. Remember going there after exams were over?

Checked in to Buffalo Wild Wings. Every football game imaginable. Besides the Cowboys.

Pic of Jasper under a denim jacket with a spoon sticking out of his mouth: "J-Fred at the campfire."

December 5, 2011

Let it flurry, let it flurry, let it flurry!

MEGAN G: *Can you please send me the recipe for your cookies?? One of the girls is asking for it.*
ME: *my recipes.com, Peanut Butter-Toffee Turtle Cookies*

Checked into Fogo de Chao: I'm such a frickin carnivore.

December 6, 2011

> It is beautifully cold and there's a freeze warning. I'm cuddled at home with a pizza and my dog. The only way this could get any better would be if I had a boy by me and a day off tomorrow.
>
> CRISTA L: Beautifully, cold and freeze cannot be in the same sentence together!
>
> ME: Uh just did
>
> CRISTA: Well my goosebumps don't like it! I'm freezing and just thinking of how cold it was out today makes me shivvvvver!
>
> ME: Grab a blanket and go curl up with your baby boy. I'd give anything for someone to cuddle with!
>
> CRISTA: Coby hates me today... and I am under a blanket!
>
> ME: Lol why does he hate you?

December 7, 2011

> ONE bad thing about the cold: getting dressed in the morning. I don't want to get out of my warm bed or move Ruby's warm little body. [I posted a picture of my dashboard saying twenty-two degrees and captioned it, "Wowza."]
>
> Watermelon Twizzlers Pull&Peel smell like bananas and taste like waterwaterwaterwaterwatermelon. Not impressed. But on the bright side, I got them for like $.46 as opposed to the normal $3.50 and they came on the side of the crackalicious Sour Twizzlers.

December 8, 2011

> It is amazing how quickly a stomach flu spreads. It's the one thing that's guaranteed to make its rounds and shoot down everyone in its path. Except me of course. Because I don't get sick. Miss you, neighbor!!!
>
> KARLA G: That includes me I feel like crap! Lol

LISA: *Thanks Courtney. I'm hoping I'm on the mend. I had toast yesterday and toast this morning. So far so good. Anyone else sick?*

ME: *Renee. And every kid in the building! And Karla. Who would have a sucky time sky-diving if she was puking.*

Wow, CJ!! Texas will sort of miss you!

ABRA N: *yeah...sort of...*

ADOLFO F: *LOL, as soon as the World Series ended every Ranger fan knew he wasn't coming back. No surprise, just a fact finally coming true.*

ME: *Totally true. No surprise, big relief. He's a cocky asshole that only got cockier once the Angels signed him. Good riddance.*

Soooo tired. If I don't sleep through the night tonight, I might not get out of bed in the morning. Fair warning, KRK peeps.

December 9, 2011

Looooong but gooooood day. I think LeighAnn and I finally found our place. I worked like a dog and my feet are barking to show for it. I got an AWESOME white elephant gift for tomorrow, and a delicious bottle of whipped cream vodka to try. Spiked hot chocolate, anyone??

December 10, 2011

Watching The Secret Circle: This show is so much better than I ever would have guessed.

December 11, 2011

Oh my god, best doormat ever. Matt's house for a little after-party! With a pic of the doormat that says "hi. I'm mat."

It's four o'clock in the morning, what did we even do??

ADOLFO F: *Not a DAMN thing!*

Excited. This place smells amazing.

Well, we have a place! Home, sweet home it will be! 5 minutes from Lake Lewisville (hello, summer!) and absolutely stunning, it's only $100 more than I am paying NOW. I CANNOT WAIT TILL FEBRUARY!!!!

Seven pictures were added to "Adventures with Roommates" folder on FB, silly shots taken by someone else. We looked happy and drunk. I also uploaded pictures with Christal and Misha at the KRK Christmas party and updated my profile picture to me and LeighAnn.
PEDRO R: *Prety girlds*
ME: *Gracias Pedro!!*

Watching Love and Other Drugs: This movie is hella sexy

December 12, 2011

Checked in at Palio's Frisco: Another holiday party!

December 13, 2011

Pedro R tagged me in a picture with LeighAnn, with Hunter doing bunny ears behind her, captioning it, "New friens."
ME: *Is Hunter doing bunny ears to LeighAnn?*
PEDRO: *jaja LeighAnn the bunny. Isa secret do not tell. Mis novias me borran porque se casan jajajaja*

Checked in at Palio's Plano. Hungry? We're open semi-late. Come seeee meeeee.

December 14, 2011

At Palio's Plano: Every time I work here I want the ice cream, and I don't even like Blue Bell that much. Come seeeee meeeeee!

I'm not afraid of thunderstorms but I am afraid of the dark. I'm not afraid of close spaces until you put a bunch of people around me. I'm not afraid of dying but I am afraid of living alone.

December 15, 2011

Antsy. I've had my fingers crossed for so long they're starting to cramp. Something good needs to happen.

DAVID A: *Don't wait for good things to happen, go make them happen! You are the master of your own destiny.*

December 16, 2011

Checked into KRK Legacy West with Lisa M and 5 others. Parents' Night Out... Lottsa kids here tonight = lottsa money!!

December 17, 2011

It is so far past my bedtime and I have a double at Palio's tomorrow, but I had two diet cherry cokes tonight, so here I sit. Y'all come see me, please!!!! I'm probably not going to be diggin' being there, so come get some food and make me happy!! Legacy location tomorrow...

MEGAN G: *Legacy and what?*

ME: *Warren*

Lisa tagged me in a picture with Allie holding up a really ugly sweater (not Christmas, though).

ME: *Looooooool!!!!! Allie's face!!!! This sweater is* AWESOME *but I need a Christmas one.*

December 18, 2011

Ugly sweaters aren't cheap!! Hitting Walmart tomorrow in hopes of finding a sweatshirt. Got my tights though, and they're tacky enough alone!!! Can't wait till Thursday!

KATHERINE H: Have you tried consignment stores? There's one here that actually rents ugly holiday sweaters—and they have some amazing ones. Wish you lived closer...

CRISTA L: I can make you one... I miss you!

ME: Kath, I'm sure I should know where a consignment store is, but...I'm not even sure I know WHAT one is. I'll be honest, wearing clothes that have been worn before me creeps me out. LOL.

AUDREY M: Try JC Penney. I got mine from qvc.com but it's a little late for shipping unless you overnight it. The quacker factory brand on qvc has some great ones.

JENNIFER M: Try Goodwill!

Man I love waking up early on a Sunday and having no need or desire to go back to sleep. It's only nine and I've already watched two shows, started laundry, and I'm headed to Target to get shopping done. I have the whole day stretching ahead to do Christmas presents and a little candy-making!

LISA M: Candy? Did you say CANDY? Will your secret Santa be getting candy?!

ME: Lol not homemade! But my parents will be.

It's interesting how some places stick in your mind and some don't. I've been to Crista's a million times but I can never remember how to get there.

CRISTA: *Just follow the yellow brick road!*

Who should be more insulted here, Crista or me?: the cashier at Walmart thought we were mother and daughter. On the off chance that I actually LOOK 30 today (which is unlikely while wearing minimal makeup and a backwards Rangers cap), the most he could have thought Crista looked was 15. AND we had Coby!!! Lolololololololol!!!!

NOT THE F——ING GILMORE GIRLS

Bummed that my fudge isn't working. Last year's was perfect; this year the flavor is good but the texture is way too hard.

CRISTA L: *Did you burn it?*
ME: *No way*
SANDER W: *Not stirred enough?*
MEGAN U: *I just made the easiest fudge recipe today... If you need a last ditch effort!!!!*
ME: *Sander, I don't think so. Megan, thanks but I think I'm just gonna do boxes of chocolate, haha*

Going redder. Re-red. Excited.
ADOLFO F: *Like EMILIE AUTUMN red rite!??*
ME: *Which is hotter, hers or Hayley's?*
ADOLFO: *Emilie's for red, Hayley's for orange.*
ME: *Well here's hoping it's like Emilie's then, cause my skin tone would revolt at orange.*

Springsteen is rad

December 19, 2011

Man, do I have a crush!

December 20, 2011

Checked in at Palio's Frisco: Werk.
LISA M: *While you are werking...go check your messages!*

When the roof caved in and the truth came out, I just didn't know what to do.

December 21, 2011

Well I'm officially dehydrated. If the crippling leg cramps at 4:00 this morning weren't clue enough, the imprint of my 2-ounce phone on my stomach (where I laid it this morning to make sure I'd hear my alarm) would clinch it.

Checked in to American Airlines Center: Go Stars!!!

I posted a picture of me and LeighAnn with Santa at the Stars, then in our new Stars hats, grinning at the camera.

KATHERINE H: Omg, two gorgeous babes!!

ME: lol thanks aunt Kathy!

Little post-game drinking our blues away (at Sherlock's)

December 22, 2011

LeighAnn and I totally just got busted at Sherlock's for a counterfeit $20. Bull. Shiz.

I'm gonna be scared to drive on 423 when it's finished. I don't know if I'll understand how to navigate a non-dark-twisty-turny-dippy-scary-shitty road. Except that EVERY OTHER ROAD IN FRISCO / LITTLE ELM WAS COMPLETED IN 8 MONTHS. And I totally had time to type all that in traffic on 423. Joy.

December 23, 2011

Listening to Bryce play. Good end to a good night.

Well last night was awesome! (Ugly sweater party at Val's.) I was drunk by 9:30, bit my lip FIVE times (ANY time I ate anything), sobered up by midnight, and then FLIP CUP. Beautiful tacky outfit was a hit, but not enough of one to win the fruitcake. Today I have a mild headache and a lip swollen to the size of a golf ball. Success!

MEGAN G: Where are the pictures of your outfit, young lady????

ME: Coming! I. Am. Not. Sober. Still

I just got told my personality matched my hair by a beautiful man with a British accent. Hope it was a compliment.

KATHERINE H: I'm sure it was a compliment unless you dyed your hair puke green.

ME: Lol true

NOT THE F——ING GILMORE GIRLS
Damn this is a high-scoring game! Go Stars!!

December 24, 2011

Sweet treats left at my door from my upstairs neighbor. Really nice to come home to! With pic of a Ziploc full of cookies and other treats, on which was written: "Happy holidays! From apartment 16306 gang. xoxo"

Watching "He's Just Not That Into You" instead of "Love Actually" because I'm already feeling too needy. Wish. This. Would. Sink. In.

LISA M: Good movie and makes sense huh? Jaclynn was right when she said you need to watch it. I wanted to read the book. Oh, and eventually it will set in.

ME: I've seen it a hundred times and every time, at different points in my life, I'm shocked at how much I sound exactly like the main character. I'm pretty sure her words have come out of my mouth to you many times.

MEGAN G: Merry Christmas Eve, Coco Crispie!!! I'm thankful for the friendship we have and feel blessed to have met you.

ME: Merry Christmas Eve to YOU, Megs!!! You're the one good thing that came out of living at the Shops. Love you!

December 25, 2011

Christmas Eve cheer. it's ridiculous how much I like this bar. And the men who come here.

In our world of plenty / we can spread a smile of joy / Throw your arms around the world at Christmas time! Merry Christmas, friends, family, and people I haven't spoken to in ten plus years.

KATHERINE H: Merry Christmas, sweet nieceling. Hope all your Cmas wishes come true.

I wish I was watching the game, but MAVS, step it up!! That is an unacceptable opening day score.

ADOLFO F: *Booooooo. Go Spurs!!!!!!*

"The kids" in their Christmas sweaters in Jimmy's kitchen: Dachshund family much?
SHELBY H: *Hahahahaha*
KATHERINE H: *Hilarious*
KIM W: *OMG!*

December 26, 2011

Sleepy and melancholy. This four-day weekend went too quickly. Hoping for a rockin' New Years Eve to top it all off. Merry Christmas, one and all.

December 27, 2011

Checked in to Bankston Nissan: Why yes, flat tire, you're EXACTLY what I wanted to spend my Christmas money (and awesome free afternoon off) on.

Whoop; a patch fixed it and it was only $18!!! Plus I got my oil changed and my car washed!! Love.

December 28, 2011

Is there ANYONE in the world with the same kind of bad luck I have? While I realize a lot of people are worse off in many ways, the kind of shit that hits me is astonishing.
JENNIFER B: *I refer to myself as a "crap magnet." Welcome to the family.*
CRISTA L: *Me!*
LISA M: *Hmmm. What happened now?!*
KIM W: *I'm having a craptastic week… let's have a pity party!*
WHITNEY R: *I'm right there with you, if it's not one thing, it's another*
KATHERINE H: *it's life, but you do have your share. What now?*
ME: *Oh, just apartment BS and red tape. It's all sorted out now and worked out for the best. Thanks for the concerns!* ♥

NOT THE F——ING GILMORE GIRLS

December 29, 2011

> *I am so thankful that it's 10:35 on a Thursday morning and I am home. I get to take sick time, get paid for the holiday, and get roughly 92 hours of pure, unadulterated free time. Miss my kiddos already, and though I'm super excited about this weekend, I'm also excited for the new year and having a full classroom and regular hours again. It'll make the time fly until I move in with LeighAnn.*
>
> *Holy God, the Flying Pig: ham, bacon, sausage link, and pulled pork. Heart attack in a sandwich and completely worth it.*
>   MEGAN G: *I'm getting chest pains just looking at it.*
>   LISA M: *Shouldn't you add nom nom nom?!*
>   ME: *Lisa… Not in this lifetime.*

I LOVE the Cookie Monster. I HATE when people say nom, nom, nom. It literally makes me want to punch something, like when I hear you make smacking noise while you eat. (I just looked up who originated it because I started to question myself. It was indeed Cookie Monster, and the article from the Huffington Post also said, "When it comes to the use of nom nom, and our bubbling hatred for it, we almost feel like we don't have to explain ourselves."

December 31, 2011

> *Complicated situations only get worse in the morning light / Hey, I'm just lookin' for a good time.*
>
> *Ready to start the new year off with a bang. Everyone be safe, have fun, and rock it tonight.*

January 1, 2012

> *Happiness lies in your own hand / It took me much too long to understand.*
>
> *I don't think I'm a fan of this Timeline thing. Aside from being able to see what was happening in my Facebook life 5 years ago. I don't love the layout.*

I hate that it's too cold outside for my ac to kick on but too warm outside for my apartment to be cold. It's gross in here.

January 2, 2012

Lisa M: I created a new Pinterest board for you, me, and Gloria for the contest. Add stuff!

January 5, 2012

It is very weird to be feeding a baby girl pears and have a face jump into my mind like a clip from a dream; I literally had to pause to figure out whose face it was. He is definitely on my mind!

January 7, 2012

Lisa M: Did you eat your Zots yet? Bring back memories?! Are you going to KRK at noon today?

Me: Of course I ate them! They're so weird. And yes I think so…for a little while.

Alas, never mind. My mom just called and I haven't seen her in like two weeks.

January 9, 2012

It's cold and rainy; great cuddle weather. Too bad I have to work tonight. And that I have no one to cuddle with except a sweetheart of a dog. Come see me at Plano Palio's tonight!!

Lisa M: Wanna go head to head with me in the Biggest Loser challenge this week?! Come on.

January 12, 2012

Megan G: Hi. My name is Megan and I'm a Cocoholic.

Well, tonight was the first time Sherlock's didn't rock. No AJ, no Brandon, no Jessi, no Jennifer!! But Daryl and Rob came and that's always awesome. And if we have one bummer night in six awesome ones? I'll take it.

Working at Palio's Plano: Is it worth it / let me work it / put my thing down, flip it, and reverse it!

Nary a charger works in my house, whether phone or computer it be. Oddly, my phone battery hasn't dipped below 58% in two days, despite it being constantly glued to my hand. My computer, I fear, will not be as lucky.

January 13, 2012

Your body is creating and killing 15 million red blood cells per second. Food for thought.

August 25, 2012

There are few things lonelier than closing a restaurant down, walking to the back, and realizing everyone has left without saying goodbye.

September 5, 2012

Pinterest makes me nostalgic for things I've never had.

I'm gonna have to be a football fan. And since I don't want to get KILLED at work or anywhere else, I'm gonna have to jump on the Cowboys bandwagon. I still hate Tony Romo. Who's gonna teach me???

September 6, 2012

Wow, a high of only 86 on Saturday!! A 20-degree difference from Friday with no rain in the forecast?? Dare I hope??

October 29, 2012

I find it odd that two of my favorite songs right now are "Kiss Tomorrow Goodbye" and "Blown Away." I sense a theme here.

November 20, 2012

>AMANDA A: *Hey woman! You wanna come to karaoke tonight?*
>
>ME: *I'm so exhausted, girl. Hopefully next time. Have fun!!*

>Day 20: *I'm thankful that a bunch of four-year-olds wore me out to the point that it's 9:10 and I'm ready for bed…after a phentermine, a couple of diet Cokes, and ten hours of sleep last night.*

November 21, 2012

>*I'm thankful that my need to have new things doesn't translate into waiting outside stores a full 48 hours (at least!) before Friday. I'm also thankful that my brain went immediately to "oh, Best Buy is selling tents now??" rather than "wow, those guys have stamina!"*

>*[I tagged Valerie C in this.] Pitch Perfect. Finally. Nobody else better throw up.*
>CRISTA L: *You two are going to love it!*

November 22, 2012

>*I am thankful that I get to spend two separate dinners with two awesome families. I love them all and am blessed to have so many people in my life. Not to mention, of course, the wonderful friends that will be joining us!! I wish everyone could come. Happy Thanksgiving, people!!*

November 23, 2012

>*Yeah, I totally just hit a Black Friday sale for Yankee Candle. Online. What, what!! Business DONE.*

November 25, 2012

>*I posted a meme of a woman in bed with tons of dogs, a man standing by the side, and a dog thinking, "Yes? Can I help you?"*

> This will be me. Ruby already takes up most of my bed and she's 19 pounds. Hahaha.

November 27, 2012

> No matter how much weight I lose, I will always be a fat girl for double stuf Oreos.
>
> ALISHA B: It's the candy cane Oreos for me. And barbecue. I'll never turn down barbecue.

> Dear God, please let it stay cold. I'll ignore the weathermen in favor of your divine intervention. It's almost December. Today it actually resembles it. Love, Courtney.

November 29, 2012

> Light up, light up / as if you have a choice / Even if you cannot hear my voice / I'll be right beside you, dear

> A few days ago I got a call from my leasing office saying they'd gotten several complaints about the noise level in my apartment. Today I got an official note saying I needed to read over my lease stating other tenants' right to quiet. WTF noise do I make at night???? All I do is watch TV and at that, it's on my computer, so it can't be that loud! And Ruby just sleeps next to me. No barking or running around or anything. I'm about to vacuum tonight... seriously, complain about me again. Try living under 20-year-old drummers.
>
> CRISTA L: I bet it's those kids above you
>
> ME: Lol, the maintenance men said the same thing when they dropped off my complaint notice... but I'm pretty sure they've moved, because I DID complain about them once (when they were drumming at four in the morning...) and the leasing lady said they were moving bc they wanted somewhere they could play their drums. Like a house in the woods...??

December 1, 2012

Happy third birthday to the cutest damn dog that ever lived!! Ruby, you've made light of my life for two years and 45 weeks. Cheers for at least 15 more years.
  KATHERINE H: We love Ruby! She's a great dog-niece to have. Happy day!

Video of Ruby climbing a tree: Super cat-dog! She was having to jump but now she's figured it out. One day she will wind up in the branches.

Tagged Crista, Valerie, and crew in a post that says McSwiggan's for MIKE!!!! Happy birthday, Mr President!

December 2, 2012

I need to go to a baseball game. Ahorita.

Crista L tagged me and friends in a pic of the tackiest sweater trophy. "You got what it takes?! This gem is up for grabs this year at our 3rd Annual Tacky Sweater Party! Bring on the tacky!"

December 3, 2012

Nothing makes me feel older than my understanding a current trend... Especially when it's well over three years old and people have tried explaining it to me. #whattheeffdoesa#signinfrontofabunchofwordsdo
  JIMMY C: #idontunderstandthatstuffeither @CourtneyCannon@lol@myhouse@
  JESSICA C: Instagram. #itscontagious
  ME: And that should say *not understanding, not MY understanding... DYA. And Jessica...that is about as clear as mud. 😷
  ANDREA P: I don't get it either... I've never even asked because I'm afraid of reality... I'm getting old!!!!

December 5, 2012

> I have no doubt that we will be alive come Christmas. But it doesn't stop me from lately panicking that I have come nowhere close to living my life the way I wish I could.
>> KATHERINE H: What's stopping you? You have the smarts, the wit, the drive and the personality... make it happen.

December 9, 2012

> Yeah that's a water slide in someone's backyard. With pic of exactly that.

December 10, 2012

> Need to sleep. But can't. Stop. Reading.

December 12, 2012

> Unorthodox Jukebox. Tomorrow. Doing it.

December 13, 2012

> One o'clock. Nearly thirteen hours of deep, solid, uninterrupted sleep. I don't know which freaks me out more, when I do that or when I don't sleep at all.

December 15, 2012

> I'm just so tired!

> Remind me never to come to Target during Christmas. I do not need my own Viva la Juicy gift set or 3 new scents of Yankee candles, no matter how cheap they seem.

December 16, 2012

> I jingle aaallll the way (with pic of an ugly sweater covered in jingle bells, two small gifts suggestively positioned).

After a WINNER WINNER CHICKEN DINNER game of flip-cup against the boys and Nathan, I am way more drunk than I intended to be tonight. I don't want to go to work.

December 17, 2012

I'm over being shocked or sad that I care about people more than they care about me. New Year's Resolution: I come first. My happiness is important to me before others'. Unless its my kids or family.
CONNER C: *Do I count family???*
ME: *Of course, Conner. All my Palio's family. And that should say it's... although technically I think it should be kids' or family's too... lol.*

I'm about to have to figure out how to be a fan of a team without most of my favorite players. YOUNG, really??? Lump in my tummy thinking about April for the first time in years... hold onto Elvis, hold onto Elvis...

She got whatever "it" is.

December 19, 2012

I never thought there would come a time when I wasn't attracted to Bruno Mars... last night's fro-look on The Voice proved that wrong... but I still adore him.

HELP, what kind of computer doesn't have a slot for a memory card???? YIKES!!

December 20, 2012

I posted a handwritten chalkboard at Palio's that said "Try our new Italian wings (while they last)" with a drawing of a chicken.
They're so good. And the chicken makes me giggle every time I look at him. Come try them soon!!!

December 21, 2012

> Is it supposed to happen at midnight in 15 minutes or do we get to live tomorrow before the world implodes? Or explodes. Or burns? Whatever?
>
> CLARISSA M: Posted a Mayan Calendar Countdown...
>
> > You've got 5 1/2 hours left. I plan on sleeping through the apocalypse.
>
> ME: LOL. Me too.
>
> With Lisa M and 4 others: It's been a good week. In light of the sadness last Friday, I spent this week really enjoying being back with kids. I might not have any of my own, but these babies QUICKLY become mine. After five months, things changed, and the kiddos who were once so close to me have all but forgotten me. But today my favorites warmed up finally.
>
> Kennedie eagerly lifted her arms for me to hold her and even buried her head in my neck when Gloria teased her. My sweet Colin, who sometimes won't even look at me, threw an all-out temper tantrum when I walked into the room today... I thought it was because he didn't want to see me, but it turned out he was sleepy, and when I picked him up to give him love, instead of squirming to get down, he cuddled with me until he fell asleep. Now that's trust: letting someone hold you, knowing they won't let you fall.
>
> After only six days of knowing me AT ALL, Connor gave his grandma his stone face when she picked him up...and followed my every move as I was getting his stuff together.
>
> Many more stories are yet to come, I'm sure. I'm just so thankful to be here again... my life is already 100 times more enriched, thanks wholly to awesome kids, their wonderful parents, and of course a staff of women (and Cody) who are incomparable.

December 23, 2012

> You keep me hanging around / my feet aren't touching the ground.

December 25, 2012

SNOW!!!! Merry Christmas weather!!!!!

I posted a picture of Ruby: Too many buttered biscuits and too much prime tenderloin. Knocked out. Merry Christmas!

December 26, 2012

Icy parking lot = Courtney's low-pressure tires careening her car into the guardrail. And then this evening, to add injury to insult, the ice AROUND MY CAR ONLY didn't melt and I just ate serious pavement, landing hard on my knees and right hand. Even my back hurts.

It's stupid that the Rangers got rid of Michael Young to "make room for young talent" and then they sign another 36-year-old... JUST RIP OUT OUR HEART, why don't you? On another note, Jessica, let's stop copying Britney NOW before you go crazy and shave your head.

December 28, 2012

If there's something to slip on, even if it's an inch in diameter, bet I will slip on it. As if the ice two days ago wasn't enough, the mis-targeted squirt of sanitizer in my classroom today provided ample opportunity for my knees to really color up.

December 30, 2012

My day started off awesome with a pay-it-forward (I suppose that would technically be backward) chain in the Starbucks line. The only reason I was able to keep it going (sixth in the line that far, with a bill double mine behind me) was because of my awesome Secret Santa, Rebekah, and her awesome girlfriend, Lluvia. Good karma to begin a pretty rockin' day, 13 hours long at Palio's, with an awesome staff (who received compliments from the dear parents of Cameron). I didn't sit down once *and didn't even notice. It would take a novel to write everything good. Thank you to all my wonderful employees and amazing coworkers at KRK (past and present) for today.*

*M*ALLORY *M: Love you!!*

December 31, 2012

Starting the new year with a new color. Dark brown is practically the only color I haven't been, and I was envisioning a deep chocolate brown. "Raspberry Truffle" was as close as I could find. Fingers crossed...

January 1, 2013

I hoped 2013 would be my lucky year since 13 is my lucky number. If this year follows last night and this morning, I'll be winning the lottery soon! Really fantastic party, sullied only once by a little scare that thankfully turned out okay, followed by a lucky stop at a gas station this morning. Not having any money to spare, I was gonna try to go as long as possible without filling up, but then my GET FUEL NOW *light came on. Astonishingly, I think I got a free tank full... I put my card in the machine and it said "begin fueling" before I hit credit or debit or anything...and filled up $25 before saying "limit reached." I don't know if some Good Samaritan turned the pump on for some lucky customer, if I just stole $25 bucks of gas off someone else's card, or if the purchase will eventually show up on* MY *card, but whatever the case, it was a really great surprise. I am so happy today, I don't even know how to handle it.*

I had so much fun at this party, I yearned to repeat it the next year. It did not go well. But this one…this one… Nathan had ghosted me most of the fourteen months since we had last made out, but some weird twist of fate brought us together for this party, and I confidently marched up to him and kissed him at midnight. I could hear our friends—mostly his friends, most of whom I had just met—whooping for him, and it pleased me.

We spent the rest of the night flirting and touching until the scare—when one of the guys passed out, and no one could wake him up. But afterward, I played Bruno Mars's "Gorilla" for him while I was in the bathroom at the end of the night; and when I came out and sat on the couch, he was on me like white on rice. We hooked up on their living room floor and were literally caught naked the next morning. It was so, so fucking fun, literally and figuratively.

> *Really cute pic of me and two friends at the NYE party, captioned, "The one flip wonders!! First round, ended heads-up against Nathan, making my score 2-0. Second round, the boys shut us out, but we got 'em in the end with a shut-out of our own."*

January 4, 2013

> *So there has been an idea for a story called "Among the Enchanted" rolling around in my brain for years (I began it in a spiral notebook working in the fitting room at Old Navy... so that's AT LEAST 7 years...) Lately I've been wanting to continue it, and I was sitting here forming ideas in my brain, and I was having a conversation between Brandon and Adrienne in which Brandon calls himself the luckiest... which I thought would make a great title too. But Brandon doesn't consider himself lucky... he's just quoting someone. He's a veteran back from overseas, and he's seen too much to handle. Suddenly it occurred to me...Nicholas Sparks got there first. Role-reversal or not, this story seems too bloody familiar. AGH!!!!!*

January 5, 2013

> *I'm so freakin excited. Five pounds off this week. First weigh-in of the year SUCCESSFUL. First weigh-in after the holiday season DOUBLE SUCCESSFUL. Bring it, 2013!!!! Here I come, bathing suit season!*

January 7, 2013

I posted a picture of me and Gabby out at some bar, where if I recall I wasn't having a good time despite the smile on my face.

I believe we were watching Bryce play. I don't remember if I started off the night not wanting to go, but I do remember leaving early and alone in anger, which rarely happened. I looked so hot. My hair was dark, long, and curly, and I was dressed completely in black. My anger was powerful, so I texted my friend and told him to meet me at my apartment. It was well past midnight, but I knew he would meet me, and he did. He even told me how good I looked (he was significantly younger and was good for nothing much more than kissing).

We had sex once or twice in our run of benefits, but he ended it real fast when he asked me for gas money after giving me head one night. (He had apparently never done it to anyone and was saving it for a girlfriend.) There were so many appalling things about that situation, not the least of which was his tongue, that I'm not sure if I ever spoke to him again. I felt like a hooker, but he was the one who was trying to sell himself, and the confusion from feelings like that will kill you.

January 8, 2013

> *Reading old diaries: not a good way to get to sleep. Although I did learn that I've been unsure of how to end my money-maker novel for over two years...*

January 9, 2013

> *On this day last year, I was 16 pounds heavier. Doesn't seem like a lot, but it's 16 pounds less I have to contend with to reach my ultimate goal. Gooooooooal!*

January 12, 2013

> *With Megan G at Cowboys Red River: All right, doing the Cotton-Eyed Joe in cowboy boots is way 2 legit 2 quit.*

> *I believe this is the first time EVER that I've had two consecutive weeks of losses... I'm on a roll!!! 3 more pounds down. BOOM!!!*

And drumroll, please, the final entry, half-finished, in a half-finished hard-copy journal:

January 18, 2013

> *I've been wanting to write about this for nearly three weeks. I didn't want to play catch up over the last year or relive the old entries, which is what I always do when I open this journal. And now the only pens I can find that work bleed through the page.*

I sounded annoyed, and I understand why now that I've connected the Facebook memories. I'm thankful this popped up, because Nathan still holds that magic for me. From here on out, it's all about social media posts. I hope I can make you guys laugh as much as I made myself laugh.

I spent a lot of time wondering if this is a story worth telling, if I'll be able to help anyone but myself. But the bottom line is, I'm trying to help myself first. I won't be able to help anyone if I can't help myself, and I want to help people. So it's at this time I'll ask, if you didn't read the note from the author at the beginning, please do now. It's straight from my heart, as is this whole book, and I need the readers to know how much I appreciate y'all even opening (or downloading, whichever you choose!) it. You guys are the magic. Remember that.

May 17, 2013

> *I posted a video of Jessalyn doing animal sounds with me, including the gorilla noise.*

July 13–28, 2013

I posted pictures with Chris and Caiohme and lots of Ruby.

Introducing Christoper and Caiohme and their mother Devon, not to mention my beautiful Jessalyn! (It must have been the summer before that I first met Christoper, but…) I got to work with the school-age kiddos over the summer, and I had such a connection with Chris. By the end of the summer, he told me he wished I were his mom, and I told him the feeling was mutual. Of course, I felt the same about all my babies, but that was the first time I really connected with a kid who talked back. And boy, did Christopher talk back.

I wrote a letter to his mother at the end of that summer, thanking her for raising such an incredible kid and that I had the privilege of being allowed into their personal lives. I went to watch the kid at football games, babysat them when their dad tried to essentially kidnap them, and watched as they bonded with my Ruby. And now Christopher is twenty-two, and we are still friends.

Jessalyn came to me at six weeks old, the most beautiful infant girl I'd seen. I don't know if I connected more to her first or to her mother, Stephanie, but I quickly became so attached to her. She became like my own. There are so many fun stories about her; her little sister, Mya, who was God's way of making sure I got "paid back" for the way I'd treated *my* mother; and their baby brother Brayden, who we'd all prayed for incessantly.

These two families by blood were so welcoming, they made me feel like a part of them just for loving their kids. And that is something I will never be able to repay. So many families over so many years, but the other one you'll read about frequently is Charlie. Between Charlie, his siblings Isabella and Jake, his amazing parents, and my surrogate fam, the Skippers, my life was full.

September 5, 2013

> *I called Ruby Pumpkin Butt this morning. It made me excited for fall.*

September 9, 2013

> *I got told I'm "not a very nice person" today. I can't shake it, even though I know quite the opposite is true.*

October 9, 2013

> *Birthday dinner at Taverna with a bunch of friends and kids.*

October 19, 2013

> *Halloween party with Devon at her sister's, dressed as a pirate again.*

October 20, 2013

> *Haunted House in Ft Worth with Taylor, Jordan, Parker, Miles in our Cowboys gear.*

October 27, 2013

> *I posted pictures of Halloween at Val's. I was dressed as a vampire, pretending to bite Maria's neck.*

November 20, 2013

Day 20: I'm thankful for babies. They remind me that there are people in the world who are completely sweet and innocent, even if they're only 6 months old.

Am I the only person who freaks out when people they're talking to online suddenly want to meet? It's NEVER been long enough!! Eek!!!!

Huh, Kins no longer a Ranger. Muy interesante.

CRISTA L: *What the what*

ME: *Lol traded for Prince Fielder. Stellar.*

November 21, 2013

I love it when I come home for lunch, lock my car, and Ruby's face appears in my window, all sleep-crumpled. She's the cutest.

I went to Target to stock up on cheap movies for my Thanksgiving with my ma, and I also caved into blue nail 3D nail polish and blue eyeliner to go with my shadow. I found Hunger Games for $10 and it was a toss up between that and the eyeliner when I exceeded my budget... I was so sure I already had Hunger Games, I left that behind. Don't have it. Epic fail.

MISHA T: *You should check into signing up for the Ipsy glam bag. It's $10 a month and you get a little makeup bag filled with fun new makeup! I always think of you when I tell people about it. I think you would enjoy it more than anyone I know!*

BRENDA C: *Kroger across the street from KRK has the blu ray & DVD for $6.99 in their Christmas DVD specials section, along with a ton of other new movies. Next time*

ME: *Misha, I heard about that!! I definitely need to check it out. Is it good makeup? Brenda, I'm buying it tomorrow. Thanks for the tip.*

MISHA T: *I will bring in my November bag tomorrow. Also, you put in your complexion and eye color so it is personalized for you!*

ME: *Oh no way. So cool!!*

KATHERINE H: *What movies did you get? Or is it a secret? Need ideas for Harper's convalescence next week.*

ME: *What is she convalescing from?? And Something Borrowed, Leap Year, Now You See Me, and 42. Pitch Perfect during my mom's nap.*

KATHERINE H: *She's having shoulder surgery on Tuesday—torn labrum, possibly torn bicep. Big owie. Will be in medieval apparatus for weeks, poor baby. Thank you, gymnastics.*

ME: *Oh wow!!! Yeah lots of movies necessary!! Poor cuz! Heal fast!*

I posted a meme of a grumpy cat that said, "What does the fox say? I don't know, but it needs to shut the hell up." HA!!! Oh God yes. Except Betsy dances to it and that's just pretty awesome.

The rain has started!!! Bring on the cold!!!

Day 21: I am thankful for my God. I don't ever post about Him on Facebook, for fear of...I'm not sure what. But the way He has provided me for this month is astonishing. And it just reminds me that He always has done, no matter what. I thank God as often as I remember to, for my friends, family, jobs, and whatever income I can reap. But I never thank Him for Him. Thank God.

KENDRA R: *I love this*

November 22, 2013

Greatest triumph so far: I really wanted Chick-Fil-A tonight. Milkshake and all. But on the drive home I kept asking myself if it was worth it. And it's just not. So I came home and ate soup. Which may or may not have been expired.

JIMMY C: *That's awesome. Keep it up.*

[I posted a picture of Ruby in a pink sweater.] How do they always know they look so silly? #ruby-duby #rubyrose #cutestthingever

Oh dear, I'm so cold I can't stop shaking. In my apartment. With my heater set to 76 because the bill is worth less than my life. It's nights like this I wish I had a boyfriend. Or that Ruby was 119 pounds rather than 19.

JENNIFER M: 76? Mine stays at 60 degrees & it's 28 degrees out. Bundle up in layers and blankets.

ME: Lol I don't know why but my heater wouldn't warm the place up. I was in blankets.

LISA M: No heater for me yet! Bundle up!

HARPER H: you need some advice from someone who lives in the north: first you need to put on leggings. then you need some sweat pants. put on a cami. then a long sleeve shirt. then a sweat shirt. and then another sweat shirt if needed. put on some thin socks. on top of those put on some thick wool socks. then put on some gloves. and finally, huddle under a few blankets and a nice down comforter.

KYLA N: Try a space heater.

ME: Kyla, that's a great idea. Those things work!! I also thought about an electric blanket. I don't need to heat my whole apartment, just myself and the Tater Tot.

KYLA: We don't have heat in our house so we've got to get creative when it gets nippy.

KATHERINE H: I was going to suggest the space heater too—cheap and they work. But you gotta remember to turn it off when you leave!

November 23, 2013

Day 22: I'm thankful that water exacerbating my rash turned into a probable diagnosis of heat rash. I don't know how I'll get rid of it considering it's freezing out and I just want to take hot baths and cuddle under multiple blankets, but I sure will try!

[I reposted a Toys for Tots flyer.] Great cause! Stop by any of the restaurants!!

[I posted a picture of Ruby with her ears perked out.] Trying to get me up. #rubyrose #rubyduby #batdog

No matter how many times I've seen it (and I've seen it more than the average person), I'm still always awed by Skylar Astin's performance at the end of Pitch Perfect. Well, really every performance.

    LISA M: Allie might give you a run for your money on the amount of times. Great great movie!

November 24, 2013

I want a Christmas tree.

[I tagged Stephanie S and Jimmy C.] Day 23: I'm thankful for silly little girls who make me laugh with every (sometimes hard to understand) word.

Day 24: I'm thankful for new mattresses and brothers who help you get one.

["Oh but for the grace of God," captioned a post from 96.3 country radio.] You do not know me but I saw that you needed some tires for your truck and I wanted to do something nice for a stranger because one day a stranger did the same for me. The receipt is in the envelope and all you have to do is go by Warehouse Tire on 3rd Street and ask for Steven Hodges and they will put them on for free. All I ask is that one day you do something nice for a complete stranger.

    HARPER H: oh my god it's like in that movie "pay it forward"

    ALISHA B: I've seen this many times before, and it still puts a smile on my face.

November 25, 2013

I'm thankful for Mondays. They always go really fast and I'm always happy to see my babies after the weekend, no matter how cranky they are that the weekend is over. I'm also really thankful for three-day weeks. Because my babies need a vacation as much as we do!

[I reposted the Book List Challenge. I had read 23/100.] Wow, nearly a quarter. That's more than I expected. #notwellreadintheclassics #lovetoread"

November 26, 2013

Day 26: I'm thankful for Lifetime Christmas movies. Just the kind of sappy cheese I'm craving.

November 27, 2013

Checked into Palio's Frisco with Blake R & Amanda A: Pre-Thanksgiving fest? Come see me! I know y'all don't want to cook tonight! Let us do it for you. I know you won't regret it.

November 28, 2013

Day 27: I'm thankful for mini-vacations. 4 days off starts now!! (Well, it started at 9:27 really!) Movies, delicious food, family, a new mattress, and fun. Minus one very important member.

AYESHA W: Cyrus said to tell you, Ms Gloria, and Miss Maria Happy Thanksgiving! Also that he misses you guys! Enjoy your time off!

ME: Awww lol!! Happy Thanksgiving to y'all. Miss him too.

With a Candy List Challenge, I'd tried 88/100 "Thoroughly unsurprised that it's so high, but quite surprised it's not higher considering not only did I grow up in the 80s, but I was as big a candy fiend then as I am now. Is it bad that I want to go TODAY to find the 12 I haven't tried?? Mom and Popcorn in McKinney, here I come!!"

35/100 ice cream flavors list: "Ew some of these should just not exist. And they spelled raspberry wrong. (Yes, this is what I do on a weekday when both my dog and my internal alarm have told me it's time to go to work.) I need to start a once-a-week Baskin Robbins outing."

I am hungry and I'm at my mom's. Is it acceptable to break into the Thanksgiving pumpkin pie

for breakfast?? She broke into the cherry one last night!!
  KATHERINE H: I say go for it.
  MEGAN U: Heck yes! Why not?!

Happy Thanksgiving. I hope wherever you are, whomever you're with, you are happy.
  PATTY M: Happy Thanksgiving to you and your family! See you soon
  ME: Patty, same to you and yours!! I sure hope so. Miss you all.
  LYN B: we were with you! That makes up happy

Omg cutest guy ever in the parking lot of my nanny Ann's. Is it appropriate to hope he's somehow heading to the same apartment? You know, someone's single relation by long distance.

November 29, 2013

Well, I caved. A little Black Friday shopping never hurt anyone. Well, anyone with a budget anyway. Old Navy for a couple of warm items (that I needed!) and Ulta for a few fun items (that I didn't!)! Yea!!

About to take a nap in my new warm memory foam bed! Climbing in was weird. No give! But let's see how the sleep is. No new pillow yet. It has a weird smell and they say to let it air out lol.

I just had an 11-year-old tell me to get a boyfriend. Seriously?? HELP!!
  LORI P: No! Seriously?
  KATHERINE H: Now we just need to find a kid to tell a cute guy to get a girlfriend and you'll be all set.
  HARPER: if I were a dude I'd date you

November 30, 2013

I've said it before and I'm sure I'll say it again: I love Ryan Tedder more than the average bear. Anyone know HIM??

SANDER W: *This one count? And posted a LinkedIn to HIS Ryan Tedder.*
ME: *Lol, that's awesome.*

OMG Paul Walker!!!! That's like (almost) Heath Ledger sad!!!
LORI P: *Very sad! I had a huge crush on him.*
CRISTA L: *It is I thought that same thing*

December 1, 2013

[I reposted Usher posting about Paul Walker: "RIP Paul Walker... our prayers go out to his family and friends #gone2soon."] Oh, this man.

I reposted Tyrese Gibson's tribute to Paul— "My heart is hurting so bad, no one can make me believe this is real, Father God I pray that you send clarity over this cause I just don't understand, My heart hurts it's broken no one can convince me that this is real... Prayer warriors please pray real hard for his only child, his daughter and family... #HeartOfAnAngel13YrsFamilyForever WeJustCelebratedYour40thBirthday... My God... My God... I can't believe I'm writing this"—with a picture of the two of them.

Oh dear. I think I missed the last six days or so for thankfulness. Bottom line, I am thankful for my life. Sometimes it hurts, sometimes it's really hard, but I love it. The people, the places, the animals... I am blessed beyond belief.

I get to see my wee bambinos tomorrow! And the two coolest co-teachers in the world. What do you get to do?
CAROLE K: *Planning three Christmas parties—one with retired MHE folks—and grocery shopping!*

December 2, 2013

[I posted a meme of three dogs in the corners of a kitchen that said, "My friend puts his dogs in time-out when they act up. This time, it was the

trash."] Omg this is simultaneously so sad and so cute. #sillydogs.

I would do pretty much anything not to have to struggle with food every day.
JAYNE W: Plexus! I can hook you up. Started almost 2 months ago and I love it
KENDRA R: Plexus! I'm 5 weeks in and never looking back!
ME: Lol Kendra I was just telling Jayne about you. I'll definitely give it a try!
KENDRA: I've had two cokes in 5 weeks and 3 pieces of candy since Halloween. I don't even know who I am anymore lol I LOVE IT!
ME: Phentermine is what does that for me. I can't convince myself to eat for anything when I'm not hungry. But when hunger hits, it hits hard.

December 3, 2013

I'm so tired and my back hurts so badly that as soon as I got home, I collapsed on my couch with my feet in the air to relieve the pressure... Now I don't think I can get up. Is bed worth it??? Would my babies care if I don't shower tonight?? (Parents, steer clear!) #spiritnight #ovenishard #paliosburnscalories

December 4, 2013

I'm so done with people. I need a few days on a desert island with my books and my dog.
TAYA B: You ok??
GLORIA G: What's wrong!?!? How's Ass do I have to Kick?!?!?

ME: Y'all are sweet lol. Yeah I'm fine. Just...aggravated! Lol.

[I reposted, "What's your elf name?"] Mine is Glitzy Sparkly-Nose. I admit this cheered me up considerably. Especially after listening to Vin's speech at Paul's crash site.

KATHERINE H: *Glitzy Sparkly-Nose fits you somehow. Poor Harper is Tootsie Tootsie. Oh sorry—she's Tootsie Sugar-Socks. Much better.*

I am obscenely excited about the weather coming to Texas. I only wish my frost-free jacket would get here NOW. I have a dilemma though. A/C on tonight??? I get so hot at night but if it gets cold enough outside, I won't be able to get out of bed in the mañana. And I know how many people would appreciate that. (Does sarcasm come across on Facebook?)

December 5, 2013

Happy Dirty 21 to my favorite brother on the planet. Jimmy > Your Brother.

Oh, my. Reason number 147,429,566 to love Paul Walker? Google "Paul Walker buys ring." Don't cry. God bless our soldiers.

Well, sitting in my very iced over car... Nothing to scrape with... Only three hours after getting back from lunch!! #texasiscrazy #godblessedtexas #lovethis

Aww Nelson Mandela! Number two...?? Sad!!

Checked in at Walmart The Colony: I am here for one reason, and that's because by the time it occurred to me to get provisions (rice, hot chocolate) IN CASE I am iced in tomorrow (by myself, all alone. Sigh.)! I had already passed Target. This place is gross. And everyone else had the same idea.
GLORIA G: *Oo that's what I forgot to get was hot chocolate!!*
AYESHA W: *I hate Walmart too.*
ME: *Gloria, oh em gee. Necessity!!! Ayesha, it gives me hives. Even the ones in nicer areas. I don't know why lol.*

Well, DISD closed!! Come on, FISD... Not that I'm hoping for no work tomorrow!

NOT THE F——ING GILMORE GIRLS

GLORIA G: *I know! Come on FISD!! I love my baby's but I want everyone to be safe.*

CHRISTY C: *Lol, FISD will not let you know until 5:30am. Then I bet it's only a 2 hr delay.*

ME: *Lol Janelle… Your husband is one who got me hoping!! I do love that baby though!!!! I hope so!!! You have got to be the busiest mom I know! He also told me about the a Cappella group Pentatonix that sang Little Drummer Boy and now I can't stop watching all their videos online. (What was the name of that Nick Lachey show that they debuted on??) So don't get sucked up in those…because that work will never get done.*

AYESHA W: *We aren't coming in tomorrow—stay safe ladies!!! Btw, you probably already know but I saw someone else posted that Frisco ISD is closed tomorrow…*

ME: *Thanks, Ayesha!! I did see that, but KRK won't announce until 6 tomorrow morning. So if you change your mind, we might be open. Enjoy your weekend!!*

AYESHA: *I'm so not going to work tomorrow—even if the roads are good, I'm still sick.*

Huh. Stuck at home with no Internet might be the worst thing ever. I get antsy enough with plenty of shows, movies, and Pinterest at my fingertips… Give me nothing and WHAT THEN????? I hate Time Warner.

I like don't think I can stop watching Pentatonix covers. (Internet is working by the way.) These people are dope.

ALISHA B: *I listen to their cover of JT's Pusher Love Girl almost every day…*

December 6, 2013

It's gorgeous and white outside. Due to it being 78 on Wednesday, I don't think it can last long, but for now it's back to bed with Ruby. Yea!!!!!

>   *[I posted a picture of the snowy apartment complex.]* #noon #stillwhite #loveit #snowday #obligatorysnowpic #babyitscoldoutside
>
>   Wow when I said going back to bed, I meant it. I slept a whole 'nother night's worth. Thankfully I have nothing to do otherwise. Today is such a blessing. Perfect ending for the crazy week. Plus I have a full-blown sinus infection. I always thought it was allergies, but perhaps it's REALLY the changes in weather. I need to find a state with four set seasons.
>
>   I am super thankful I am not one of the many with no power. I would literally go crazy. On another note, I slipped as soon as I stepped outside. Be safe and stay home!!! The high is 27, so this isn't going anywhere for a while.
>
>   Two musical proposals today. Grey's Anatomy, which I've been watching singly for months now, and Glee, which I put on hold for months to watch Grey's. Weird.
>
>   Reposting this gem in the happy news that these two are now engaged! So much love in this picture. So happy for y'all, Kevin and Kelsy! Even your names look good together! Love you both. *With pic of K & K nose-to-nose and grinning at each other.*
>
>   KEALEILANI S: Love it!
>
>   DANIELLE S: Sweet love!
>
>   *[I shared Vin Diesel's post with a picture of him and Paul Walker.]* "When I heard, I immediately flew back to California, and went directly from the plane to his mother's house... I thought they needed my strength, but realized when I got there and broke down before his family, that it was I who needed theirs. His mother hugged me and said I am so sorry... I said sorry? You're the mother who lost a son? She said yes, but you lost your other half..."

Ten years later, I still bawled like a baby reading that. This one will never not hurt. Oh, and great, it's followed by this. This day ten years ago was an emotional wreck!

Finally watched the episode of Glee where they honor Finn. In a puddle on the couch. So now I'm playing Wii Glee Karaoke to make myself feel better.

It is entirely too strange to walk on ice over grass. It looks like snow. But it's not and it sounds like gun shots.

Ohhhhhh my GOSH Adam Lambert on Glee!!! I forgot about this!!!!! So excited.

Ruby and I just trekked across the Antarctic to get to my leasing office to pick up my new winter jacket. She had a grand time, sledding in the tire tracks, bounding up to people trying to get their cars out (thankfully they were all dog-lovers). But me? I probably burned off every calorie I consumed these last 36 hours, and that was only in the final climb back to my apartment. A climb, mind you, that at most inclined about 5 inches. Oh, Iceageddon! This is fun!!

Safety tips. It even works for walking! "Don't drive in the ruts created by other drivers' tires, drive outside of them. Better traction, no black ice."

Watching Bachelorette with my girl Brenda. Watching a movie at the same time as someone else and texting through it makes me feel so much more connected. Almost as if she was actually here!! This is such a good idea!!

December 8, 2013

Wow, I'm watching SNL because its host is Paul Rudd and musical guest One Direction (although the reason I started watching was because I thought it was One Republic) and I only recognize TWO names from the cast... And one of them is from my childhood!! WTH??

I want ice cream. Every time it's cold. Calories you eat while iced in don't count, right?

Well I am starving so test run, here I come. I'm not sure how to even start chiseling my car.

So that was fun. I made it to Target a mile down the road because it seemed the safest route. Any fast food around here has a major hill. So at least I got a lot of food (and ice cream!!) for nearly the same price I would have spent at a restaurant on one meal. But this shit better quit if you want me to leave my apartment again.

AYESHA W: They better de-ice the parking lot at school tomorrow morning! It's basically on a hill too! Jason just went to Kroger to buy whatever was left (not much) and he had one helluva time getting the car back up the driveway!

ME: Yeah... that's how I wrecked my car last year. KRK parking lot. And I made it all the way home and got stuck going back INTO my apartment complex!!! It's still scary.

[I shared a post.] "When we sleep, they are awake. When we are warm, they are cold. When we can stay home and safe, they must brave the elements. We wanted to pause to say 'thank you' to all of the first responders who risked their own safety to keep north Texans safe through this winter storm! If you have a responder who is special to you, please be sure and comment so we can recognize them!"

December 9, 2013

121, which I live off of, is closed down. Somehow I'm more nervous to take the back roads. I hope there are some babies there.

ANGELA H: Mine will be. be safe
CANDICE L: Be careful!!!
AYESHA W: Be careful!!!
AMY W: I thought you guys followed Frisco closing?
JIMMY C: Why was 121 closed?
ME: Amy, we make our own rules. Janelle, your baby is the only one not here. Well except Brinklee, and her mom works far away. Stay sane girl!! Jimmy, because they're having to use a monster to break up the ice. [I added a picture of an insane-looking machine after Jimmy posted a picture of all the Monsters University crew.]

I posted a cartoon of an old couple sitting by each other. The man said, "My butt fell asleep!" The wife replied, "I know. I can hear it snoring."

December 10, 2013

Wow, Tom Hanks makes a killer Walt Disney. Seeing this movie is an obsession. #savingmrbanks #tomhanksbiggestfan #disneygirl

I posted a cartoon of two birds sitting on a branch. The skinnier one said, "How's your diet doing?" The fatter one answered from the end of the bending branch, saying, "Fuck you."

December 12, 2013

Wow I'm hungry.

Hahaha!! Florida Georgia Line wants to collaborate with Garth Brooks because "apparently he's making some kind of comeback..." Next artist they named was Wiz Khalifa. Oh, man, how can you pretend to be a country singer and not have more respect for Garth than that??? Lmao!

I got a "tall" from OldNavy.com and look what I get! A sweatshirt that comes over my hands! #longarms #newfave

Oh Lord, I have to stop watching Lifetime when I'm babysitting! Even the COMMERCIALS make me cry.

KATHERINE H: You are the cutest thing ever. And I totally get what you're saying... sniffle.

December 13, 2013

Florida-Georgia Line's new song "Stay" sounds just like 3 Doors Down. Happy Friday the 13th!!

Bruno Mars Billboard Artist of the Year: Very well deserved. Love this man.

December 14, 2013

#topone #howmanycalories #iwish #bottomone #hurrytheeffupthen #wannaberich with pics of fortunes from cookies: "Three time a week, treat your-

self to dessert!" and "Your talents will bring you the highest status and prestige."

Wow, I think this is officially the longest Ruby has ever gone... Took her out at lunch at 12:30, and now just getting home. Champ. At this point, I should probably just stay awake, go shopping when the stores open, and come take a long nap till the parties start.

I also left my phone charger in my car. I'm at 18% but I had to park in BFE because it's nearly five and a whole block of parking is closed so I'm not going back out there. No one freak out if I don't answer my phone.

I'm sitting here trying to do the math, thinking there's no way I left her alone for longer than twelve hours; sixteen hours. I left her alone for sixteen hours? No wonder we have such bad separation anxiety; I tortured her as a baby! This dog is going to have the best rest of her life.

KRK West Frisco holiday party! Let's get crunk. [I tagged Lisa M.]

Holy shit, I won a week's paid vacation. Holy. Shit. If I had Paul and Tammy on here, I would tag the crap out of them. THANK YOU!!!!

AMY W: THATS AWESOME!!!!

MEGAN U: *If this is for real... This is AMAZING! You totally deserve it!*

KELLY M: *Where? How? I want one too!*

JIMMY C: *Wow! How'd that happen??*

AYESHA W: *Yay!!! Congrats!*

ME: *Raffle at our holiday party. I put 5 tickets in, knowing it would have by far the most tickets in it, and spread the love elsewhere too. But I won!! Yes!! Lol.*

KELLY: *Enjoy it!*

JACLYNN H: *Yay!!! You deserve it.*

LORA M: *Awesome!!!!*

PATTY M: *Congrats!*

December 15, 2013

Jessica C tagged me and eight other friends in family photo time, where for once I was smack in the middle rather than pushed to the edge somewhere.

I posted a meme of a dog and a cat in Santa hats, the dog eyeballing and licking the cookies, the cat drinking the milk. It's ok, they will just think Santa ate them.

Finally watching the live Sound of Music. I'm not that sad. Carrie is stunning, if not the best actress in the world. Stephen Moyer kinda just…is blah. The kids are less annoying than I figured they'd be (some of them are less annoying than the originals).

December 17, 2013

Most current obnoxious commercial: "pear; apple; hourglass; everyone's got a shape, do you like yours?" LIKE YOURS. At least enough to love yourself.

Only know you've been high when you're feeling low / Only hate the road when you're missing home / Only know you love her when you let her go.

GLORIA G: An you let her go!

I took my headphones off and my chain was hanging from them, clasp broken and cross missing. I've had that cross for 14 years. It was a gift for all the departing seniors in my church choir. And I lost it once at my old job and the cleaners found it!! And now… Now it's somewhere in the Target abyss. So. Sad.

> PATTY M: So sorry Courtney—I have had mine for 24 years yesterday. Randal gave it to me on our wedding day. I know how sad I would be if I lost it.

December 19, 2013

The wind just blew me over. And I think a rat made a nest in my hair.

December 20, 2013

> 5-day weekend peeeeeeeps. Followed by two really short days at work and then two more off!! What WHAT!!
>
> Hmm I want one, with a meme of a man in a cowboy hat and jeans: "Find her, protect her, spoil her, dance with her, and never stop loving her or someone else will. —The Cowboy Way"

December 21, 2013

> Last night "Rise of the Guardians" with my big kid, tonight "Santa Clause" marathon with my littlest munchkin. No matter how grown I get, I will always believe in magic.

December 23, 2013

> Just watched the silliest little musical Christmas movie, "Mistle-Tones." It was a surprise to find out Tia Mowry can sing like that, but not unbelievable, but there's no way that was Tori Spelling singing.

December 24, 2014

> TimeHop of Ruby 3 years earlier, looking eagerly at me to wake up, "Pretty much the same thing happened this morning. She must be excited for her cousins to come over. #christmasevelover"
>
> MEGAN G: Ruby!! I miss that face.
>
> Merry Christmas Eve!! This is my virgin champagne with pomegranate seeds floating in it!! #mykindofalcohol [with a picture of apple cider in a champagne flute].
>
> LYN B: Had such a great time with you. ♥
>
> ME: Me too. Too much fun. ♥

December 25, 2013

> Merry Christmas, everyone!! I love seeing all these pics of kids. I hope everyone has a thoroughly blessed day!!

NOT THE F——ING GILMORE GIRLS

December 26, 2013

> Well, it was a pretty awesome day. I love it when people play games with me!

December 27, 2013

> Who wants to go to IHOP with me this weekend? Cause I really want it. For like two weeks now. And I figure better to do it before I get my treadmill and start to feel guilty if I eat something to undo my workouts.
>
> KATHERINE H: You're getting a treadmill? Awesome! Check out the used ones on Craigslist... you can get a really good bargain.
>
> ME: That's what I did the first time. The belt shifted and stuck in the tread and ripped to shreds. Pretty much as I ran. It was not a pleasant experience. Nor a good use of $100. I'd rather get the warranty.
>
> Anyone want to come help me get this treadmill out of the back of my car? My door is roped open and I don't want my car battery to die. There is a set of stairs and $20 in it for you.

Y'all, I must have had a plan that fell through. Otherwise, why in hell would I go buy a treadmill that I didn't know how to get up the stairs? I do remember, my friend Jeff came to the rescue that time, but the idea of carrying a treadmill these days already hurts my body.

> [I posted a picture of the treadmill.] Uh, yeah-uh!! (Think Lil' John!). Thanks to a very sweet friend for helping me out. Now if I can just get the belt to run... Thank God for warranties!!!
>
> Man this is just my luck. Troubleshooted (troubleshot?) from every angle. Still can't get it to work. Anyone have any suggestions? Display works, even counts down, just the belt won't move.
>
> AMY W: Do you have an emergency stop pullout? If so is it plugged all the way in?
>
> SANDER W: Blown fuse?
>
> AMY R: I think the one you have is just like mine... there is a little plastic red round thing that

> has to sit in the middle below the display on a metal circle…
>
> ME: Yeah, I got that lol. Everything works but the belt. I'm gonna call Gold's Gym tomorrow, see if there's something obvious I'm missing.
>
> AMY R: Lol! Well mine ended up under the couch when Jonathan dumped the box out… I didn't know it existed at first.

December 29, 2013

I posted a meme that said, "I'm going to make sure that 2014 is my year, so…bring it on!"

December 31, 2013

> I hate it when people slow down in the intersection of a 4-way stop when they think the person coming up on them isn't going to stop. Why wouldn't they speed up to get out of their way?

January 1, 2014

> While the start may not have been the best, I'm hoping for a great year. Happy 2014, y'all.
>
> KATHERINE H: I hope 2014 brings you all the love and affection you deserve. You really are very special to many people.
>
> ME: Thank you, Auntie. And back!
>
> LYN B: Hey! What about me? Love you tooo.

I'm thankful I didn't write anything negative. It was almost as bad a night as the year before had been excellent. But that story rests in the past.

> When you feel my heat / look into my eyes / it's where my demons hide/ Don't get too close / it's dark inside / it's where my demons hide

January 3, 2014

> I just found out someone died this morning that was sweet and caring and too young. He texted me on Thanksgiving and I never remembered to reply. I don't know if he was okay at the time…

He had a rough time of it over the last few years. But I do know I wish I had found out. I don't often make resolutions; I always say if I want to change something, I don't need a new year to do it. But this makes me resolve to be there for my people when I can. I've always been almost too PRESENT. I try to stay in touch to the point of annoyance sometimes. But you never know when someone is going to just need to know you're there. God knows I do.

CRISTA L: I seriously can't believe it.

KATHERINE H: Oh, honey. Sad day. I'm sorry to hear about this, but you're right—it can make you live YOUR life differently.

Yikes, watching Dumbo with a 2-year-old is not the cure for sadness!!

January 7, 2014

Checked into Varsity Club in Frisco. Karaoke after work. Too much pizza, not enough beer. Need to be drunker!!!!

January 9, 2014

Why does red hair dye NEVER wash out? I've probably washed my hair 7 times since I went red and there are STILL red stains on my pillowcase.

Somebody PLEASE come unscrew this stupid treadmill for me!!!! HELP.

January 12, 2014

Well I borrowed a power drill from my bro to try to unscrew this thing. It ate the screw. And it's still holding the treadmill together. Grrrrrrrr!!!!!!

July 4, 2014

I went to the splash pad with Maria, Gloria, and bunch of kids—theirs, Kennedy, and Mason. This is a core memory for me. I don't know how many years we did it or what memories belong in what years, but spending the Fourth at the splash pad with Maria and as many kids as we could wrangle was always so much fun. The splash pad was in the neighborhood of some of the families we babysat for, so it was free and mostly, usually, pretty empty. We would pack sandwiches from the eighties, which always hit so hard after a pool day.

August 12, 2014

Pudge Rodriguez bobble head night at Ranger Stadium!

September 6, 2014

Ended up with (Christopher) for the night. Not a bad change of plans!! #lovehim #greeneyes

With Devon H at Olive Garden: Treated to dinner for hanging out with two of the coolest kids on the planet? Deal!!

Happy first birthday to mi favorito cacheton. I love you so much, Charlie! With my fav pics of him.

September 9, 2014

When is it going to be my turn? I'm tired of being unimportant.

September 19, 2014

Bowling with KRK friends, after a really hard week where we all posted that we needed drinks on Facebook.

October 23–28, 2014

California for Kevin and Kelsy's wedding.

October 31, 2014

Dressed as Rainbow Brite during the day, pics with Rhett (he made me take off my wig) and baby Bella. Night time, dressed as a flapper. Pics of car wreck (Snow White) and bruises. Stayed at the Legleiters' with the dogs, house sitting.

Whew, y'all, this car wreck. The one and only time I was involved in a wreck with someone else, I knew it was coming. I had had Snow White for less than two months, and she was my first white car. I didn't want white. It was after two in the morning on Halloween night, and I saw the driver on the other side of the road speeding to make the light to turn in front of me. The woman in front of him shouldn't have even gone, and yet he basically pushed her into the intersection. He was drunk. So I took my foot off the gas, slowing enough that when he plowed into me, it was into the nose of my car rather than directly into me. It was the worst sound ever. If you've never heard a car wreck, it was wild. Thankfully, the lady he was tailing stopped, and she was my witness for the cops.

A friend who had been at Val's party with me saw me on the side of the road, shivering in my flapper dress, and stopped too. When he came to hug me, I immediately burst into tears, the shock giving way to fear and relief. Andrew took me home that night, the drunk driver got off with a ride home from an equally drunk-looking friend, and I spent the week house-sitting and recovering from some super intense bruises but otherwise okay. Thanks to Stephanie and some other amazing friends and insurance, I had a new car within the week. I will never again drive a white car.

November 21, 2014

> AMY W: *[She posted a meme of a onesie indicating shoulders are created to roll down when there's a blowout.] Courtney, did you know this???? Facinating...*

November 22, 2014

> *Watching a special on Disney cruises. Disney theme park and resorts just ended. I thought I wanted to go badly an hour ago... Now it's an obsession.*
>
> ANNETTE W: *Welcome to my world*
>
> ME: *I haven't been on one since I was 10. It doesn't look like much has changed... And I totally want to experience all that as an adult.*

November 23, 2014

> *[I checked in that I was watching Mockingjay at Cinemark West Plano with Audrey.] Opening*

weekend WHAT WHAT. Adolfo, come see me soon and we will have a marathon.

[I shared a video of dogs in shoes.] No matter how many times I watch it, this remains nothing but absolutely hilarious. I must find shoes for Ruby asap.

November 26, 2014

[I posted a picture of Mason asleep on top of me, his hand over his eyes.] Got his baby brother this year. Heart full. ♥

I am so dizzy I literally feel sideways whether sitting or standing. Walking is an adventure. #sinusproblemsmuch

They need to make a "diet" plan for an ADD girl. I lose focus much too quickly.

November 28, 2014

[I reposted Toni Braxton's post on Black Friday.] Here ya go, Brent: "Did you know: Black Friday stemmed from slavery? It was the day after Thanksgiving when slave traders would sell slaves for a discount to assist plantation owners with more helpers for the upcoming winter (for cutting and stacking fire wood, winterproofing, etc.), hence the name...

> ME: Lol right?? They should just call it SALE Friday. Duh.
> AYESHA W: Working in retail, not sure I believe that—it is the day we go from being in the red (losing money all year) to in the black (making money). Most retailers do 10-20% of their annual sales from Black Friday to Cyber Monday! Shop away Karen! Lol.

November 29, 2014

My weekend of dogs. #dogpower #lovethisdog #coltrane #cookie #monte #tootsie #cuddlebuddies with pics

This is the lost weekend. I lose time so quickly in my little Woman Cave (no windows!). I'm usually ready to go back to work on Mondays... I could use another few days off this time around.

November 30, 2014

[I reposted Ruby.] Tomorrow is this little girl's birthday! How cute is she?

Happy 5th birthday to this munchkin. #rubyrose #sillydog #lovethisdog #notreadytogetup with pics

December 2, 2014

[I tagged Audrey in a picture with Grace and animals.] Cuddling with all kind of mammals. And Ruby's ear.

December 3, 2014

[I posted Tootsie with a tiny stocking across her face.] The #tootsie who stole #Christmas. #sleepypups

December 5, 2014

Nightmare Before Christmas onesies with KRK fam, Gordita Mya pouting at camera with shirt off.

December 6, 2014

Checked into RoughRiders Dr Pepper Ball Park for Kids R Kids holiday extravaganza, tagged Maria, Lisa, and more.

It's funny how some people's eyes disappear when they smile, even if they're quite round and big when they don't smile.

December 9, 2014

I am not nor will I ever be a Taylor Swift fan. But she's best friends with an Angel. So that's pretty cool. #vsfashionshow

I was so sure that I was right. She bugged the heck out of me. But I am a recent—within-the-year recent (I blame TikTok and "Anti-Hero")—bandwagoner, and there was a kid who used to come in my lives and ask me to play Taylor. He schooled me in all her best songs, and I've had the pleasure of getting to know her lyrics. She's fantastic. So is Jack, the kid who turned me on to her. He calls me Mother Goose and is just the cutest thing. I wish him the best in life.

December 10, 2014

> *Watching Dave: This is such a great quote about jobs: "It's not about the paycheck; it's about respect, it's about looking in the mirror and knowing that you've done something valuable with your day!"*
>> *Katherine H: And you certainly are doing a valuable service—one of the most important.*

December 11, 2014

> *Haaaaa ain't it the truth [with a meme that said, "The best things in life either make you fat, drunk, or pregnant"].*
>
> *Is there anyone who doesn't hope or plan for the future, but successfully lives day-to-day who can share their wisdom? I'm tired of... Getting my hopes up. #livefor themoment*
>> *Brent C: Rich people. You have to have money to be successful and live that way. Or incredible luck.*
>> *Me: Lol!! I think rich people probably hope for the future too...*
>> *Brent: Greedy ones, yes. But if you have the money to do whatever you want in life, your failures are your fault. When you're a normal person who can't just do anything they want whenever they want, life is a lot about luck.*
>> *Me: Lol oh kid. You should know better than anyone exactly what I'm referring to in this post... While having money certainly would make life easier, as the cliché goes, it doesn't buy happiness.*

BRENT: *Then you're just being dumb. Don't fault someone else for blatantly showing you that they're stupid, but you keep ignoring those signs. When you choose to ignore the glaring signs they're giving you, hoping that they're not true, then that's on you...not them. When people show me that kind of stuff I cut it off, just like I did today.*

ME: *I am being dumb lol. And I'm looking for advice on how to cut it out. It's not that easy for me.*

BRENT: *Simple: When someone acts like an idiot, get rid of them.*

DANIELLE S: *I understand what you are saying. When I was younger, I was always waiting for that "something" to make me happy. Being content in your circumstances is key for me. Every time I start thinking of things I don't have, I have to think of the things I do. Blessed beyond...*

ANGELA W: *Self evaluation! Figure out what it really is u want in relationships, career, life, etc... and then don't accept less. If u allow things to come into your life below your standard then u will never be satisfied. You are worth all the happiness in the world*

MARCUS R: *Here is my advice. Happiness does not come from any outward source. Nothing you have or do will give you happiness. You may experience a moment of joy but that is fleeting. People disappoint and that includes self. That is a fact of life along with taxes and death. I separate my judgment from my disappointment and just try to be satisfied with being a good person. That is the source of my happiness. I only judge if I'm fulfilling by current capability for goodness. When I find myself lacking I forgive myself and correct but do not chastise or punish. Everything that is outside my control I decide is not worthy of a happy rating. What I am able*

> *to accomplish is only material to my happiness if I've been able to maintain goodness in the process. People that do not help you be a good and better person but hold you back and want you to do things that are not in your good should be put in perspective if not pushed away. Hope these words are helpful. It's all a mind game in the end lol.*

I got told recently that I was trying to play mind games, and it made me stop and think because of whom it came from. Rereading that post, I understood it in a different way and immediately turned to message the person who had said that. If trying to maintain happiness for everyone I love is playing mind games, then okay, I'll take it. All I want to do is smile and make other people smile, love and be loved. I hope that makes me the Olympic gold medalist for mind games.

December 12, 2014

> *TimeHop of my Diary of a Stranger post: It's been four years and STILL this is my dilemma... Think I should start writing. VOTE!*
> *LISA M: Irish guy. You can't go wrong!*

I wonder if I'll ask again in nine years—nine years to finally understand I don't need other people's opinions on how to live my life or how my characters should live theirs. I value them, but I don't need them. My life and my characters' lives, my decision.

December 13, 2014

I love the view from up here / warm sun and wind in my ear / We'll watch the world from above as it turns to the rhythm of love.

December 14, 2014

> *Finally played the game which I've heard so much about tonight! Cards Against Humanity = #winning*
> *JAYNE W: That game is hysterical!*
> *STACI M: Awesomely inappropriate.*
> *MARIA V: It was fantastic!*

December 16, 2014

    [I was tagged in four photos from Ugly Sweater by Valerie.]
  Hamilton BK: *Merry Christmas!! A big hug from all of us.*

December 16, 2014

    [I shared a video of a woman grabbing a foul ball from a little girl.] Wow. Some people. Shame on you, lady. Boy, that girl gave her a dirty look though!!
    I shared a video of a unique traffic stop in Kansas City, Missouri, where cops handed out one-hundred-dollar bills to unsuspecting drivers.

December 18, 2014

    Minnie Mouse just took my order at Chick-Fil-A.
    YEAH!!! Hour long drive for an 8-second decision, but charges are DISMISSED!!!! Hallelujah, and thank God!!!!!
  Maria V: *I'm so glad they let you off for murder. I kid i kid*
  Me: *Haha might as well have been for as stressed as I was about it.*
  Kealeilani S: *Was that for the washing machine?*
  Me: *Yup. Big relief.*
  Katherine H: *Justice prevails! You were really courageous to stand up for yourself and the truth... not everyone would have done that.*
    [I posted a Timehop from 2010: "I'm getting to the point where I dislike weekends. I can only take so much down time."] Baaaaaahahaha. How much changes when you hit 30... Seriously. #wanteverydaytobesaturday

December 19, 2014

    I wish I had a man to buy Christmas presents for.

[I was tagged by Michelle B. with pics of Easton and Jackson.] Took the boys to see their teachers! Sorry we miss you, Tricia!

Beth C wrote, "I want to wish a very Merry Christmas to the most amazing girls that take care of our little guy every day, and also did so with the twins! Thank you, Courtney, Gloria, and Maria... you make it so much easier to transition back to work knowing my babies are with you! Thank you for our gifts and the best Christmas pictures of baby Victor! [He was dressed in a diaper and Santa hat and Santa bib!]

December 21, 2014

Went to a Christmas party tonight and came back out 13 years ago... #gaspricepicturebandwagon #fillerup (with pic of prices at $1.39!)

Watching Gilmore Girls: Super weird. When you've watched a show 409 times, you can keep your eyes peeled for guest stars... Just saw Schmidt from New Girl in Dean's wedding party and the vampire who can control the elements in the last Twilight.

Funny, I still don't know Schmidt's real name, but that vampire became Freddie Mercury. Rami Malek, way to glow up.

December 29, 2014

Lol 4 years later, and little has changed [with Timehop from four years earlier]: "I want to be a Dallas Cowboys Cheerleader. And the next J. K. Rowling. And a girlfriend. And a mom."

December 31, 2014

Happiness lies in your own hand / It took me much too long to understand

Here's what I've learned since then, to add on to these marvelous lyrics. You can't blame anyone for your station in life. Yes, my mother broke my heart and sent me into a black pit of despair, but she was not responsible for the fact that I stopped looking for work or that I stopped showering. I stopped. I stopped for almost a year. And now I get it, why I was so happy even when my heart was breaking. I know how to make myself happy (not like that, dirty birds), and other people will come and go. I want to love them as long as I get the chance to, but sometimes, that just isn't very long. I will always love them from afar.

January 1, 2015

> Happy 2015!! #newyearseve #sparkles #wishyoucouldseemyskirtandtights #tiaras #fabulousfriends
> Watching The Interview: Watching this with the most awesome friends a girl could have. Already laughing a lot and it's only 5 minutes in. Hope this continues!
> SHELLY T: Loved it.
> SANDER W: Worst movie ever.

January 4, 2015

> Stephanie Skipper: Tomorrow is my official return to work and Mya's start of daycare. I've already had 2 mini breakdowns tonight. Good thing I LOVE our daycare and completely trust Courtney Cannon and Gloria, but it's still so hard!
> ME: If it's any consolation, I can't wait. I've been thinking about her all weekend.

January 5, 2015

> I posted pictures of silly, pouty Mya to compare to baby Jessalyn.

January 7, 2015

> Watched He's Just Not That Into You: "This needs to become a monthly viewing until I get it through my head. #whenwillilearn

January 9, 2015

> My mom pointed out to me once that Hollywood kisses always take action with the man's hands on the woman's neck. Every once in a while, I don't notice because the chemistry is too good. But mostly

I think, who actually kisses like that?? I don't dig it at all. Watch. It's a thing.

January 10, 2015

Watched Jersey Boys at Mom's: FINALLY watched this. It was stellar. Took me a while to warm up to Frankie, but I was in love with Tommy and Bob from the get-go. So. Good. Want more of the closing credits!!!!

What's the record number of times to have seen a movie over a nine-year period? I bet I shattered it with this one.

March 5, 2015

Snow in Texas!! Playing outside with Lani and Audrey at 1 in the morning.

March 9, 2015

Mom, Jimmy, Audrey, Grace, Lani, and me at dinner, Mom's hair is super short and she looks happy.

May 5, 2015

[I posted Mya and Charlie's Mother's Day pictures.] Good moms have sticky floors, messy kitchens, laundry piles, dirty ovens, & happy kids.

June 12, 2015

[I posted a video from parents' night out where everyone was screaming.] Late nights were hard for those babies at school hahaha.

July 10, 2015

Parents' Night Out with Ayva and Mya, who I did a series of Squish Face photos with, and when I stopped playing with her chubby cheeks, she started crying.

July 28, 2015

> *Very sleepy Charlie stacking his cars in my lap. I asked him if I was the parking garage, he swiped some cars off my lap and exclaimed "oh no!" and then continued stacking.*

July 31, 2015

> *Took Jessalyn and Mya to Palio's for dinner, spent the night, and took them to IHOP for breakfast...*

The first time I spent the night at the Skippers', Jessalyn was only about six months. I had a blast with her and I then broke their guest bed, which was super fun to explain. (My pants got caught on the end of the bed and completely pulled the footboard off, total freak thing that would only happen to me.) That weekend, she fell off the couch, and I got to experience the terror of dropping a baby. The weekend when I had her sister too, Jessalyn managed to pull an entire cup of coffee into Mya's lap. I ripped her from her high chair and unzipped her onesie immediately, and no real harm was done. But man, that was scary too.

I can't tell you how many times I had the privilege of playing parent to those kids, and my heart smiles at every memory. I wish y'all would get the same joy out of it as I did if I shared every one, but it doesn't quite work that way. I just hope that you have kids in your life who bring you cheer the same way all my little wonders did. The Skippers became my family.

October 3, 2015

> *State Fair with the Skippers...*

This was absolutely one of my favorite traditions. This particular year, I stayed with Mya while Steph took Jessalyn on the rides. We went through adorable, kid-friendly displays where they pretended to grocery-shop and other things. Jessalyn got chosen to be onstage for something, and the pictures of her posing were hysterical. We met up with Maria, Leo, and her kiddo. Mya looked thoroughly confused as to why she was there. More shots of Jessalyn posing in front of Big Tex ended this group.

October 11, 2015

> *@ 2:22: On the DART with Adolfo, headed to the State Fair again...*

This was another tradition that was precious. Who would have ever known that the kid I had such a crush on at Pizza Hut would grow into my best friend for years? I have so, so many good memories with this man, but most of them revolve around food and movies and baseball.

November 20, 2015

> *Pinking out for Ms Lisa. #cancerhasnomonth #faithgivesmestrength [I posted this with a picture of me in a pink shirt, hair braided.]*

November 21, 2015

> *Hanging with an 8-year-old and a 5-year-old for a bit...*
> *ME: You guys thirsty?*
> *H: Yeah, I saw some Pepsi*
> *E: I want Pepsi!*
> *H: E, you can't have Pepsi, you need Sprite.*
> *ME: Can YOU have Pepsi?*
> *H: Yes. I'm 8. (With all the scorn in the world.)*

November 22, 2015

> *Pleeeeease we have to stop this madness. Thinking of working retail and being forced to work on one of the few holidays everyone closes for DISGUSTS me. I saw an ad for "Happy Thanksgetting" today and it broke my heart. We need to go back to the meaning of the holiday. Accompanied by post of "The Dirty Dozen" opening on Thanksgiving: JC Penney, Kohl's, Toys R Us, Walmart, Target, Sears, Macy's, Belk, Sports Authority, h.h. gregg, Dollar General, and Best Buy.*
>
> > *AYESHA W: It's not going to happen—for every upset person, there's another one who's excited. We are now operating in a market where this is necessary to keep in competition and make your sales projections—every major depart-*

> ment store is doing it and will continue to do so. They can't afford not to. I totally agree, but working in retail, the reality is... unfortunately this is the new norm.
>
> KELLY N: My company is on this list. However I can tell you that working on thanksgiving is voluntary and comes with double pay not time and a half. Also, all Store management and VPs and above are required to work in the stores. For some families the double pay will make a difference. Not saying I agree with being open but at least we are trying to make it better for our people.
>
> AYESHA: same with my company who is also on the list.

November 24, 2015

> Ugh. Humanity. In the best and worst situations.

November 26, 2015

> [I reposted Ayesha W's meme of Friends.] Monica & Chandler's twins would be 10 this year, Emma 12, Phoebe's triplets 15, and Ben 19. Let's just take a moment to let that sink in.

Let's add to that: The twins are now eighteen, and they had to say goodbye to their dad this year. Emma is twenty, and it was her uncle. Phoebe's triplets, who are twenty-three, got named for him. And Ben, who's twenty-seven, is old enough to date.

> [I watched Macy's Thanksgiving Day Parade.] Thanksgiving with my sweet Logan and two awesome girls. Spending the holidays with kids is such a blessing. (Asking them what they want for Christmas is NOT!! Lol!)

November 27, 2015

> Ruby just ate half a Chick-Fil-A milkshake while I was washing dishes. The whole thing. Thank

God it wasn't chocolate, but I feel like she has a fun night ahead of her (and me).

NICOLE O: In the rain!

November 28, 2015

[I reposted a family picture originally captioned, "I love that Anne's arm looks like mine."] Five years ago...and I still think Anne's arm is mine every time.

KEALEILANI S: What a great pic. Gma and all her grandkids.

ANNE A: I would not have noticed! Lol it does! Lol how funny.

[Someone who no longer has FB pointed out Rosie wasn't pictured.] LANI ADDED: Or Jimmy.

I love Jennifer Garner. She's just about as cute as a person can be. But she just really isn't that great of an actor! That said, "Miracles From Heaven" looks awesome and like a movie I will most likely need to see alone.

Checked in at Hobby Lobby: Normally madness on a Saturday. Saturday after Thanksgiving? Utter chaos.

NICOLE O: Yeah, I was there this morning

SAMANTHA K: The one in San Marcos was nuts today too, and I had to make two trips!

[I shared a post from Jennifer M.] Maturity is learning to walk away from people & situations that threaten your peace of mind, self-respect, values, morals, or self-worth.

On a cold night, it would be nice to have a human cuddle buddy. But this girl does an awesome job. #rubyrose #whatafatty #cuddlebuddies

[I shared Donnie's Daddy Daycare post and pictures.] I can't believe how adorable our son's pictures with Santa came out. After falling asleep in line waiting, Santa asked us not to wake him and the outcome was the cutest thing I've ever seen.

November 29, 2015

> [I posted a picture of Ruby eyeballing some tamales.] She would really like a bite of these amazing tamales. #rubyrose #cutestthingever #whatafatty
>
> [I captioned a picture of a snow-covered dog that said, "If you are cold, they are cold. Bring your pets inside."] Y'all.
>
> [I posted a picture of a painting I started.] Interesting... #sunset #blending #prettysofar #partoneanddone

November 30, 2015

> There she is! #parttwoanddone #prettyalldone #dowhatyoulove #artistiam [with a picture of the finished painting]

December 1, 2015

> Hey guys, if a girl you like shows you something she created, tell her it's pretty, even if it's not your thing. If she tells you she's in a bad mood, ask her what you can do to cheer her up. CARE. Just care.
> JESSICA R: You can't change him!
> HALLIE W: Good luck with that.

I am watching Hallmark Christmas movie *A Dickens of a Holiday!*, and one of the men said "Good luck with that!" right after I typed it. #clairaudient

> Happy birthday, honey pie. #sixthbirthday #rubyrose #cutestthingever I would happily stay home and take you to get ice cream [with a black-and-white picture of Ruby]

December 2, 2015

> Weird how today is supposed to be sunny and the warmest of the week, yet my car is frozen over and there is frost on the ground. Come on, Jack!! Stay with us!!!
>
> I still believe in Santa. [This was my caption to this post: "Dear Ryan, You asked a really good question, 'Are Mom and Dad really Santa?' We know

that you want to know the answer, and we had to give it careful thought to know just what to say. The answer is no. We are not Santa. There is no one, single Santa. We are the people who fill your stocking and choose and wrap the presents under the tree—just as our parents did for us, their parents did for them, and you will do for your kids someday. This could never make any of us Santa, though. Santa is lots and lots of people who keep the spirit of Christmas alive. He lives in our hearts—not at the North Pole. Santa is the magic and love and spirit of giving to others. What he does is teach children to believe in something they can't see or touch. Throughout your life you will need this capacity to believe: in yourself, in your family, in your friends, and in God. You'll need to be able to believe in things you can't measure or hold in your hands. Now you know the secret of how he gets down all those chimneys on Christmas Eve: he has help from all the people whose hearts he has filled with joy. With full hearts, people like Mommy and Daddy take our turns helping Santa do a job that would otherwise be impossible. So no, we are not Santa. Santa is love and magic and hope and happiness. We are on his team, and now you are too. We love you, and we always will."]

December 3, 2015

> KATHERINE H: *While the world goes crazy and our country sinks to its knees (cheerful opening) I wanted to write a note of appreciation for all my amazing nieces. Kealeilani, Anne, Courtney, Jocelyn, Megan, Rozie, Alie. These young women are trying so freaking hard to help make the world a better place—working with kids, helping people figure out their finances, working in an ER, helping people be healthier, studying, studying...trying to be a better person. If more people were like you guys—there'd be peace on earth this Christmas. (This is me, being auntiesque.)*
>
> ME: *Aww thanks!!!*

MEGAN U: This gives me goosebump a lil... I love this! Amen to making this country/world better despite all of the horrid things happening... Treating people like people not things/objects!!! Harper added to this list... She's gonna do great things too!!!

KEALEILANI S: Wonderfully said. I got tears building up while trying to read. Love all of you amazing women.

MARK E: You are a special individual. Lani told me about you.

ELLEN Z: Inspiring. I love girl power. ♥

December 5, 2015

[I posted a picture of me and Jimmy at Dad's in Ohio. I was wearing a sky blue tank and hugging the stuffing out of him.] Happy birthday to the best brother in the world. Through thick and thin, I'll stand by you.

ANNE A: Omg. That is sooo cute!!

KATHERINE H: Gosh you guys were adorable.

December 6, 2015

I tagged Jimmy "Happy birthday!!!!" in pictures with Kaitlyn at Phillip and Claudia's house.

DAVID P: That's a lot of candles!

Being an adult is mostly being exhausted, wishing you hadn't made plans, and wondering how you hurt your back.

December 7, 2015

[I tagged Lani, Harper, Anne, Jocelyn, Alie, Patrick, Ryan, and Megan in a post.] I need a Cuz Jam. Can y'all come to Texas??

Watching The Voice: Man, what a season. I want to be friends with Jeffrey Austin soooo badly. I cannot STAND Shelby. And Zach Seabaugh is. I mean. Come on. Jail bait. One of those two boys HAS IT.

So something fun about me is, I was a rock star when it came to picking the winners of these shows. I was the best at *American Idol*. I called top two since auditions for, like, four seasons. And Javier Colon from *The Voice*, he was special. I have no idea what makes me feel the magic, but I trust it. However, neither Jeffrey nor Zach won that year, though I think Jeffrey got pretty close.

December 8, 2015

> Watching The Voice: All right, I lost Zach but Jeffrey and Barrett are through! Jeffrey for the WIN!!!
>
> JAMIE W: Who all made it?? I was working...
>
> ME: Oh girl!! Jeffrey, (YEA!!), Barrett, Jordan, and Emily Ann. Zach was so close. Woulda been funny for Team Blake to dominate. But I'm still hoping for Jeffrey.
>
> JAMIE: Good choices! Jordan or Jeffrey for the win!
>
> JAYNE W: Lexi screamed when Zach didn't make it. I'm team Jordan. He's insanely talented.
>
> ME: I'm just not a Jordan fan. Jeffrey or BARRETT all the way. (I'm Team Blake, but Jeffrey is better than Barrett lol).
>
> [I posted pictures with Dad.]
>
> NICOLE R: You look just like your dad!
>
> ME: You think so?? I'm the spitting image of my mom, so that's funny. My bro looks just like my dad. Except the nose. I have a 100% Cannon nose.
>
> NICOLE: Yep the nose stands out as a match and the smile/eyes. Now I want to see your mom!
>
> BRENDA J: I see a beautiful blend of the two in you!
>
> KATHERINE H: Wow, your dad looks GREAT! And you know how pretty I think YOU are.
>
> AMY M: Beautiful. You do look a lot like your dad.

December 10, 2015

> No I would NOT like to play chicken at midnight, dumb ass coming the wrong way down Lebanon. Nothing like cresting a hill and thinking, is that a car coming at me??
>
> SHANNON M: Yikes!! That's scary.
>
> BRENDA J: Very scary! Glad you were alert!

> "Good reminder: Commitment means staying loyal to what you said you were going to do long after the mood you said it in has left you."
>
> Watching The Tonight Show Starring Jimmy Fallon: I've started recording this just so I don't miss the games... Claire Danes from a few nights ago was AWESOME. I can't stop laughing when I watch this man. He lifts my heart.
>
> BRENDA J: He is so funny! I love watching him too.
>
> Bernie Sanders on Jimmy... First thing I've watched having to do with anything about the election. #jimmymakeseverythinggood #feelthebern
>
> Love, love, love this!! [I posted this with a cartoon of a stick figure holding a heart in front of Jesus, saying, "It's all I have." Jesus answers, "It's all I want."]

December 12, 2015

> I don't understand chefs who smoke. Doesn't it ruin your palette?
>
> KATHERINE H: It is kind of weird, isn't it? They all drink and do drugs too. Did you read "Kitchen Confidential?" It's really a tough life.

Leave it to my aunt Katherine to be the empath. I clearly need to read that book, but I still don't think chefs should smoke. I don't know what drugs do to your palette, but I could tell when a smoker is in the kitchen for sure.

December 12, 2015

> Singing "Little Drummer Boy" with a two-year-old may be my favorite thing ever.

December 13, 2015

> Watching Wicked City. I can't believe this was cancelled after three episodes. I haven't been watching because I was saving them up... It only just occurred to me that I only have two!! I need some Ed Westwick SOMEWHERE ELSE.

LISA M: *Oh no!!!! I wondered why it hasn't been recording. I loved that show.*
STACI M: *I liked it too! It was cancelled?*

December 14, 2015

After her bath. She's so mad at me, she's sitting on top of her cage rather than on the couch. #sillydog #rubyrose #cutestthingever [with a picture]

Just got done shopping at Target and Five Below and came to two conclusions: 1, I am a wicked good Secret Santa, and 2, I am extraordinarily excited for this week and subsequent weekend. Secret Santa, Christmas Craft Night, KRK holiday party, and Tacky Sweater!!! YEA!!

MISHA T: *Oh my gosh! I forgot about Secret Santa. I better get back out.*

#selfiesunday #greeneyes #sofairdontcare with pic

Will y'all vote for my friend's tree? All you have to do is go click "like" on the picture that says Samantha K. She's in second right now; let's push her into first.

SAMANTHA: *Thank you!!!*
MEGAN F: *Done and done! Beautiful tree!*
SAMANTHA: *Thank you Megan!*

Aww Stephanie, look how gorgeous you look!! Everybody donate [with a post of my friend Stephanie on WFAA news 8]!!

December 15, 2015

I have a non-rhetorical question, particularly directed at those without kids! Is it better to love and have lost than never to have loved at all? (I ask y'all with no kids simply because the kids make a different spin... If you'd never loved their (other parent), you'd likely not have them.) HELP!!

ASHLEIGH M: *Better to love and lose. I've lost in a relationship before and have learned what better love is.*
BRENDA J: *LOVE is always the better choice. I know I have kids, but I had to weigh in on this.*

Favorite Charlie-isms of the night:
(Baby commercial comes on TV)
Me: *Charlie, what are you going to do when your baby comes?*
C: *Help!*
(Now whether he was talking about he will help mommy or HELP, don't give me a baby!, I am not sure.)
(After changing a particularly stinky and painful diaper)
Me: *It's okay, Charlie, it's because you ate so many oranges!*
C: *Lots of oranges.*
Me, while putting Desitin on: *Yup!*
C: *Giant poopy!*
Thanks, kid. I needed to know just HOW big it was.

December 16, 2015

I watched the animated "Little Drummer Boy" with Charlie last night and it made me hear the song in a whole new light. I know the lyrics but I'd never really listened to them. And now I can't hear the song without crying.

December 18, 2015

When the world kinda sucks, at least I have this. What a way to start my weekend. Love this sweet boy [with a picture of me cuddling a Davis baby].

Man, why does food make everything feel better? Just had an incredible sandwich from a new place and I'm like truly sad it's gone. #needtofindanothercomfort
Ayesha W: *What's this sandwich and from where?*
Me: *Grilled cheese with Turkey (or ham) from Norma's in Frisco.*

Surprised this sneaked up without warning, but this was the last time my mother went into the hospital. I remember eating Norma's for dinner at the school, feeling loved as my bosses listened to my woe as I held babies and ate good food. She was so angry at us. Jimmy and I went to visit her that time, and it was terrifying being there for twenty minutes. Living there would have been an actual nightmare.

December 19, 2015

> KRK Christmas party, Lisa's first day back.

December 20, 2015

> Ugly sweater party at Val's.
>
> That moment you look in an old wallet and find five unspent gift cards.
>
> [I posted a video of us doing the wobble at the KRK Christmas party.] Baha. Proof I look just as good as I thought I did.

December 21, 2015

> Yes: "Dear Santa, this year I would like a slim body and a fat bank account. Please don't mix them up like you did last year."

December 22, 2015

> Stress manifests in the oddest of ways sometimes. Over 90% of the last few days, all I've wanted was to curl up on my couch with "FRIENDS" playing and nap. The other 10%, I just want someone to hold me. Or hug my fat butterball babies.

December 23, 2015

> Money is wonderful. Not having it (or being able to access it!!) sucks.
>
> [I checked in at Studio Movie Grill with Valerie C.] Sisters with my girl.

December 24, 2015

> I posted a picture for Ugly Sweater: red tights, green velvet elf shorts, black boots, and Santa socks; the sweater was made by Crista.
>
> CAROLE K: Love your style!

December 25, 2015

Another year of making googly eyes at all these amazing kid Christmases. Trying not to be so jealous I actually turn green. Merry Christmas to all of my sweet friends and their incredible families.

December 26, 2015

Rearranged my living AND bed rooms because one guy SUCKS. It actually looks bigger. Pleased.

Okay. What's with the sirens???? No!!!

Lights flashing and sirens still blaring. Someone please make it stop. I am not cut out for this.

LYN B: *Stay safe.* ♥

JENNIFER M: *Oh dang, sister. Hope you're safe!*

KIM M: *Me either!! I'm such a weenie!*

December 27, 2015

[I tagged Audrey.] Finally got this beauty hung up. A year after receiving it. I just gave up on the support hooks... Hopefully it doesn't tear holes straight through the wall [with a picture of my nail polish shelf organized in rainbow order].

Birthday FaceTime with my favorite teenager turned into a detailed explanation of how a hover board works... These things. #backtothefuture #thefutureisnow #hesapro #iwoulddie

December 28, 2015

AMANDA A: *Dearest karaoke friends, How I long deeply for the day we shall karaoke again. My heart mourns and yearns for the sound of Ralph Dixon's mad karaoke skill. Willst thou join me for some gay camaraderie tomorrow's night?*

Why does ice cream have to be so cold? It's all I ever crave when it's cold outside. And I'm literally shivering on my couch.

GLORIA G: *So cold but so good!!!*

> MISHA T: *Kaili and I just discussed having a big bowl of ice cream!*
>
> AMBER S: *I'm doing the same thing!*

Whyyyyy are dogs in sweaters so funny? She's miserable, but maybe this will make her actually go to the bathroom.

December 30, 2015

I just can't believe tomorrow is New Year's Eve. I'm just. Blah.

January 2, 2016

Brought Jessalyn and Mya home to see Grace and meet Audrey. Grace loved cuddling the baby. Must have spent a couple of nights with them, lots of sleeping Mya pics and dinner and bath time.

[I reposted "The Weight Loss Diaries, Day 1."] Six years ago, and I'm back at square one. So much work undone in the blink of an eye (or let's be honest, in the repetitive motion of a hand!). I will try this again.

> LU B: *You can do it!*

January 3, 2016

Back to the grind in a hardcore way tomorrow! Three new babies and a full work week. I've forgotten how to do this!! But I sure am excited to have a full class again. Gonna miss my sweet Ellie but can't wait to get to know the new babes.

January 5, 2016

How do you tell a friend who has been served more hard knocks than anyone deserves in ten years who doesn't believe in God that you're praying for him? How do you help support him, help him look on the bright side, when he truly doesn't believe there will ever be a bright side for him?

> LISA M: *Just being there is one of the biggest things you can do. Be his friend. Listen and support. Life can throw you some pretty crappy things*

and just knowing I have friends and family who care means so much.

MEGAN G: Just say it. He will hear it but whether he listens depends solely on God. God will reveal himself to him in His time. Until then, all you can do is pray and let him know that you're doing it.

LU B: Actively listen without trying to solve the problem. Sometimes people just want to be heard.

VALERIE C: Just because someone doesn't believe in God doesn't mean they automatically don't see a bright side or see a purpose in life. Having supportive, loving people in your life is worth more to some people than leaning on an imaginary friend. And when you have religious friends who keep trying to cheer you up with something you have openly said you don't believe in, it is more infuriating than anything. The best thing you can do it just be supportive and listen.

January 7, 2016

Watched American Idol: Dalton Rapattoni. Dallas representing BABY!! This kid is SICK.

TRACY F: Aww, he used to take lessons where I taught in Dallas a few years ago. Sweet kid!!

I just belted "The Star-Spangled Banner: in my shower. It was amazing. #iamthenextamericanidol #betterthanwhitneys

January 8, 2016

That moment your Bubble-Guppies-obsessed kid tells you he doesn't want to watch it because "Buppies is broken." Omg. And just for the record, "Mickey Mouse is broken" too. And then you can't figure out what ISN'T broken because when you change it to something else, he cries and said, "I don't want that one."

Zac Efron giving an interview about a phone conversation he had with one of his heroes, Michael

Jackson, and MJ ended the call with something along the lines of: "Hey Zac, isn't it awesome. (I was like, what?) Dreams really do come true, don't they?"

January 10, 2016

Watching "Grey's Anatomy": The Derek death. Didn't want to believe it till I saw it for myself.

January 13, 2016

Baby Victor trying to learn how to "chew" on me and copying tongue and mouth sounds: "a new trick with the cutest kid in existence."

October 22, 2016

I posted about Halloween at Val's. I was dressed as Rainbow Brite.

This is the weekend I remember understanding that my friendship with these guys had come to the end of the road. I walked up on Laura, whom I was living with, and Val talking about me at what was supposed to be doubling as my birthday party. I don't know how I hung in for another six months, unless it was out of complete necessity. It's hard to live with people who don't like you. I had surgery (you'll read about that) in March, and they didn't ask me once if they could do anything for me. It was shocking. And sad. And not uncommon for me.

As I write this, it sounds like I'm begging for pity: "Oh, poor little girl never knew real friendships." But that's not the truth. I'm asking you to remember that people come into our lives for a reason, a season, a lesson, or a lifetime. I'll admit, I need some more life-timers. But I don't doubt that at some time, these people loved me despite how our situations ended up.

November 11, 2016

I posted beautiful selfies in a Disney villainesses shirt. Weekend with the Skippers, accompanied by favorite pics of Mya...and videos of the girls singing, Mya the alphabet in a restaurant at breakfast and J "We Will Rock You" loudly and off-tune in the backseat of my car, wrapped up with a video of me straightening J's hair.

November 20, 2016

    Sweet Jesus, I didn't think this man could get any sexier. #bruno #vesrsaceonthefloor
    [I reposted an article on WBC from Jay Pritchard and tagged Mark Winfield and George Mason.] A great surprise to end a beautiful day at Wilshire Baptist Church. #OneWilshire [with a picture of steps with chalked words: "Thank you for loving all people"].

November 21, 2016

    Almond Joy cookies recipe http://gimb.co/2cNEWrl

November 25, 2016

    Me and Isa [with a picture].

November 25, 2016

    [I reshared the announcement that Florence Henderson died.] Awwww!!
    [I posted about watching Gilmore Girls: A Year in the Life.] Logan. #winter
    GG: AYITL. Phew Jess looks hot. He could have gone totally the other way. #summer
    Delish post Thanksgiving in a Blanket: http://dlsh.it/tdBLleW
    Baby girl was so cuddly tonight, she somehow managed to slip a car in my shirt pocket. #whatthewhat #howdshedothat #sneakybaby And big boy told me I wasn't going home with Ruby; that I was staying there. #lovehim #thatboy My heart is full.

November 27, 2016

    Baby stringrays look like raviolis stuffed with tiny damned souls, with pic.

COURTNEY CANNON

KATHERINE H: Creepy

November 28, 2016

> *Checked into Crest Nissan: Well, came in for my regular oil change and an inspection and found out I need new tires, which was my biggest fear. And this is exactly why I say my luck will never change… I get somewhere almost good and then it all goes down the drain in one fell swoop.*
> *AYESHA W: Don't buy from the dealer!!!! Go to somewhere like discount tire!*
> *JAMIE W: At least you found out that way… instead of one blowing and leaving you stranded on the side of the road…*

What Jamie said. I did indeed have a blowout before—two, as a matter of fact. The first one, I was on the phone with my friend Adrian, who was supposed to have gone with me to Dallas. My van started shaking audibly, and Adrian made me start pulling over. It was me and one other person on the highway at the time, and when he saw me start to shake, he stopped his car. I blew out in the left lane; my van's rear fishtailed to the right, followed by the nose, and then spun a complete 180, traveling back across the highway and careening backward several feet before coming to a stop inches from the guardrail. Shocked, I waited until the guy who had slowed out of my way came running across the highway and pulled my door open to burst into tears.

The second one came years later, after two in the morning on the road home from Cowboys in Arlington. Thankfully, I had a friend with me that time, because it's scary enough in the daytime. A Good Samaritan pulled over to put on my spare, and a cute but married cop parked behind us to keep us safe. Then the Good Samaritan asked us to breakfast, and we followed him for about twenty minutes before we decided he might be leading us to doom. So we swerved off, sending up thanks and good blessings for him. Oh my goodness, the guilt I still feel about that!

So apparently, I still have a lot of guilt about that. I can almost guarantee that guy didn't give us a second thought once he realized we weren't behind him. If I was talking to one of you, I would say let it go. People are allowed to do good deeds for you with nothing in return. Say that out loud: I do not owe people more than thanks for being kind.

November 30, 2016

>There are four ailments that literally drive me to the brink of insanity: sinus headaches, stomachache caused by acid reflux, restless leg and/or phantom body aches, and unstoppable itching. I don't remember what it's like to teethe, but as an adult, I have experienced ALL of these others in spades, and I can't imagine being a baby and being able to do nothing. My fingernails are my best friends right now. No wonder my poor babies just cry all the time. #lotiononthosebabies #winteriscoming

December 1, 2016

>I posted birthday pictures with Ruby, Piggie Pie snuggling behind me on the couch: Ruby and I would both like to know why this pig has his face buried in my couch and his entire weight dumped onto my thigh and hip.
>
>Celebrating 7 in style. #birthdaydog #happybirthdaybaby #rubyrose with pic

>>CHRISTY V: My aunt's dog turned 7 today, too. It's a small world! Happy birthday, Ruby!
>>
>>ANNE A: Ruby!! So cute. Our families love dogs so much it's crazy! Lol

>I just can't stand the cuteness. Birthday overload. Love her so. #rubyrose
>
>Why do birds suddenly appear / every time you are near? Just like me, they long to be / close to you! #piggiepie #gordonwarden

December 3, 2016

>[Lisa M posted a company called Grateful Bacon that lists glitter, unicorns, and rainbows with a picture of a sparkly phone case.] OMG. Does this company know you?! It was made for you!
>
>So sad to be missing the KRK Christmas party for the first time in six years, but this. THIS. Football

is tiring [with pictures of Kaiser, the boxer, passed out with the football in his mouth].

 Every child must be made aware / Every child must be made to care / Care enough for his fellow man / to give all the love that we can. Peace on Earth... Can it be?

December 4, 2016

 Yum with Delish recipe for Funfetti cheesecake: http://del.sh/6004BUYoQ

December 5, 2016

 [I posted a picture collage of me and Jimmy as kids.] Happy birthday to this guy. We've had some ups and downs, but through it all, there's no one I trust more to be there for me. I hope this year is magic... it's time.

December 6, 2016

 [I posted a picture of Ruby curled pitifully under my sheets and blankets.] I have a very sick dog. I hope she's okay. I don't know what to do for her.

 CHERI F: What are her symptoms?
 STEPHANIE S: Oh no, I hope she gets better soon.
 MARIA V: Did you take her to the vet?
 ABRA N: Vet??
 ME: No, she's never been that sick thank God. Usually I can stop it with some chicken and rice. I'll have to see how she is when I get home.
 DAVID A: Awe poor puppy.
 ASHLEIGH M: For dehydration mix some Gatorade with water... she should want it because of the flavor. Also pumpkin.
 MARIA V: We give Harley pumpkin purée before she gets boarded due to anxious tummy issues. Works like a charm.
 KELLY M: What breed is she? She looks like my Molly girl [with a picture]

NOT THE F——ING GILMORE GIRLS

MARIA: *That looks more like Valerie's dog*
LYN B: *Swine flu?*

December 11, 2016

Why have I forgotten how to drink water?

[I shared a meme of Neil Patrick Harris: "Can someone please explain how words like 'turnt,' 'fleek,' and 'bae' are now universally understood but people still don't know how to use 'you're' & 'your' in a sentence?"] So true.

December 13, 2016

I am not someone who professes to hate Brussels sprouts (in fact, the couple times I've had them, I actually really liked them), but these should make a lover out of anyone!! #baconrulesall with video of bacon-wrapped Brussels sprouts with creamy lemon dip: http://www.foodtv.com/5abhf

December 14, 2016

I need this like I need air. #always with a link to an "awesome color changing Harry Potter mug!" https://www.theloomfactory.com/products/always-color-changing-mug.

MARIA V: *Love it! FYI Courtney and Jessica…I'm finally reading the books. Finished the first last week and halfway through the 2nd. When I'm done…WE WILL FINISH THE POTTERTHON.*

ME: *Yesssss. Are you liking them?? Clearly they get better… the first couple are so easy and short.*

MARIA: *I am. It's tedious sometimes due to the similarities but I love it when I get to parts that weren't in the movie.*

Money is literally the worst. Can't live without it but can't keep it to save my life. I want to barter. Groceries for a massage? Sounds like a winner.

KYLA N: *Find small local shops. Then you can trade all you want! I used to get a free CSA veggie box in exchange for babysitting the founder's* kid. You might be surprised how many people would be open to it.

I miss the good old days of going in and picking up candy and a movie from Blockbuster.

December 16, 2016

In case you didn't already know she's the cutest. (Does that not hurt her little shoulders??) [I posted this with pictures of Ruby sleeping awkwardly.]

[I posted a video of a little kid: "When you get a hold of your idol's hand, you don't let go, especially if it's Leo Messi."] Adorable.

When you wake up at 5:30 completely unprompted, there's only one thing to do: post on Facebook four hundred times.

[I posted another picture of Ruby.] She must just be cuter on Fridays.

I get to do this for a living. #blessed [with pictures of James asleep on me, then sitting with a grin and a ponytail]. This is what happens when you wake up before your mom is ready to go... you get a ponytail. #realmenrockponies

CHRISTAL K: He loves his Ms Courtney.

HEATHER H: Oh my! How cute!!

CHRISTAL: So funny! His hair is longer now. What was the gel again?

Live on FB with DJ Shawn Solo: "Check out the new trio!" Doing "Hell on Heels" with Mandy Joe and Britt, then "Take 2!! CMB!" Taking lead on "Let 'Er Rip" while Mandy did harmony.

Charlie and Isa's comparison Christmas lights photo.

December 17, 2016

OMG I'm doing this. Crock Pot Cinnamon Bun Casserole: http://wishesndishes.com/crock-pot-cinnamon-roll-casserole/

Val's dog Patches spent the night with us: "I stole Patches tonight because my friends went bar-crawling and I just wasn't feeling it. So here I lay, with three big fat animals (Gordon's the red lump) and a cup of hot cider. #mykindofsaturday #needsomeonetoshareitwith #butdontknowhowanyoneelsewillfit"

What. The. Hell. This is not okay. I mean, I always knew they weren't real results... but I figured they just used people with naturally thick or long lashes. This is like...false advertising. No. How do I ever trust an ad again?? [with a picture of a magazine ad that had "Simulation of product. Results on lashes enhanced with lash inserts" written in the corner]

[I tagged Ayesha W, Stephanie, and Beth C in an Elf in the Shelf post where the Elf broke his leg and was on strict orders not to move.]

AYESHA: Yep... I'm almost to that point...
STEPHANIE: Great idea! Lol

December 19, 2016

Watching Honey, I Shrunk the Kids: OMG. Thank you, Netflix!!

December 21, 2016

[I posted a picture with Ruby's face against mine, her head through my necklace chain.] She was so excited to see me, when she jumped in my lap, her big ol' head went through my necklace. Try as I might to push it back the other way, she didn't get it and the chain snapped in two places. Anyone have a James Avery connection?

December 22, 2016

Singing with Maddox, who fell asleep, with Ryan, who hit me in the face, and James, who laughed at me the whole time.

"This year's Christmas gifts... the first year we've ever done four photos, and they all turned out beautifully. Love my job so much" [with Jackson's finished photo collage].

Y'all, these pictures were amazing. We were such good teachers. I remember spending an entire day baking and cooking for my first class's parents.

I want to be able to do this for people still; I'm thinking about having a small studio at my house! It was so easy; all we needed was a sheet at the school.

December 23, 2016

Watched Robin Hood: Prince of Thieves. Best Christmas movie there is.

Watched The Fast and the Furious. This is where it all began. I hope they have all of them, because I've only seen one of them.

December 24, 2016

Scratching lottery tickets with the family at Lyn and Michael's.

December 29, 2016

Checked in to Crest Nissan. I feel like I've been living here lately. Come on car, I'm being an adult and actually servicing YOU; why you gotta disservice me?

With Delish recipe for fried lasagna. Holy yum, Batman: http://dlsh.it/iUnex9e

"Not gonna cry in the Nissan lobby" [with a video of shelter animals picking out their Christmas gifts].

December 31, 2016

At 22 hours awake with a bad sinus infection, I can only consider myself delirious. #mustsleepnow

Another tattoo possibly?? #nodaybuttoday

January 1, 2017

2017, y'all. What in the world?

[I posted a beautiful picture of my alarm clock, which was glowing pink at 3:33 AM] Good omen?? #2017willrock.

January 2, 2017

Y'all. Every year since I was about 30, I resolve not to make resolutions. It puts a bunch of unnecessary pressure on you when you inevitably stop resolving. If you want to change something, it shouldn't be because it's a new year. Change it because it's important to you. That said, there's nothing like a fresh date to make it the perfect time to start a book. So this is my year; I say it a lot, but this time I'm setting reminders. I will write every day. 2017 will rock.

AYESHA W: I feel the SAME WAY about resolutions. Well said!

CANNOT believe I didn't know The Bachelor premiered tonight. And that is MY MAN. Uggggggghh.

CRISTA L: Mine too. ♥

[Kealeilani S posted a unicorn cheesecake to my wall.] This tastes just as magical as it looks. Full recipe: http://dlsh.it/AS8K3a7

January 21, 2017

I posted a video of Mya, just beginning to get hair, telling me in the silliest little voice that she had a poopy butt.

February 4, 2017

Out with Kaitlyn, had to be the Tavern on Main. Is this the night I left early because my stomach hurt so much?

February 22, 2017

Trying to get Charlie to say "happy birthday Courtney's mom" turned into a conversation about my tongue ring and whether I ate it like candy or it stayed in there all the time.

February 24, 2017

Out with Kaitlyn again, super dressed up.

March 10-ish, 2017

>I have the oddest feeling about this, the fact that there seems to be zero indication leading up to it—my intense stomach pains, pictures at the hospital, anything? If it wasn't for my scars and Stephanie's memory, I would wonder if I ever had surgery at all. The brain is weird. I remember recovering at home with roommates who weren't speaking to me and Stephanie bringing me food when she was about to pop with Brayden. I remember not eating at all the week leading up to my final attack, and my blood work coming back clean again and again; even the sonogram didn't show anything. But the doc said the gallbladder looked much worse than they had expected, and I should be happy they removed it (thanks, of course, to my doctor-dad, who believed me when I said how bad the pain was).

March 16, 2017

> Brayden was born, and I posted pictures of Jessalyn and Mya holding him at the hospital.

March 25, 2017

> Onstage at the Tavern, it was the first time I sang sober, only a couple of weeks after surgery

April 29–30, 2017

> Video of Shawn and Jon doing "Blue Moon" and Bonnie doing "Dear Future Husband" for Shawn. Mike doing "Drive" and Jon making a toast to his best friend, Shawn Solo.

I was already crying watching them do the Eagles. But, y'all, this weekend was so precious. I had barely met these guys—if pictures are proof enough, I spent every weekend with them after my gallbladder surgery, and y'all know music and alcohol bring people together—but they already felt like family. Mandy Joe was at her bachelorette party, and I was too new to the group to be hurt that I wasn't invited to that, not to mention Bonnie and Laurin were at the bar too, and they were supposedly close with Mandy. I was just praying for a way to be invited to the wedding.

So it was just a lot of fun. We did marriage and wedding songs for Shawn. Then we went over to Laurin's when the bar closed. Somehow, the three of us girls did "Seven Bridges Road" and pretty much killed it. We spent weekends thereafter battling the boys at the bar, with Mandy Joe, for most applause. I remember Shawn was super cuddly that night, and because I didn't know him, I assumed it was because his woman wasn't there. But it turned out she didn't care and was, in fact, just as cuddly herself. I would keep gushing about these guys, but they were my family for, like, three years, so I'm sure more stories will crop up.

This was also the inconspicuous beginning of Bonnie and Jonny, as I loved to sing about them. It's funny to look back and think about the prayers I had even then that were coming true before my eyes, just not for me. (I prayed real hard for a karaoke romance. I was dreaming of my own John Hughes movie. It happened, complete with jealous friends and brothers. I just watched as it again happened to someone besides me.)

I was set to babysit the night of their wedding, likely in an effort to distract myself since my new regular was them and the bar. Shawn called me hours before, saying someone couldn't make it, and they would love if I could come. Of course I did. (I'm pretty sure it was the Skippers I cancelled on. I had fun, but it was a tiny bit awkward; it was Bonnie and Jon's first public appearance, and Laurin was boycotting the wedding because she didn't approve, if I remember correctly. The hole was massive.

May 23, 2017

Hanging with the Skippers, including baby Brayden. My first favorite shot with them was Jessalyn lying on my shoulder, Mya on top of her, and B in my lap.

June 15, 2017

Perot Museum of Nature and Science with the big kids.

My babies were my heart. Everyone knew that. But I loved getting to go on field trips with the school-age kids during the summers. The kids always loved me because I was firm but insanely loving and funny. They used to clamber to be in my group. So I got to form amazing connections with kids who could speak, and I got to see cool stuff that I normally wouldn't have seen!

September 6, 2017

This song got me this morning. "I'm hard to love, hard to love, I don't make it easy. I couldn't do it if I stood where you stood."

I looked up at a plane and wondered how many people inside were heading somewhere they were excited about. How many were heading to sadness. I wondered if anyone on board was truly carefree. If anyone was contemplating a way out. I also wondered how many seats were full. If anyone had missed the flight at the last minute because of tragedy at the takeoff. How many screaming babies were aboard. How many stressed-out parents were deflecting angry stares. How many people were terrified of crashing. How many people were terrified of someone having a heart attack or throwing up. How many people were calm and worry-free. How many planes were following that one.

I wish I could be on a plane. Filled with worry (mostly about someone throwing up or having a heart attack), I want to head somewhere I'm happy about.

September 29, 2017

State Fair with the Skippers; this year Mya went on the rides too, and I stayed at the bottom with Brayden. Mya looked so proud, Jessalyn looked bossy and all-knowing, and Brayden looked grumpy and sleepy. Some of the best times ever.

October 18, 2017

State Fair with Adolfo.

October 19, 2017

> Dinner where Adolfo and I both wore Star Wars shirts without planning it.

October 21, 2017

> Mya's 3rd bday, Brayden and me hanging out, her blowing out her candles; me and Jimmy at my bday at The Tavern later that night, me and Adolfo (I remember being so thrilled that he got to see me sing), me and Bonnie.

November 20, 2017

> My friend Jamie did this and the answers have been adorable. Let's do it!! Mine are posted below. [I posted this with a meme of a turkey in a microwave that read, "Text your mom and ask how long it takes to microwave a 25 lb turkey. Post results below."]
>
> ME IN TEXT: Hey Mom. How long would it take to microwave a 25-pound turkey?
> MOM: Gack. I have no clue and why would you do that?
> HEATHER H: Hey Mom! How long would it take to microwave a 25lbs turkey?
> MOM: Lol. I have never done it. Really???
> ABRA N: Mine was kind of boring but it's still funny. How long does it take to microwave a 25 pound turkey?
> MOM: lol you're kidding right?
> WHITNEY R: Mine said I already saw the meme... nice try.
> MANDY P: How long does it take to microwave a 25 pound turkey?
> MOM: Number one you just don't microwave a turkey and a 25 pound turkey would feed a small army.
>
> This. Always [with a screenshot from Plenty of Fish].
>
> HIM: U im carrollton
> I wanna give u babies honny

ME: *Lol no thanks*
HIM: *Jiji ok*
So i will like to see u
Be with u
Love u baby
 [*I posted a video from Delish of Thanksgiving in a blanket: "The most genius thing to do with your leftovers. Full recipe: http://dlsh.it/tdBLleW."*] *Omg. I'm doing it. I need ALL the leftovers.*

November 21, 2017

 [*I posted a video of a mom pushing her baby's face into her birthday cake and the baby turning around with her fist in the air, captioned, "Why did my little sister square up at my mom?"*] *Omg hahahaha. This will so be me as a mom. (And honestly, probably my kid too!!)*

November 23, 2017

 [*I posted a meme of a turkey predictive text: "I stuffed the turkey with…"*] *The meat and the turkey and the cheese was yum meat was yum I was sent home and I had to get it back in my mouth.*
BONNIE A: *I stuffed my turkey with a lot more fun.*
LAUREN Y: *I stuffed the turkey with my little boy he is my husband!!!! Wtf!?*
TAYA B: *I stuffed the turkey with the chicken in my mouth. Hmmm what the hell!?!?*
JENNIFER M: *I stuffed the turkey with the teacher is a stressful time and do not want to add more stress.*
ME: *Omg new winner!!!*
BETTY W: *I stuffed the turkey with you when I get back to killing of a little bit more than words can say. Lololol*
ASHLEY B: *I stuffed the turkey with the lid on it and it looks good but it looks good on the wall.*
WENDY M: *I stuffed the turkey with you guys for coming out and about. Haha!*
HEATHER H: *I stuffed the turkey with the cheese stuffed turkey and I was just getting off Twitter.*

I've never understood scenes in movies or TV when people are golfing off a rooftop. Don't they think about where the balls would land?? And on the flip side, can you imagine being beaned in the head by a rogue golf ball??

VALERIE C: Are you watching Gilmore girls?
DAWN L: Or Grey's Anatomy?
ME: What the heck??? How did y'all know?? These are exactly the two shows I've been watching today…

November 24, 2017

Well, it's that time again. Possible impending move to happen in January. Anyone know of someone who needs a roommate or has a room to rent? (Someone who's cool with dogs!)

November 25, 2017

I posted a video meme that said, "Don't forget that maybe you are the lighthouse in someone else's storm."

[I was watching Forrest Gump.] Bill Murray, Chevy Chase, and John Travolta were considered for this role… NO.

November 27, 2017

I think it's gonna be a long day. Had trouble falling asleep, then got woken up at 3:50 by an absurd amount of sirens. Finally had to turn on my TV to cover it up. Woke up again at 5:02 when my TV turned back off. Then my alarm goes off at 5:25… I managed to fall asleep AND DREAM in the 10 minutes between that and the second alarm at 5:35. I'm groggy.

[I posted a Boomerang of Ruby digging and dancing on the bed.] This is my new favorite app.

November 28, 2017

>Omg, it smells good at my apartment complex! Can whomever is cooking please add some for me?? I'm so tired, all I have in me energy-wise is chips and beans for pretend nachos!
>
>Reading Simple Perfection: This is the worst book I've ever read. Do yourself a favor and don't read it. Ever.
>> Holly C: Woman! For the love! Read A Court of Thorns and Roses!
>> Alyssa M: omg I second the comment above!!! Such a good series and she's writing more! The Throne of Glass series is amazing too if you like A Court of Thorns and Roses. And I always have to recommend my absolute favorite series... Red Rising by Pierce Brown.

November 29, 2017

>Opening night at Cedar & Vine, pictures with Britt W and Jimmy C

December 1, 2017

>[I reposted a LADbible video of a dog in a sweater.] It's getting colder and colder, so make sure your children are wrapped up warm.
>
>[I posted a picture of a candle and aromatherapy bubble bath.] This is happening in a big way.
>
>[I tagged co-teachers in a meme of Cinderella that said, "Most days while at work, I'm this close to losing my shit."]
>
>I didn't take a picture today because...I was home for maybe an hour. Happy 8th birthday to this sweet, silly, funny piece of my heart. We'll party it up right in Austin for your birthday!! [with a picture of Ruby]

December 2, 2017

>[I posted a picture with Britt W and Ruby.] Five days off got us like... #austinherewecome #roadtrippin #rubydidnotwanttoholdstill #lastnightslipsense

With Britt W at Texas Ranger Hall of Fame and Museum: Stop one on our road trip!! (I thought it was THOSE Rangers. It's not.)

At Magnolia Market. Stop 2. And Ruby got to go in, and she didn't know what to do with herself! She never gets adventures like this!

At BUC-EE'S Temple: THERE IS A BUC-EE'S!!!! I'm in heaven.

December 2, 2017

[I posted a picture with Britt at a table with the Beatles on it, drinking and singing karaoke at the Common Interest in Austin, Texas.] Karaoke somewhere else… this is strange, but the table speaks volumes… I went straight to it naturally!!

December 3, 2017

Checked in to Magnolia Café South with Britt: Taking her to all the Austin staples. It was a toss-up between here and Kerbey Lane, but in truth, Kerbey queso always wins over breakfast. So tomorrow it is.
LISA M: Kerbey Lane has awesome gingerbread pancakes and migas!

Checked in at Texas Toy Museum: So so so cool.

Checked in at Amy's Ice Cream: Another staple. Chocolate peanut butter Oreo and Drumsicle (dreamsicle and chocolate chips… so amazing).

Checked in at Z'Tejas 6th Street: So many years. Y'all. Five cheese macaroni with some kind of spice on the chicken. And of course the shrimp tostadas. Legit.

December 4, 2017

Checked into Lone Star Café in San Antonio with Britt: I guess when you're on the River Walk, you can charge whatever the heck you want. This place looks (and smells) amazing with decent prices.

I posted pictures on the River Walk (Paseo del Alamo) at Christmas.

December 6, 2017

    Cool! I wanna work there [with a video of Lisa Frank being interviewed about a new coloring book].
    I reshared a post of Texas jokes by Jeff Foxworthy:
* If someone in a Lowe's store offers you assistance and they don't work there, you may live in Texas.
* If you've worn shorts and a parka at the same time, you may live in Texas.
* If you've had a lengthy telephone conversation with someone who dialed a wrong number, you may live in Texas.
* If "vacation" means going anywhere south of Dallas for the weekend, you may live in Texas.
* If you measure distance in hours, you may live in Texas.
* If you know several people who have hit a deer more than once, you may live in Texas.
* If you install security lights on your house and garage, but leave both unlocked, you may live in Texas.
* If you carry jumper cables in your car and your wife knows how to use them, you may live in Texas.
* If the speed limit on the highway is 55 & you're going 80, and everybody's passing you, you may live in Houston, Texas.
* If you find 60 degrees "a little chilly," you may live in Texas.
* If you actually understand these jokes, and cannot wait to tell all your Texas friends, you definitely have lived in Texas.

December 7, 2017

    Can y'all imagine driving past this?? What do you do?? Please continue to pray for Cali [with a video of the California wildfires where a man stopped to save a baby bunny from the flames].

December 8, 2017

> *Omg [with video of a Twix pie]. Full recipe: http://dlsh.it/g3W99DN.*
>
> *[I shared this post.] Just let this sink in for a second: New Year's Eve, 2017, will be the only day when every adult was born in the 1900s and every minor was born in the 2000s.*

December 9, 2017

> *I posted a picture of me next to the Jenny Craig I Can Do It sign. [Checked in at Jenny Craig Weight Loss Center: so. Psyched.]*
>
> *[I posted a picture of Charlie holding my hand as I stroked his leg.] I love that he still wants to cuddle, even if it's from clear across the couch. Boy do I look white next to him.*

December 9, 2017

> *Me reading my own posts: "She is so damn funny I love her."*

And now you're writing the book. Hopefully, other people will find you as funny as you find yourself.

> *Everything hurts.*
> *BRENDA J: Working out?...or sick?*

Glad to see (relieved?) that it was pre-COVID that I felt that way. There was speculation that having COVID woke up autoimmune diseases but didn't appear to be so. Likely, I was more high-risk than just being overweight, though I would have never admitted it. "I never get sick" was my mantra after years of working with kids. Autoimmune disorders were not catching.

> *Jenny Craig Day 2... I had to rush to eat everything I was supposed to yesterday, so I didn't get everything in. Today, we are starting fresh. Plain Greek yogurt (GROSS!!) with pomegranate seeds that I hope will make it edible, and a chocolate JC muffin [with pictures].*
>
> *KATHERINE H: Pom seeds aren't sweet. Do you have to eat JC yogurt? Some kinds are pretty good.*

Lu B: Could you add vanilla extract to yogurt so it's tolerable?

Brenda J: I know that plain Greek yogurt is not that great tasting by itself, but on the up side—it is so filling! I'm not hungry for hours!

Lauren Y: Can you eat honey? It really helps the Greek yogurt!

Alexandra P: Yum! My kind of snack

Tenesha I: Hang in there! Soon, won't think much about it. Results are on the way!!!

Cris A: Try drizzling agave on the Greek Yogurt make sure your yogurt has high protein (at least 12g) and low sugar with lots of berries! Trader Joe's has a great GY!

Abra N: The only kind I'll eat is (Dannon Light &Fit). My dietician recommended it when I had gestational diabetes. Delicious flavors!

I shared a video of Hanson singing Christmas songs at the Bowery: Omgaaaaah.

December 12, 2017

Day 4 and going strong. I'm already burned out on yogurt, so I'm gonna have to figure out a sub there. Tonight is orange chicken with rice and veggies (JC-provided) and browned garlic cauliflower rice. All together about 320 calories (give or take a few for the butter I browned it in!). Sooo hungry tonight so hoping this cauliflower helps fill me up [with pictures].

Kara S: Looks yummy!!

Ashley B: Good job girl.

I don't remember how it came up, but one of my co-teachers said dog feet smell like tacos or Doritos. I told her my mom used to say the same thing. Just smelled Ruby's, and IT'S SO TRUE.

Lauren Y: I third the Fritos comments—so weird!!!

Jamie W: Really? I smell Froot Loops.

Heather H: Lol! We always say my dog, Bella, smells like Doritos. Haha

December 13, 2017

> I ♥ USAA.
>
> [I tagged Jimmy Cannon in a Fox News post about a meteor shower.]
>
> This. So much this. I freaking love Yoda. He's adorable [with Jimmy Fallon's post of Star Wars characters reedited to sing "MMMBop"]. #fallontonight

December 14, 2017

> [I posted a video of a dappled dachshund puppy getting her first bath.]
>
> Dude I haven't been to the doctor since I was a kid. I'm kind of scared lol.

December 15, 2017

> Sooooo cuuuuuute. Joey was like 10 (with a throwback video from 1988, when New Kids on the Block wowed the Apollo Theater in New York City with their first Top 10 hit, "Please Don't Go Girl.")
>
> I just don't know that I've ever been more proud [with a picture of Jimmy, Brandon, and Sam and a post from Lake Highlands Advocate]: "People are eating in all these restaurants in Uptown, downtown, and Lower Greenville," says Cedar & Vine—Community Kitchen + Cocktails' Brandon Carter, "and they're going to really cool bars and asking 'where is that around here?' It just didn't exist, so we created it.

December 15, 2017

> There is nothing like Christmas with kids. It makes everything so magical.
>
> LORI P: I guess I'll need to rent some then.
> BETTY W: Yes it does
> HEATHER G: Yes it does! ♥

December 15–17, 2017

> Weekend with the Skippers... This was a fun one. We went out to eat, of course, and had lessons and

baths, but we also went to some bowling alley that I can't remember the name of. Brayden slept in his car seat most of the time, and I got the privilege of feeling like a mother as I chased the girls around with a car seat in tow. Those things are heavy AF. But then we had a photo shoot outside, where the girls got to be silly and show-offy, presenting the prizes they had chosen from game tickets, which they loved to do. It was just pure fun.

December 16, 2017

Checked in at Jenny Craig Weight Loss Center. 3.4 pounds down. Whoop. Off to a good start.
ANGELA W: Good job!!
HEATHER G: Congrats! Good for you! Great start!
TAMEKA G: Good job Courtney you can do it... I know for a fact it's a long road and you've got this! Having a good support team helped me a lot so I'm here to cheer you on girl

I'm officially useless at plunging a toilet. No idea.

I tagged Jimmy in a video of a sausage dog walk in London.
JIMMY: Love how our neighbors across the pond call them sausage dogs. Makes me laugh.

I really want Alexa. And a place in which to wire her fully. "Alexa, sing me a lullaby."

December 18, 2017

Oh em geeeeee. WANT IT [with a video of a glittering white Mercedes-Benz].

Do I have any friends in the airline/airport/traveling business who know how to get deals on tickets? I'm trying to find two tickets to California in February.
KEALEILANI S: I'm trying too
DANIELLE S: Clear your cookies and browser and try booking on Tuesday am.
SHANNON M: You should download the Hopper app! It has a picture of a bunny on it. You plug in

your dates and it'll tell you when prices drop. I've used it a lot and have found some steals!

Watching Gilmore Girls: Every time I watch the series finale, I bawl and want to start it all over again.

December 18, 2017

> MY BODY: WHAT DO WE WANT?
> MY BRAIN: SLEEP!
> MY BODY: WHEN DO WE WANT IT?
> MY BRAIN: AT EITHER 2 PM OR 3 AM
> MY BODY: *hey wait—*
> MY BRAIN: LITERALLY NO OTHER TIME.
> MY BODY: *no that's not—*
> MY BRAIN: WE ARE UNWILLING TO COMPROMISE

December 19, 2017

This has never actually happened to me, despite the bunch of winners I've encountered over the years. I knew in my gut... #trustnoone #whatanactualidiot...

Ahh, the first time I almost got truly catfished... his name was "Wayne Porter" (at the moment) and he was posing as a very handsome white man with nice teeth and a military uniform...

> WP: Lol, just to know more about you. Are you single or married?
> ME: I'm single...and I believe I answered that with "do married people really get on dating sites?" I'm not looking to talk to anyone in a relationship.
> WP: Yes am not in any relationship right now. Well am single and that's why am on that site looking for serious and honest relationship. Did you have any special man right now?? And what's your idea in true relationship??
> ME: Sorry, left my phone at work. No. I don't have a man. Special or otherwise. Which is why I'm on a dating site. I'm not sure quite what you mean by the last question. I hope this

> *doesn't sound rude, but is English your first language?*
> WP: *Yes. So what are you looking for in a Man?*
> ME: *Kindness, loyalty, a sense of humor, confidence, an ability to go with the flow. A fondness for karaoke and a deep appreciation and love for music. Someone who loves to cook would be amazing. And who would be happiest at home on our couch with our dogs and a bunch of movies.*
> WP: *Oh that's really perfect and I think that's lot of me. I really want that to be and I will be happy to have you as my soul mate and future partner. How's your relationship with you and your parents?*
> ME: *Haha well good... but while it sounds like you on paper, chemistry is a big deal. Let's slow down and just chat. We will learn more about each other.*

My intuitive ass is insane. If you don't believe empaths can get energy through texts, befriend an empath.

> ME: *It's okay. My mother and I have had our problems, but we are okay now. I love my dad; he's the best.*
> WP: *Yes, that's good. Well my parents are old and I pray for them always. I'm a military man and my father also... he's retired. What's your work? You there?*
> ME: *On the phone with a friend*
> WP: *Okay. Text me when you're free.*
> ME: *I'm always free lol. Just might take me a minute to answer. And I'm a preschool teacher.*
> WP: *Okay. Can you care for your man when he needs your help?*
> ME: *Well, I guess. I'm a very caring and loving person. In what aspect do you mean?*
> WP: *Yes that's really what I mean. [He sent pictures and even had Porter on his military uniform.] Can you tell me do I really look like the kind of man you want in a relationship??*

ME: Well you're very handsome. But again, chemistry is important. You could be the cutest guy ever and we have nothing in common. In what ASPECT do you mean will I care for my man? Do you have PTSD or are you in a wheelchair or something?

WP: Lol. No but can you do anything to make your man happy with you. I have been looking for that special woman that will love me with all her heart…and I need a woman that I can wake up in the morning and tell her that she's the most beautiful woman in the whole world… I let her know that she own the key to my Heart…

ME: No… happiness is a 2-way street and I won't change who I am to make someone else happy. I'm very loving and affectionate and I'm the most generous person ever, but I won't give and give and give without getting something in return.

Yay me for having my own back. Man, I love it when I stand up for myself, but I bet someone had just broken my heart.

WP: Yes that's true. What are you doing for living?
ME: Sent snarky screenshot where he'd asked before, and I answered.
WP: Lol. Yeah I said that. What's your work?
ME: I don't understand why to keep asking me the same things over and over.
WP: Sorry. So what times it there now where you are?
ME: Huh?? What time is it??
WP: Yes
ME: 6:43… the same time as it is where you are.
WP: No I am on deployment right now in West Africa country. And I will be back home soon. What's your favorite colour?
ME: Oh, I have an army friend who's in Africa too.
WP: Oh that's really nice.
ME: Purple. And rainbow.
WP: Am single right now and I will be happy if you can be the woman of my dreams

Me: Haha well again, thanks. But you don't know me. I'm not a Dream woman, I'm a real woman. I have flaws and so do you. What time is it in Africa? No wonder you were texting me at three in the morning the other day.

WP: It's 1:48 AM right now. Can you trust me?

Me: No, not yet. Why?

WP: Oh okay. Do you have a pet?

Me: Why do you ask if I can trust you? Do you feel you've earned my trust yet?? And yes I have a dog.

WP: Same here. [He sent me a picture of him shirtless in bed with a dog.] Lola. What do you do in your free time?

Me: That's a great picture. She's beautiful, and so are you. I am a homebody. I like to binge Netflix and watch movies. And most weekends, I'm at my karaoke bar. [I sent a picture of me, Britt, and Ruby.] There's my little girl lol. Clearly did not want to take a picture.

WP: Oh you're looking beautiful. That's gorgeous. Sorry I fell asleep. How are you doing.

Me: Lol well thank you. We were on our way to Austin. Super excited. Why do you stay up so late? You need to get some sleep.

WP: Thanks. How are you doing?

Me: Thanks?

WP: Yeah. Well I need your help right now. I don't know if you can really help me.

Me: Lol how can I help you, you're in Africa?

WP: Yes you can help me out. I want to upgrade my phone and the apps on it, you just need to help me get 50$ iTunes gift card for that. That's the help and I hope you can.

Me: I'm sorry, I haven't had any signal. Sure I can help, send me your bank account number. I'll need a checking account and a routing number, plus your date of birth and social security number. Oh, and your mother's maiden name.

WP: Oh you can get me the iTunes card at the store. Go to the Walmart store or the nearest store to you and buy the 50$ iTunes card for me okay. It's not necessary I gave you all that you ask okay. I hope you understand me. You got nearest store??

ME: I mean, this is a joke right? Do people actually fall for this crap? You out of your ever-loving mind.

WP: Well it's okay if you can't help me. Thanks for your time. And thanks for deceiving me.

ME: You're kidding. Deceiving you?? The only reason I haven't blocked and reported you right now is because I'm going to blast you all over Facebook and let people see this crap. I'm literally laughing out loud right now. We've been talking for two days, what makes you think I'd be stupid enough to send you money? In any form or fashion. No more replies, eh?

WP: You're telling me shit.

ME: Lol. Okay then. You need some professional help.

ASHLEY D: This happened to a friend of mine as well. Can you make it public so I can share it please.

DANIELLE S: So sorry you went through that, but good thing you are wary of this.

KELLY M: I knew within the first few texts that he wasn't a real person.

JENNIFER H: Yup has happened to me too, lots of cat fishers out there...

JENNIFER M: What's sad is the poor guy whose photo he's using

JOCELYN G: Giiirrrl that's a catfish lookin' for some $$. Def don't fall for that. Also, I LOL'd at "is English your first language" haha. It's most definitely not. Your responses are amazing though, I'd date you!

DESTINY O: What the heck!

BRANDY R: People are such jerks!!!

LAUREN Y: *I'm still laughing at the "is English your first language" line*

ME: *I like literally can't believe this. I've watched the show Catfish and am like...at least they make someone fall for them. This guy tried scamming me after two DAYS?? #holdyourhorsesbro*

JEFF K: *Good job nailing that criminal. As a cyber security guy, I love to see people do what you did. Super cool.*

Why am I so tired???

ASHLEY B: *Probably from all that messaging with the crazy guy lol*

December 21, 2017

After seven long years, my career at Kids R Kids has ended. I will miss (almost) everyone, most of all my babies, but this is God's plan. I can't wait to see what is in store for me. (And guess what, now I can babysit!)

CAMBRIE R: *WHAT!!! Charli is not going to be okay with not seeing her Coco... but go ahead and PM me that number*

LAUREN Y: *What!? So excited to see what the future holds for you!*

ILSE S: *What!!! Whyyyyyyy?? Love! are you ok??*

HOLLY C: *WHAT?!?!?*

STEPHANIE: *Such sad news, it won't be the same without you.*

KARA S: *What?!?!?!?!*

ALEXANDRA P: *Oh no!!!! I am so sad. God has indeed great plans if you trust Him! I will contact you for babysitting. Will sure miss seeing you everyday*

STEPHANIE W: *Say wha?!!! We'll miss seeing you everyday, but I'm sure I'll see you on Mariner soon enough*

ASHLEY S: *I'm so sad to hear this. We will miss you but don't be surprised if you hear from me about babysitting*

JACLYNN H: *What?!? God definitely has a plan my friend.*

NOT THE F——ING GILMORE GIRLS

Lu B: *Hopefully you found a new position that helps you reach your goals!!!!*

Kelly N: *I just saw you this morning. What's up?*

Kelly M: *So surprising! But I know God has great plans for you!*

Lyn B: *Thinking about you—can't wait to see you this weekend* ♥

Ashley B: *I hope you are ok!*

Josh M: *Well you were one of the great ones and one of the few reasons we stuck around for Greyson! I know you'll do great on your next journey. We will definitely be in touch for babysitting!!*

Julie M: *Totally agree. Your love for those babies helped all of us moms be able to leave for work a little bit easier just knowing how much you loved and cared for them while we were away!*

Paige E: *I'm shocked. Thanks for all the love you gave my babies!!*

Nicole R: *No!!! My baby isn't even with you yet. When is your last day??*

Tenesha I: *Oh no! You (and a few others) was why we held on as long as we did! You will be missed.*

Jamie W: *Come be my live in Nanny!!!! I'll cover your room and board, groceries, and pay you weekly!*

Hallie W: *What on earth???*

Janssen A: *Their loss. Xoxoxo*

Kristen M: *So sad to hear this! Thank you for always loving on my girls!!*

Kimberly M: *I can't even begin to express my feelings on this... you were exactly why we brought Grey to KRK at 3 months! We trust you with our babies and I'm heartbroken and honestly in complete shock about this. KRK has changed a lot since we first started with Ayva and it has never been as good as it once was... you know you'll be missed Coco*

[I posted the trailer for Mamma Mia! Here We Go Again.] *Yesssssss.*

ILSE S: *I died a little when I saw this.* ♥

December 23, 2017

Recipe for Dill Pickle Soup from Noble Pig: http://bit.ly/2dp2plW

Feeling Christmassy. It's (finally) cold outside, I dyed my hair without worrying my bosses would hate it, and I have this adorable shirt from Whitney. #dontstopbelievin

LYN B: *You may be the big winner tomorrow night too! #dontstopbelievin*

You guys, I was!!! It was my first time playing bunko, and I was the big winner. Everyone put it down to beginner's luck, but now reading this, it was #cocomagic. Thank you for the extra confidence, Aunt Lyn!

December 24, 2017

Give them to me nowwww [with a video of pickle mozzarella sticks]. Full recipe: http://dlsh.it/gRV95tk.

Dad came to Christmas Eve dinner, we took Snaps, pic of delicious looking meal. Nanny Ann bought Ruby a stocking full of rawhides.

PATRICIA S: *Merry Christmas, love from us*

KATHERINE H: *Your dad looks great. You have awesome genes.*

December 26, 2017

Watched The Greatest Showman: "Musical double feature today. This was so good, I'm not even checking into Pitch Perfect. I just. Wow. Hugh Jackman is fucking fantastic. And Zac should only ever do musicals. He's adorable. #criticssuck

December 27, 2017

[I posted pictures with Mason and Logan.] Finally able to post when I watch these sweet boys. Logan told me he loved me and Mason's reply was "and I love Ruby."

NOT THE F——ING GILMORE GIRLS

[I posted old pictures with Christopher.] How is he 16?? I am just...getting too old. Happy birthday, sweet Christopher. Love you.

December 29, 2017

Amen.
Checked in at Jenny Craig Plano: When you go in for your weigh-in and find a job opportunity. Fingers crossed and prayers please!!! This would be so awesome. (.9 pounds down too.)

December 31, 2017

NYE at the Tavern with Mandy Joe, Laura, and crew. We played a "new song" bingo game that took us outside our comfort zones with song choices.
  Bonnie A: I absolutely loved playing this game with y'all!

January 1, 2018

What a fantastic night. Thanks to the best DJ on the planet, Shawn Solo, the bar was the place to be. Love these people. Happy New Year.

I don't make resolutions. They're much too easy to break. Instead, I pray. I pray this is my year. God has already taken me out of my comfort zone by pushing me toward leaving my job. I pray I will find an amazing job (hopefully within the next week or two or I could be in major trouble) which will afford me the opportunities to meet new people, and most especially a man. I also pray it brings me the opportunity to start saving for my future. This paycheck to paycheck thing is for the birds. I pray I can stay focused enough to stay on Jenny Craig for the year...which would easily bring me to my goal weight by next NYE. And I pray that I can cultivate the relationships I currently have. My friends and family are so important to me, and time is so short (how is it 2018????). Happy New Year to everyone. I pray it brings massive blessings. Last year was hard.

HEATHER G: *You got this! Wishing you many blessings and successes on your journey in 2018!*
KELLY M: *Goals are much better than resolutions IMO!! I have a long list of goals for my YL biz!! And plan on hitting every one of them! I wish you the very best 2018 possible.* GO GET IT!
ABRA N: *Best wishes for your 2018!*
KARA S: *Happy new year!! Many blessings and great things to come!!!*
BRENDA J: *Be strong, Courtney! You can do this! "I can do all things through Christ who strengthens me." Phil 4:13*

January 3, 2018

My dad gave me a daily devotional book for Christmas. I'm a few days behind, but this. This has always been "my" verse. Saw me through a lot of tough times when I was younger. And here it is, front and center, the hallmark for a new year and a new life. I hear you, God. Wow. Jeremiah 29:11.

January 4, 2018

I posted a picture of a T-shirt that read, "Superwoman: single. Batwoman: single. Wonderwoman: single. I get it now... I'm single because I'm a superhero."

Oh my God. The guy who tried to scam me the other day was going by the name Wayne Porter on kik and is now going by Charles Farrar. How I can still see that after blocking him, I have no idea, but more to the point... why hasn't kik punished him??

[I posted a video of the TGS cast practicing for the show. Hugh Jackman had just had nose surgery and wasn't supposed to sing.] Okay, not sure what Jeremy (Jordan) is doing there since he wasn't in the movie (I had to look it up to make sure he wasn't one of the freaks!!) but OMGGGGG. I need to see this again ASAP. Hell, who am I kidding?? I need to be IN IT.

January 6, 2018

> Today I feel like a million bucks, despite allergies that are kicking my ass. Even being jobless, my quality of life has improved so greatly. I'm happy and optimistic and hopeful. I want to thank every person who has given me referrals or offered to be a reference. Every interview I've gone on so far has been... well, interesting, to say the least. But I'm optimistic the right person will appear soon. One day, ten applications, and three interviews at a time... please keep sending prayers my way. I'm feeling every one of them.

January 7, 2018

> Watched "Grey's Anatomy": Alex Karev is my favorite character ever written (aside from Jamie Fraser possibly). I just started crying unexpectedly with a mouthful of shake. It was hard to swallow.

January 9, 2018

> [I posted a picture of Brayden asleep in my arms, me pouting at the camera.] Sickie babies make the most amazing cuddle buddies. He's in such a good mood, but passed out hard.

February 1–5, 2018

> *Camarillo for Grandma's ninetieth.*
> It was all about the lips on this trip, and I felt confident, although I do remember things being awkward with my mother; whatever I did, it wasn't right. Jimmy wasn't supposed to come, but I imagined him surprising everyone and just showing up, and that was exactly what he did (just as if I had written it). I suppose that means he didn't surprise me.
> I don't remember why I was able to do it other than the Skippers were taking care of Ruby, but I drove home with my aunt Beth and got to see Vegas for the first time. Then we all got super sick—some kind of crazy flu that put my grandmother in the hospital and knocked over half of the rest of us on our asses. So I didn't enjoy Vegas the way I would have otherwise (I'm embarrassed I even went to see shows, feeling as

horrible as I did, but it was pre-COVID, and I was convinced I only had a sinus infection). But we saw the Blue Man Group and Criss Angel, and it was just great.

April 28

Mya giggling over pizza, then trying to say a word in Spanish that Jessalyn and I had to guess.

This is one of my favorite videos. I can watch it over and over. She was so patient with us, simply repeating herself and then getting happy for me when I finally understood her. I went from thinking she was saying something with four syllables to estrella and finally escuela. We then talked about how to say "Sit down." Then she burped, so I taught her con permiso. There was no end to the laughs with this kid around.

June 5–10

Road trip with Britt.

This trip started off great; we were driving to Cali for a wedding where Britt was doing the bride's makeup. She made us special T-shirts that said The Wildlife Wedding Roadtrip, which we wore for our photos at the Grand Canyon. I will tell you what, I suppose it was an experience I needed to have, but it was certainly not one I would ever do again. I was terrified. It took over an hour just to get into the park. Ruby, on her stretchy leash, took off after a squirrel and ended up dangerously close to the edge of the canyon. I literally reeled her back in, shrieking at her.

Then we went to Vegas, where we stayed at a hotel off the strip but super nice, called Westgate. We went to see Impractical Jokers with Beth and ate at one of Gordon Ramsay's restaurants, but we still didn't get to eat at a buffet. We continued on to Cali, where we took my grandma (or she took us) to Applebee's.

It was on the road home that things fell apart over—you guessed it—money. The hotel the bride had booked didn't allow dogs, so I told her Ruby and I could sleep in the car (I meant it; I didn't have money for another unplanned hotel). But she booked a Motel 6 instead, and I was simultaneously so pissed and grateful (she told me she didn't have money either), but we slept upstairs with her. To me, it seemed martyrish.

Anyway, the rest of the trip was tense. I could tell she was angry, as if I had forced her to do it, and when she pretended not to feel well and asked to drive straight home, I complied even though it put us driving long hours late at night, and it ended up storming. I remember making an effort to keep in touch for a few weeks after that, but then our friendship completely disappeared—over one hundred dollars. Sad.

July 31

Jessalyn and I went to the movies in the afternoon (we saw Mamma Mia! Here We Go Again) and I had Charlie and Isa in the evening.

August 25, 2018

Attended Rascal Flatts: Back to Us Tour with Bonnie, Jon, Mandy, and Shawn: "Trent Harmon, Dan + Shay, and Rascal Flatts with my favorite people."

September 8, 2018

Dallas Chocolate Festival with Kaitlyn.

I'm about to get weirder than normal, y'all. Have you ever heard of astral projection? It's a term I only recently learned (or if I'd heard it before, I'd forgotten it), but it applies really well to a lot of my life. To save you from having to look it up, I'll fill you in: Basically, it's "an intentional out-of-body experience that assumes the existence of a subtle body, known as the astral body or body of light, through which consciousness can function separately from the physical body and travel throughout the astral plane" (thanks, Wikipedia).

I don't know if I fully believe it, but I definitely don't not believe it, and the way I got through some of the things

I did all my life is amazing. Despite near-constant physical body pain, not sleeping well, and being alone, I pulled off Coco mode a lot. Working the Chocolate Festival annually was some of those times. Don't get me wrong, I had a blast. I wouldn't have done it otherwise. But it was hard work and long days, and keeping up the Coco energy was tough. That was why I started asking if I could bring a friend. As long as I wasn't alone, I could handle anything. I do think there was always some guardian angel energy there, but astral projection? Who knows?

October 3, 2018

> Mya showing off in the dance lobby, eating noodles at Cici's and me trying to get her to say "Oh-wah-tah-goo-si-am." There's also a comparison picture of her wearing my rainbow sunnies when she was a baby and "now," and a video of Mya telling me that men had to wear glasses to be married. My point to her was her daddy didn't wear glasses. She kept arguing that he had to, or he couldn't be married. I told her she better tell him that.

October 12, 2018

> Us at the State Fair, J and me on the haunted house, me with Brayden at the bottom of the rides, and the girls tearing into turkey legs.

October 13

> Hanging at their house, silly face pictures, B sleeping on me, and the girls knocked out on the couch.

November 27, 2018

> Babysitting baby Jake and the Legleiters at their house, always some of my favorite things to do; bring all the people I love into one place.

November 28, 2018

If there was ever a reason to get back on Facebook, this girl is it [with videos of Mya in her blue ballerina outfit, videos of her singing Halloween songs a month late, and songs from TGS, totally my kid].

My personal troll doll watching The Greatest Showman…which of course, she lives daily.

I'm watching Jane the Virgin: Does anyone watch this show? I stopped for a long time because I couldn't get used to Jane with Rafael, but now I want to stop again because I HATE Rafael's sister so much. She's the worst. Character. Ever. Written. Someone please tell me something permanent happens to get her off the show.

November 30, 2018

Movie night with the kids.

December 3, 2018

Baking apple pie from scratch with J for her daddy's birthday and reading out loud from Harry Potter.

December 5, 2018

Mandy Joe and me with Santa at the Winspear Opera House.

Shawn couldn't go to the Christmas party for some reason, so Mandy asked me to be her date. I even wore Shawn's name tag. We had a good time, taking pictures with Santa and seeing Hillary Scott from Lady A. We looked like a couple in most of these pictures, and often, people at the bar thought we were until they saw her kiss Shawn. Honestly, that was the first time I ever considered polyamory. (Sorry if that embarrasses y'all, but I loved you both enough to make it work if that was what we had chosen to do!) But it never went there!

December 6, 2018

Facebook test results: "Courtney is Merida. You are strong and brave, and you fight for you what you want. You desire freedom, and that is the force that drives your every action." Hey I'll take it!!! Another red-haired princess!!

December 7, 2018

Practicing "Bridge Over Troubled Water" in the shower, which I had a solo for later in the year... did I know that already??

December 9, 2018

[Mandy Joe tagged me, Bonnie, Jon, and Shawn.] Dr Shawn performing surgery at The Tavern on Main Street. (Jon got something in his eye, I held the flashlight lol.)

Facebook quiz: "Which three movie roles suit your face: Mia Thermopolis (The Princess Diaries), Ariel (The Little Mermaid), and Rosie (Love, Rosie)?" Ariel. But really... why does Anne Hathaway have to be making that face??

December 10, 2018

[With a reshare of the Pet Collective's video of a service dog making a cute mistake and bringing her owner a bottle of ranch instead of a water].

Jessica S: ♥

I believe milkshakes make sore throats better. #notgonnalosemyvoice

Mindi W: *Absolutely!!*

Carol B: No you are not!!

Yesss [with a Facebook quiz that said, "@simon-cowell said 'I would have to say that Courtney has the best voice I've ever heard. Without a doubt, she has the voice of an angel'"].

December 11, 2018

Doing tricks with Ruby.

Omgggg this is the truth (with a meme of Kermit looking in a mirror, one of him in a black hood: "Courtney: That's a nice picture. I should give it a like. Evil Courtney: Have they ever liked any of your pictures?")

[I posted a meme of Jonathan Taylor Thomas and Devon Sawa.] *If your boy-crush had this haircut, it's time for an eye cream.*

MEGAN U: *Waaahhh* ♥ *and started this year*
LAUREN Y: *Nooooo!!!!!!!!*
CHRISTAL K: *Not cool bro*

December 12, 2018

The newest Mya Chronicles. In the first, she wanted me to read my book to her ("Falling for Christmas"), and instead I asked her to read to me... y'all need to hear this one. (Also, she had the most adorable habit of saying "y" instead of "and"... those are not typos, she was the Spanglish queen...

"There was a house and people lived in the house. And the mom said 'it's 24 days and Christmas, kids!' Y then the dad says 'get upstairs kids, it's bedtime!' Y then the kids go upstairs, y then they get into bed, and they turn on a movie, y then mom comes and knocks on the door, y then the kids say 'Come in!' And then the mom comes in and sit on their bed and 'oh my heavens, what are you guys doing watching the tv when you're in trouble? No you guys cannot watch the tv!' Y then the mom just turned off the tv and comes and lays with them for a little bit. (She paused to eat some Goldfish, where I asked her if that was the end.) No. Y then um I really do not want to read this book. (Me: Okay. The end then.)"

Continuing her performances, she sang some Christmas songs, including "Feliz Navidad," which she sang almost perfectly.

December 12, 2018

Watching The Great British Baking Show: Can't stop. So good.

STACI P: *Oh gurl! I binged that so hard!*

COURTNEY CANNON

LAUREN Y: I love Prue and Joel!!!!!

December 14, 2018

Christmas with the Chorale performances: Dress rehearsal!! So sparkly!!!!! This is my dream costume.
AMOS H: Go have a ball, looking good
MELANIE J: Is that Candy Cane?
ASHLEY B: Super pretty
KATHERINE H: What's the dress rehearsal for?

December 14, 2018

Today was a hard day for my brother... he had to put his sweet daughter dog to sleep, suddenly and unexpectedly. As Jimmy wrote, to know her was to love her. This dog was everything a man's first dog should be... sweet and loyal and funny and caring and compassionate and stubborn and funny and infuriating and cute and oh-so-funny. Her sweet heart loved everyone and her dirty looks could kill. She was the ultimate dachshund, and she was wonderful to the Norah Bone. The picture Jimmy took of her so many years ago has hung on my wall, over my own sweet pupper's crate, for as long as I can remember. We love you, Norah, and we will miss you so much. We will celebrate your sweet 16 thinking of you... rest well, dear one. We love you so [with pictures].

MELANIE J: So sorry to hear. Hugs & Prayers for your Brother on the loss of his Fur-baby
JESSICA S: I'm so sorry for your family. My puppy mama heart hurts for you all.
QUINN C: We are a dachshund family too. So sorry about yalls little lady, you'll see her again
AMOS H: They are hard to let go. Just like children to us while they are here with us.
KATHY H: So sorry!

December 15, 2018

[Lyn B checked in to St. Barnabas Presbyterian Church, attending Christmas with the Contemporary

Chorale.] Ready for some holiday music with this girl 🖤

>ME: Are my eyes closed??? Thank you so much for coming. Love you!!!!
>
>KATHERINE H: I'm so jealous! I want to hear you sing. This makes me so happy.

Stephanie, in case you get bored [with a picture of Elf on a Shelf frozen in a block of ice, Elsa standing outside, her hand pointed at Elf].

December 17, 2018

This is literally my favorite way ever to sum up having kids. #patienceisavirtue: "Moms forcing their kids to take pictures… They'll be like sit your butt down and smile. And then post it saying 'the reason I breathe.'"

>MARIA A: Guilty
>
>ANGELA W: Hahahaha.

Ruby is obsessed with a blue squeaky ball. Her obsession over this ball is so dog. She uses it as a back massager and then brings it to the bottom of the couch and stares at it. Like… who taught you to play fetch that way??

December 18, 2018

Oh God. I remember losing my baby blanket when I was a kid. Worst. Ever [with a post of a lost teddy bear (the bear made it home, thanks to social media!)].

December 20, 2018

[I added thirteen pictures to "Old School Pics."] Christmases past. Man we were cute. [I tagged Jimmy.]

>KATHERINE H: You were SO CUTE. And your parents were a really good-looking couple.
>
>BRENDA N: Love the family photos!

December 23, 2018

As a special Christmas treat, because her mama was too lazy to go into Costco on the weekend before Christmas, Ruby got Rachael Ray food. She is now busily picking out all the vegetables.

December 25, 2018

Ruby wearing Max antlers from The Grinch.
Watching Aquaman at Studio Movie Grill: It's a little absurd how beautiful this man is. #khaldrogorulesthesea

December 26, 2018

[I tested the 3D picture effect on Facebook with a picture of Ruby.] Yoooooo. Neat. Don't mind the dribble from her lip.

December 27, 2018

[I posted old pictures of Christopher.] 17 today. Like. Not allowed. Happy birthday, Chris!!! Love you.

December 28, 2018

Facebook survey where nothing has changed, but one notable question: Favorite TV show: Gilmore Girls ♥

December 29, 2018

Hard lessons to learn: Things everyone (a.k.a. me) needs to come to terms with: *No response is a response. *If they wanted to, they would. *Timing will not always be in your favor. *Not everyone has the same heart as you.

LISA M: So very true.

KATHERINE H: These are hard lessons. Important ones too. Figuring out how to be YOU in a hostile world ain't easy.

NOT THE F——ING GILMORE GIRLS

December 30, 2018

FOOD today!! 7.9 pounds down to jumpstart this thing off. Already know I'm having blueberry pancakes and sausage for breakfast. Jenny Craig ROCKS. And trying Hello Fresh tonight… we will see how that goes.

[Pictures and videos were added to Facebook folder "Adventures with Charlie, Isa, and Jake."] Catching up. Jacob Edward, the spitting image of his dear brother Charlie. How I adore him.

Omg [with meme that said, "I honked at the car in front of me, and this angry Alpaca popped out, and now I'm not sure what to do"].

December 31, 2018

Katherine H posted "Top 10 Dog Breeds." 10. All 9. Dogs 8. Are 7. Beautiful 6. It's 5. Cruel 4. To 3. Rank 2. Them 1. Dachshund

I posted pictures of NYE upstairs at the bar, me in a silver tank top, short skirt, and knee-high boots. We looked hot.

January 1, 2019

[I posted an LADbible post of a dog leaping in excitement at the vet's desk.] If this doesn't make you smile, you have no soul.

FB quiz: "What's your word for 2019?" "Change: Courtney, get ready for your life to change in incredible ways in 2019. You've always been a dreamer and this year you'll see the payoff of all of your hard work manifest itself in a beautiful way."

January 6, 2019

I posted the six names game on FB. 1) Your actual name: Courtney 2) Your soap opera name (middle name and street): Elizabeth Leora 3) Your Star Trek name (first 3 letters of your last name, first 2 of middle, last 2 of first): Caneley 4) Superhero name (color of your shirt and item to right of you): Black Sharpie 5) Goth name (black and name of one of your pets): Black Ruby 6) Rapper name (Lil' + last thing you ate): Lil' Chocolate

January 9, 2019

Practicing tricks with Ruby.
"You know what makes me sick to my stomach? When I hear grown people say that kids have changed. Kids haven't changed. Kids don't know anything about anything. We've changed as adults. We demand less of kids. We expect less of kids. We make their lives easier instead of preparing them for what life is truly about. We're the ones that have changed." —Frank Martin, SC Head basketball coach.

January 29, 2019

Jessalyn said she didn't like a cover of "Wrecking Ball" because it was too slow, and it wasn't entertainment; the real "Wrecking Ball" was entertainment.

January 30, 2019

[I posted a video of Ruby trying to chase a duck and of Mya over at Charlie and Isa's with me. She loved their dogs.] "I want them to live with me. Um, Ruby's on their couch." [I also posted another video of Charlie, Isa, and Mya all sitting around Charlie's table, eating dinner.]
MYA: That's because you're eating it
CHARLIE: Mm-mm
ME: Charlie, who's really in charge? (Charlie looking at me with popsicle in mouth and eyes wide.)
CHARLIE: not me; at the same time Mya says "your dad"! And then NOT ME again louder, over Mya.
MYA: Your dad (again, this time looking at me.)
ME: Who? genuinely confused.
MYA: Your dad.
ME: My dad?

MYA: *Ms. Courtney! Ms. Courtney!*
ME: *There you go! Did you mean Charlie's dad?*
MYA: *Yeah.*
ME: *Well Charlie's dad just went out of town, so who's really in charge now?*
MYA: *Ms. Courtney (while Charlie stays silent sucking his popsicle)!*

February 2, 2019

I posted videos of Ruby on whipped cream, chattering her teeth to the rhythm of me squeaking her ball.

February 5, 2019

Jessalyn and Mya passed out on the couch, J with a book open in her lap and her chin on her chest, M with her blanket up to her chin and her mouth open.

February 6, 2019

Ruby was eating a pickle, trying to power through the sour and finally giving up, glaring at me over her shoulder.

February 13, 2019

Mya eating her Hawaiian rolls on the couch because she was definitely sick… video of her "taking her ears," and then checking her "pempature"; video of her telling Ms Lisa she heard she was in town and she might get to see her…and then…

February 14, 2019

MYA: *Hi, my name is Mya Alysse Skipper. Why won't you let me be a queen? By the way, I am not a drama queen, just a regular queen. Bye!*
ME: *Okay, what do you think Jessalyn is gonna do when she sees all those presents?*
MYA: *She's just gonna flop down on the floor and just pretend she's dead.*

Me: *And what are you gonna do?*
Mya: *When she gets home, I'm just gonna, I'm just gonna be in a hiding spot and when Jessalyn and mommy and daddy get home...*
Me: *Well, we're going to get Jessalyn right now, goofy. That's why I said you have to keep it secret.*
Mya: *Okay, yes, okay. So when Jessalyn gets home, I'm gonna jump outta my hiding spot and say SURPRISE.*
Me: *Honey, you're going to be with Jessalyn.*
Mya: *With Jessalyn? Oh.*
(When we got home a little later...)
Jessalyn was very excited, but said she didn't know who Cupid was. Guess they'll never know who brought the Valentine's gifts.

February 15, 2019

Jessalyn and Mya teaching Brayden how to be sumo wrestlers in the (blessedly empty) waiting room of their doctor's office.

February 20, 2019

Brayden holding my fingers like a security blanket while he sucked his paci and we watched tv.

February 21, 2019

Movie night with Skippers and Trevor and Troy.

February 23, 2019

Ruby being guilty because she tore up the trash; Jake having a bottle in my lap.

February 27, 2019, 3:33 PM

Jessalyn feeding Ruby her puppy snow cone, then home for a snack and video...

Jessalyn had huge dreams of being a YouTube star. In this video, she was walking her audience through how to make toast, and she was such a natural.

She showed them every step, from plugging in the toaster to buttering the finished product. In the next video…

Jessalyn is sitting next to me, on top of Brayden, who was covered in a black sheet and patiently cooing at us while we giggled. Mya came in, and I asked her where her brother was, and she said, "He's in the bushes." And I said, "Well, you better go get him!" And she said, "No, he's going to live his life in the bushes." Finally, we heard a protest from Brayden, and he began climbing out from underneath his sisters, strong like a machine.

March 5, 2019

> Mya being a brat when Steph came home with Grandma Kay Kay as a surprise; me telling her "Look who's here" and her saying "I don't care" with a little smirk at her mother, and then a "What, I didn't even see her!" when she saw her grandma.

March 13, 2019

> Lisa came to visit from Colorado and we went to Buc-ee's.

March 19, 2019

> Ruby was acting guilty; I asked her why she thought she was in trouble, and she looked at me sadly. "Is it because you have an upset tummy?" I asked, and she flipped to her back, thunking her tail. "I know, I know it! Don't worry, we'll figure it out," I told her as she meechily crossed the couch to get a scratch.
>
> At the vet later, swapping pics with Mom, who had Monte and Cookie at the vet too.

March 21, 2019

> Lily (a huge Bernadoodle) and Ruby playing; Brayden trying to say "boom, baby!" and saying pretty much anything but: "bubby, be Bobby, be-bah"; trying to get the kids to dance to the Chorale's version of "Come Alive," Mya got super awkward and said she couldn't dance without the movie, so we put the real soundtrack on; Mya glar-

ing at me after I'd taken her braids out and her hair went wild.

March 26, 2019

Mya making up a song called "Flowers," the main lyrics being that she wanted some flowers and always had, then making up another one called "This Is Me" (not The Greatest Showman one, as Jessalyn had instructed her), getting louder and louder as Jessalyn grew bored and began dancing in front of her.

March 29, 2019

Baby Jake in my lap, Brayden, Mya, and Isa on the couch next to me as Jake stared at them; outside playing T-ball with them; slow-mo video of Mya and Isa dramatically telling Brayden not to do the roller coaster; Brayden passed out on the couch, surrounded protectively by dogs and his sister.

April 3, 2019

Trying to get Ruby to carry my keys by hanging them on her collar. She did not want to.

April 5, 2019

Six Flags with the kids and Jessalyn's best friend Tori, as a way to tide us over till the fair:
Video of the three girls on a smaller version of Superman Tower of Power, Mya's shriek and subsequent giggle was hysterical. Tori had some kind of allergic reaction and we had to go to a gift shop for Benadryl, poor baby. They even rode Shockwave while I stayed at the bottom with Brayden.

April 23, 2019

Video of Jessalyn telling me that a toot was small and a fart was big.

May 10, 2019

> *Spring Concert with the Chorale, dress rehearsals leading into the concert, and interviews with people afterward...*

This was when I had my first solo. I don't know if I owe more thanks to my choir director, the illustrious Melanie Moore, or karaoke, but being able to belt out "Sail on silver girl" to a crowd of (almost) three hundred people was insanely thrilling. I was on a high for a long time after that, a high that continued late into the night.

May 11, 2019, 4:44 PM

> *Tommy and Becky Haines, dear friends from Jenny Craig:*
> Me: *What did you guys like about the show?*
> Tommy: *The postiveness.*
> Becky: *Well we liked Courtney the best but we loved the Street Choir... that's fantastic.*
> *Jessalyn and Mya:*
> Me: *Same question*
> The girls, simultaneously: *Ummmmm*
> Jessalyn: *That you were in it!*
> Me: *Good answer! What'd you like, Mya?*
> Mya: *Um, you had a pretty voice.*
> Me: *Aww thank you.*
> Mya, being shy: *You're welcome.*
> Me: *Did y'all like the dance from The Greatest Showman? That's your favorite movie!*
> All 3 Skipper women together: *We missed that one!*

May 14, 2019

> *Mya "flossing" in the lobby of her dance-costume store while we waited for her shoes to be fit; the girls pretending to do a YouTube on new toys, then Jessalyn being a brat and losing the toy... J: If I do my homework, can I have the toy back? Me: That's up to your mother. The decision wasn't to take the toy because you wouldn't do your homework, it's because you were being a brat.*

> *Brayden began growling and made moves to jump on her, and she complained about it.*
> *ME: He's two, J. That's a normal two-year-old response to someone who's bugging them.*
> *J: Well, tell him not to be two; tell him to be 17 and grown up.*
> *ME: You wouldn't like that because you'd be 23.*
> *J: Ooh, then I can drink alcohol.*

May 21, 2019

> *Played with portrait mode while the kids decorated and ate giant cupcakes. Some gorgeous shots here.*

May 29, 2019

> *Mya singing "Mamma Mia" while Brayden tried to get my attention, completely making up her own lyrics, then saying "Yisten, yisten!" and switching songs to "I love you babysitter."*

June 5, 2019

> *Mya making a video for Grandma Kay Kay...*
> *"Hi, Grandma Kay Kay! I'm gonna wear this on stage (she gestures to the tutu she's being fitted with) and also it comes with yittle unicorn headbands but we're not gonna wear that on stage because we are learning about mermaids, not unicorns. BYE!"*

June 12, 2019

> *Photo shoot with Mya in her ballerina costume, posing, pretending to laugh so her smile looked natural and beautiful.*

One of my favorite parts of helping raise this kid was her flair for the dramatic. At forty-two, I'm 99 percent sure I'll never have kids of my own, but I sure got mine with this one, sass and all.

NOT THE F——ING GILMORE GIRLS

June 29, 2019

> *I love my job. Love it. But I love karaoke nights more. I would do anything to be independently wealthy and be able to take care of the kiddos and watch Netflix. This has been a great (almost) two weeks, and I just. Don't. Want. To. Go. Back. Being able to stay out without stressing about the amount of sleep this 37-year-old body needs to survive a packed schedule is wonderful.*

July 3, 2019

> *Live band karaoke with Bonnie, Jon, Mandy, and Shawn; plenty of patriotic selfies.*

July 10, 2019

> *Snapping with Mya while we waited for Jessalyn, who was doing camp at the Dallas Cowboys stadium with the Cheerleaders.*

July 27, 2019

> *Doing "Bye Bye Love" with Mandy Joe...*

I have a boot on my foot in this video, which means I already fell down the stairs. So let me use this time to tell that story. I was carrying a box of trash down the stairs, Ruby's leash in one hand, my phone in the other. I was counting the stairs, and I have no idea how, but I missed the very last step and went careening forward, the box flying out of my hands and scattering everywhere. I thought I might throw up from the instant pain, so I crawled around, picking up the trash as best I could, pulled myself to my feet, and tried to rally.

I managed to get through the hallway door and the secondary outside door (somehow, I don't think I was carrying the box any longer) and knew I was gonna pass out. I did, hard and face-first, right into the dirt. The rest of my body ate pavement, but at least my face was saved. It was something like ten in the morning on a Tuesday, so there was no one around, and I sat against the wall of my complex, crying quietly, wishing for the millionth time that I had someone in my corner.

I don't know how long it took me to finally convince myself to crawl back upstairs (yes, I crawled up three flights of cement stairs), but I managed to get back into bed and called my dad. He told me to come to the office for X-rays, but there was nothing alarming. We ordered a little boot on Amazon, and I continued abusing it for an additional five weeks before I decided something was still wrong. More X-rays at a foot specialist revealed a Lisfranc fracture, which I had likely given to myself by abusing my foot. Surgery was indeed recommended.

My optimistic little heart took it in stride. The Skippers took care of me better than blood family would have, and my mother made it clear she would have been there if she could. I was not alone. And yet rather than ask for more help or put people out for the sake of my comfort, I had such bad panic attacks that my doctor recommended a six-week leave of absence from work. So a sweet friend who lived down the road came over twice a day to take Ruby out. I only left my apartment once a day, and I had to crawl or put weight on my cast to get back up, which meant my toes did not heal, and I was left with hairline fractures there too.

August 12, 2019

I posted black-and-white shots for Facebook, nominated by Brenda J: "No explanation, just pictures." The first one was at Texas Health Presbyterian, a picture of "Someday, Someday, Maybe" by Lauren Graham (I just got butterflies reading that title) sitting in my lap, my IV-riddled hand on top of it. In the second one, Ruby's face on my blanket-covered knee, my new walker and my new cast at the edge of the photo.

In the third one, Jessalyn and Ruby lying on the foot of my bed, J playing with her iPad with her arm thrown over Ruby, *Gilmore Girls* frozen on the screen. In between, color shots of the kids decorating my cast.

Looking at these pictures, I feel so blessed all over again. I hope those kids have half the love for me that I have for them, because just looking at their faces makes me smile. The memory of all three of them piling into my bed while I recovered is too precious. The memory of their mama bringing me food and not getting upset when I couldn't eat it (I didn't eat normally for, like, a week after that surgery). Thank you, God, I have known love.

In the fourth picture, walker outside in the living room, *The Bachelor* on TV. In the fifth, Ruby sitting on the rug in the bathroom with me, her head hidden behind a hanging towel. In the sixth, my poor, beautiful legs standing next to my crutches, Ruby sniffing the toes of my cast. Moments later, I had to pull myself up those stairs again, only on crutches. I ended up sitting and doing them on my butt, which seemed doable at the time. I was covered in a slick of sweat; I had never sweated like that before in my life.

On August 19, a week after my surgery and the day after I braved my stairs, I had a video of Mya doing "You're a Grand Old Flag," which means I tried to do both Jenny Craig and the kids that day. Fail. I ended up panicking at work, so convinced my leg was swollen they had to remove my cast (quite a bit earlier than normal) and give me a Doppler. It was not swollen, nor was there a clot. I was just alone, and that was that. But I did get a sweet rainbow cast after that.

August 25, 2019

> "Please explain to me why you'll buy candles from Yankee Candle, but not from a Scentsy or Country Scents rep? You'll buy skin care & makeup products from Ulta and Walmart but not from a Senegence or Mary Kay rep? You'll buy supplements, protein bars, vitamins, or shakes from GNC and Walmart, but not from a Le-Vel rep, Modere rep, or RevitalU rep? You'll go to the nail salon, but not buy an $11 set of nails from a Color Street or NZ Nails rep? You'll buy clothes and bags from Target, but you've never tried a friend's online boutique, Thirty-One or Style and Sass? Why are we as a society, so apt to support... Yes, I realize sometimes pricing is the factor, but remember you get what you pay for. Direct sales companies sell the best of their products, and the purchase comes with great customer service through your rep! I challenge each of you to purchase one thing from a friend this week instead of from a store! That one thing is helping your friend support him/herself. Also, post your link in the comments." I loved this so much.

August 27, 2019

> Mya pretending to read a thank you card from my mom:
> "From Gus. Dear Mya. I just wanted you to know, Gus brings this to you. You just have to ask God if Gus is doing okay in heaven." (Gus was their dog, and he had recently died.)

August 30, 2019

> Another new cast, this one hot pink; Ruby whining sadly while Gilmore Girls played in the background.

September 29, 2019

 Mya trying to scare Ruby with a Halloween mask, instead pissing Brayden off so that he kept trying to hit her with a drumstick.

October 5, 2019

 Singing "Boondocks" with the band, I was off my crutches and in a boot; next night Leo filled in for Jon and it wasn't nearly as fun.

October 9, 2019

 Jessalyn peeling the skin off a grape with her teeth before eating it.

October 12, 2019

 Selfie at the Billy Joel concert (bucket list!!), red lip gloss all over my teeth. [I posted a picture and video with Leo, who went with me.]

October 16, 2019

 State Fair with the Skippers, including my favorite pics in sunset by the Ferris wheel, and the kids and me enjoying turkey legs.

October 18, 2019

 Birthday weekend at the Tavern.

October 19, 2019

 Mya's costume birthday party (she was Maleficent).

October 23, 2019

 Photo shoot with Mya; the girls dancing to Bohemian Rhapsody so I could show them where to headbang.

NOT THE F——ING GILMORE GIRLS

October 26, 2019

>Halloween at the Tavern, I was a cop (my last Halloween "out").

November 20, 2019

>WHY is it November, my AC is set to hold at 68, my fan is going full blast, and I'm SWEATING???
>KEALEILANI S: That's how I was when I lived there. Sweating all the time.
>I was up earlier today than I am on a work day, and all I could think was YOU HAVE TO WRITE. The pup is forlorn in the Love Sac without me [with a picture of Ruby], but I'm slogging through the beginning… it's always the beginning and the ending I have the most trouble with. GETTING IT OUT. #sureillchangeitlater #writersblockbegone #justdoit
>[I reposted a video of dogs being silly.] Tommy's little face omg.
>KATHERINE H: Tommy is sitting next to me right now. We're BFFs.
>My week in car: Tuesday, engine light comes on. Take it in, diagnosed, fixed. Wednesday, headlights stop working. Both of them. Take it BACK in, one decides to work. They changed the bulb on the other. Saturday, other one goes out again. Saturday afternoon, take it in for an air check bc one tire looks low. Find out have two leaking tires. Get air to last me through Sunday (cause they're closed). Engine light comes back on. Call the shop AGAIN, hoping maybe they just forgot to reset it. Find out they're also closed Sundays and Mondays. Now sitting at Discount Tire, hoping it's JUST A NAIL in the front tire (and a tiny piece of metal he could see in the back tire) and that this will be free, because it's back to the muffler shop tomorrow.
>[I posted a link to Charlie's Helping Hands.] It started like any Hallmark Christmas movie… but it's real life. An 8-year-old wants to help the homeless. Can we help him get there?? First goal is $83 to buy a box of food. MREs to take to a soup kitchen.

Anything over that will go to buying and creating toiletry packs and winter packages for the homeless. Thank you all. ♥

    Waiting for Mya and an older lady walks in:

RECEPTIONIST: "Hi there, we have cookies out if you'd like one!"

LADY: "Are they fat-free?"

RECEPTIONIST: (Pause, where she's likely trying to convince herself not to be sarcastic) "Isn't everything around the holidays?" in such a sweet voice, I almost applauded.

    The lady ate a cookie.

ASHLEY P: That is an amazing level of restraint!

November 21, 2019

    Secret Santa name-draw in two days!!!! Who else wants in? I'm tagging a few more people I thought might be interested, but please no negativity. I've got people from all walks of life signed up, wishlists being made, so you'll have no guesswork, just a surprise from someone you may not know.

    DAY 20: (anyone think I can complete the month without skipping another day??) I'm thankful for the weird burst of energy I had yesterday morning. My apartment is 80% clean and it made me feel less guilty about giving into my Love Sac for the morning.

    DAY 21: I'm thankful for Advil. Every. Part. Of. My. Body. Hurts. But I'm thankful for that too... because it means I'm alive.

    [I posted a meme that said, "Tis the season to be crying uncontrollably over a Hallmark Christmas movie."] Currently, A Grandpa for Christmas.

DEBORAH G: A Grandpa for Christmas?? I haven't heard of that one! Was it good?

    Guess there's a #decadechallenge happening, and y'all know I'm all about those. The black hair is EVERYTHING, but I'd definitely give some of the wrinkles back [with a picture of me with black hair and a red shirt versus 2019 in a rainbow shirt].

SHERI B: Beautiful for 10 years.

November 22, 2019

>Crying at a meme of Sandlot family that said, "At some point in your childhood, you and your friends went outside to play together for the last time, and nobody knew it." I think about this quote a lot.
>STEPHANY N: My gosh... that's really sad. But true

November 23, 2019

>Dammit, I couldn't even make it through another day, much less the rest of the month...
>DAY 22: I'm thankful for Mucinex Night Shift. I slept like 14 hours yesterday lol.
>DAY 23: I'm thankful for food. Because, come on.
>Ashley D posted, "Fuck a sugar daddy. I just need my actual dad to gimme all the money he didn't pay in child support."
>"What will you look like when you're 77 years old [with a picture of an old lady in a pink spandex bodysuit with a rainbow on the bib]?" Damn straight.

November 24, 2019

>I drove by a bank today that I drive by every day, but for some reason today I noticed a sign on the building that read "since 1906." I was impressed until I got closer and saw it really read "since 1986." Not impressed. 1986 is not historic, y'all. Because if it is, then I'm ancient.
>[I reposted a tweet from Shanny from the Block: "A lady in the store tried convincing my daughter to buy a doll because dinosaurs are for boys. So my five-year-old roared at her. I'm not even embarrassed."] Good for the kid. I would have roared at her too. #toysarenotgenderbiased #norarecolors
>I'm thankful for Sharpies. Nothing makes my heart as happy as an excuse to use them in rainbow order. (Yes, that may be an exaggeration. Lots of things make my heart that happy. But I need y'all

to understand the importance of rainbow order to this OCD brain.)

ASHLEY B: Girl... My closet is in ROYGBIV order. This OCD brain understands.

MELANIE J: I have No Idea what Rainbow order is! Lol. I can Barely organize my jeans from socks lol.

[I posted a meme that said, "At least I'm a fun hot mess, like a train wreck full of pizza, fireworks, and glitter."] Spot on.

[I posted a picture of a big hole in the clouds.] God's eye? #bluehole #nofilterneeded #texassky #godseyeview

November 25, 2019

[I posted a map showing the favorite Thanksgiving Day pie by region: "Discuss. Weird choices: sweet potato, blackberry, coconut cream, pecan, and key lime across Texas and the southern states. RT if you live in the yellow area and have never had key lime pie on thanksgiving."] Oh please.

STACI P: [She commented a meme of Trump that said "Fake news."]

SAMANTHA K: Key lime pie is gross.

JENNIFER M: Yeah pink isn't right either. This whole map is suspicious.

Ruby had clearly had enough of being left in the car (while I went to ring the doorbell to get J, while I pumped gas, and finally while I checked the mail), so she jumped out of the car. I told her "no, get back in," closed the door, and said, "two seconds, dude." A guy came into the mail house laughing and told me, "You can't leave your man like that, he's watching you out the back window." It literally made my day. Teach me not to call her dude, lol!!!

Day 25: It's been a rough evening, and I can't stop crying. Hallmark movie bingeing, zero appetite, and my mind is spinning. But I am thankful for, and will always be, the wonderful people in my life. I'm 99% sure I've used that one before, but...

sometimes it's necessary to remind yourself you're not alone.
  Laura Lu: Love you
  Ashley B: You are not alone and you are loved!
  Katherine H: Keep sending your pure light out into the universe, honey. It will be returned.
  [I shared a post of musicians' faces.] Mick Jagger told me that "you can't always get what you want, but if you try sometimes, you'll get what you need." John Lennon told me that "you may say I'm a dreamer, but I'm not the only one." Robert Plant told me that "there are two paths you can go by, but in the long run there's still time to change the road you're on." Eric Clapton told me that "there'll be no more Tears in Heaven." Bob Dylan told me that "the answer, my friend, is blowin' in the wind."

November 26, 2019

  [I reposted Charlie's Helping Hands.] December 3 is #givingtuesday. It's a big holiday thing, this giving game, and it makes my heart smile. I just came from a memorial of one of the most giving men I've ever known. One of the speakers mentioned never letting a day pass without letting people you love know you love them. I wish I had the ability to do more, but raising funds is never something I shy away from. Every dollar helps. Click the link for the story behind the fundraiser. Love you all. Thank you.
  Day 26: I'm thankful for the Contemporary Chorale and "Stars I Shall Find." Come see us sing December 14, directed by the incomparable Melanie Craighead Moore, for whom I'm also incredibly thankful, because it's gonna be gorgeous.

  [I posted pictures of me and the girls and a video of Brayden getting tongue-tied over "Coco" and "KayKay."]
  [I reposted my prayer to God for it to stay cold.]

Tear 'im up, beat 'im up, get 'im!! #rubyrose #cutestthingever #dogsofinstagram #tearthestuffingoutofhim" [with pictures of Ruby with a new toy].

November 28, 2019

Day 28: I am thankful for family, friends, and food. Not necessarily in that order. What a wonderful, blessed day. Hope everyone had a fantastic Thanksgiving.

Thanksgiving Number Two with my amazing surrogate family. and yes, we are a little addicted to SnapChat. (Mya's exact words when we'd exhausted them all: "it's over?")

November 29, 2019

Excuse the insanely swollen left eye...platinum glitter and glacier glitter on lids, lapis glitter lower line; lips are one layer each of plum, peacock pearl, and chocolate copper topped with ultra gold glitter and glossy [with pictures].

This is where my insane allergies started and the majority of why I stopped wearing eye makeup. I would be driving, and my eyes would start to burn so fiercely that I couldn't keep them open, and more than once, I had to pull off the road. I still have no idea what was truly causing it, but it was miserable.

November 30, 2019

Day 30: (and I think I forgot yesterday too!!). I am thankful for leftovers. But really. It's been a blessed month. I've been getting to know a guy who SEEMS great. I've seen the true colors of some people. I've watched tons of wonderful happy movies. December looks promising. It's a fine line around the holidays of being happy and excited because it's a beautiful time of year and miserable and depressed because, well...holiday blues. I heard Garth Brooks today and remembered to thank God for the unanswered prayers too. I am blessed. I am thankful.

I posted a video of me doing "Alone" by Heart simply because Mandy Joe told me I should, and it was her last weekend at the bar (still wearing my boot), then doing "Will You Still Love Me Tomorrow" with her.

December 1, 2019

[I posted a meme.] I am (your name) God/dess of (predictive text) bringer of (predictive text). Fear me because (predictive text): "I am Courtney, goddess of the day I love, bringer of all the best ways of music. Fear me because I'm a little bit too hot." Yesss.

ALISHA Y: I am Alisha, goddess of the time, bringer of the year. Fear me because I have to do something to do with it and I don't want to go back.

BONNIE A: I am Bonnie, goddess of course, bringer of the week. Fear me because y'all have been so excited about the school year.

ASHLEY B: I am Ashley goddess of the skincare. Fear me because you have a lot to be happy about. Could that have been more perfect? Hahahaha.

HEATHER G: I am Heather goddess of wine. Bringer of all. Fear me because you know that I'm going to be a good friend. I'll take Goddess of wine

I was too sleepy to go to a #doggiebakery today, so she's celebrating 10 with prime rib. #rubyrose #happybirthdaybaby #tenthbirthday #cutestthingever #dogsofinstagram

SHERI B: Happy Birday Ruby!

Phew, this evening has been emotional. #tryingtoworkforgod #amidoingitright [with a picture of my devotional]. "Whatever you do, work at it with all your heart, as working for me, not for men. Half-heartedness is not pleasing to Me, nor is it good for you. It's tempting to rush through routine tasks and do them sloppily, just to get them done. But this negative attitude will pull you down and lower your

> *sense of worth. If you do the same tasks with a thankful heart, you can find pleasure in them and do a much better job.*
>
> *It's helpful to remember that every moment of your life is a gift from Me. Instead of feeling entitled to better circumstances, make the most of what I provide—including your work. When I put Adam and Eve in the Garden of Eden, I instructed them to work it and take care of it. Even though it was a perfect environment, it was not a place of idleness or total leisure.*
>
> *Whatever you do, beloved, you are working for Me. So give Me your best efforts, and I will give you Joy."*
>
> MARCI S: *If you're trying, you're on the right track!!!*
>
> *[I posted a picture of Ruby passed out.] Birthday bashed. Belly full of prime rib, likely dreaming of her Doggie Bakery treat she will soon get. Look at those crossed paws!!*

December 2, 2019

> *Oh God willing. Facebook test on Zodiac said, "Scorpio, Your strength and determination have gotten you through every struggle you have faced, but in 2020, you will finally experience a turning point in your life. You will shed many tears in the next year, but it will be tears of joy most of all. A big dream will finally come true for you, but most importantly you will..."*

It's cut off, but the first part is enough, because it came true. I moved to Connecticut, which had been one of my biggest dreams for a very long time. Now will you choose to believe it's a self-fulfilling prophecy that was bound to happen no matter what some silly Facebook test said, or will you choose, like me, to believe that signs are everywhere?

December 3, 2019

> *So now it's Rudolph that's offensive. It's sexist. And it's terrible for one of the reindeer (Comet?) to tell his wife to stay home while he looks for their son*

because it's "a man's job." Y'all. This is a 55-year-old cartoon. It's a classic. I understand things have evolved. Moms would be looking for their kid too. But come on. Teach your kids better, and they'll act better.

Oh WOW I hope this is real!!!!! The Hallmark movie I watched last night was so incredibly touching… this would mean so much to those guys!!!: "When sending out your Christmas cards this year, please consider taking one card and sending it to this address: A Recovering American Soldier c/o Walter Reed Army Medical Center 8901 Rockville Pike Bethesda, MD 20889 You may also help by copying and posting this message on your wall. Thank You and God Bless!"

> JESSICA H: Omg which one did you watch? Because I watched two in a row, but it wasn't that one. One was Stephanie Tanner and some candy canes and the other was about some neighbors. Both super cute!

Some of the words J "learns" in Spanish are super foreign to me. (Excuse the pun.) I've had to use my translator more than once, and every time I'm like, YES, THAT is the word I remember. Curious if they're learning slang words or if she's just pronouncing them differently? Usually she's very good at Spanish.

December 4, 2019

Thirty pictures with the kids were added to Facebook, not the least of which was baking an apple pie from scratch with Jessalyn for her dad's birthday; we also went to the Star in Frisco to take pictures with the big blue Christmas tree.

> ILSE S: Brayden! Omgggg! he's so cute! And big!

December 5, 2019

[I shared the Contemporary Chorale's performance of "Jingle Bells."] This year's Christmas show is in 9 days!!!! Get pumped and buy your tickets!!!! It's gonna be GRRRREAT.

WHY has no one learned that she doesn't say "SHIT" in "Rolling in the Deep? #donteditstuffitsdumb

December 6, 2019

[I shared Contemporary Chorale's video of Jennifer Wheeler, our amazing guest artist that year.] Y'aaaaaalllll. This girl can SANG!!! Come see her live at our concert next Saturday!!!

J is quickly tiring of my picture obsession. What a fun evening. I love when I get to steal her [with pictures].

We met the Adams family at the mall for a book reading of the Polar Express with hot cocoa at Barnes and Noble, while we waited for our table at Cheesecake Factory to be ready. At dinner, Charlie flirted with Jessalyn while Jessalyn remained completely uninterested. It was a wonderful night spent with good friends.

December 7, 2019

[I shared a post.] "Another time, my dad gave 50 bucks to a guy who said he needed to buy medicine for his kids. I told my dad he was probably going to spend the money on alcohol or something, but my dad said that 'whether he was lying or not says something about his character, but hearing someone in need and choosing not to help when I have the means to says something about mine.' I never forget that." Wow!!!!

KATHERINE H: Exactly.

Christmas PJ/ onesie night... watching a new Christmas movie (thanks Disney+!!), eating popcorn, and snuggling in our warm pajamas on this balmy December eve.

December 8, 2019

Scottish Twitter is literally in its own world:
RYAN B: Asked the burd in Krispy kremes for 5 Nutella donuts and she says "have you got

any nut allergies?" aye pal I'm planning suicide by donut.
MONTYFUCK: Never understood why acts at festivals shout "are you ready" aye two seconds pal a needty tie my lace pause the tunes.
UNKNOWN: Why dae folk ask babies stupid shite lit "ur gettin big arent ye?" As if the wee cunts gony be like aye Moira yer spot on am oan the protein.
UNKNOWN: Just got 4 drinks at the drive thru n that guy asked "do ye want a cupholder." Obviously a do ya fucking reprobate am no a fucking octopus.

RENEE B: Took me so long to read those lol.

December 9, 2019

Ruby is annoyed that J isn't paying attention to her [with videos of Ruby standing behind Jessalyn, who was lying on her stomach, painting her nails, tossing her ball repeatedly at her].

I just watched a (Hallmark) movie where Lacey (the star of every Christmas movie Candace isn't in) is pitching an idea for Christmas 365. It instantly made me think of Charlie and his sweet heart... some people DO do good all year round... December is very tight for some people, myself included... but aren't we more blessed than the next person? Everyone is struggling. But we can help. Again, if you can't donate, please share. Four more days, but I'm likely going to extend it... we can get to $500, I know it!!

December 10, 2019

THIS. Omg. I love their replies [with a video]:
QUESTION ASKER: What are you looking for in a man now?
RIHANNA, IN THAT BEAUTIFUL BAJAN ACCENT: I'm not looking for a man. Let's start there.

QA: *You're gonna walk home with more than maybe just a trophy tonight. I think lots of men.*

TAYLOR SWIFT, LOOKING DISGUSTED: I'm not going to walk home with any men tonight; I'm going to go hang out with my friends and then I go home to the cats.

QA: *Were you able to wear undergarments?*

SCARLETT JOHANSSON: Since when did people start asking each other in interviews about their underwear?

QA: *Is it inappropriate?*

SCARLETT: Did you ask Josh what kind of underwear he wears?

QA: *No, no...*

SCARLETT: What kind of interview is this?

QA: *There's one subject we didn't discuss... What was that? Everyone's talking about it...*

BRITNEY SPEARS: What?

QA: *Your breasts.*

BRITNEY, SOUNDING HORRIFIED BUT SMILING: My breasts.

QA: *If you could use make-up or your phone one last time which would you pick?*

ARIANA GRANDE: Is this what you think girls have trouble choosing between?

QA: *How do you balance your career and having a personal life?*

KEIRA KNIGHTLEY: Um, are you going to ask all the men that tonight?

QA: *Are you not worried they'll pick up the sexual references and not care about the music?*

LADY GAGA: No. I've got 3 number one records and I've sold almost 4 million albums worldwide. If I was a guy talking about how I make music because I love fast cars and f—— girls, you'd call me a rockstar. Because I'm a female, you are judgmental. I'm just a rockstar.

First Secret Santa delivery arrived!!! I'm so excited they were so excited. This is gonna work.

RICH A: *I got mine yesterday too! Thanks to the Skipper family for my awesome gifts!*

NOT THE F——ING GILMORE GIRLS

December 11, 2019

> *I tagged Ashley D in an Awkward Yeti cartoon:*
>
> BRAIN: *It's time to move on, Heart.*
> HEART: *I'm not ready!*
> BRAIN: *You'll never be ready. But the longer you stand still, the worse it will be.*
> HEART: *Onward to good things?*
> BRAIN: *Onward to good things.*
> ASHLEY D: *Damn, Heart, why you gotta be so stubborn??*
> BRYTTANI D: *My professor used all their cartoons for anatomy & physiology lol*
>
> *Wow such a cool picture. #stronger #thick-skinandanelasticheart [with a gorgeous picture of a woman lying on her back, exhaling the purple and blue universe, with the words "I hate that my past has made me harder to love, but I will not be broken again"].*

While my past has definitely made me harder to love (in theory, as we all have baggage, people), I realized something when I burst into tears reading this: I will be broken again. You know how I know that's a fact? This post is four years old, and in that amount of time alone, I've been broken several times over. And I'm about to start reliving the most recent years, which is going to be awesome (sense the sarcasm).

Anyway, the point I'm trying to make (over and over) is to open your heart to love. Don't be afraid to be hurt. It's going to happen no matter how careful we are, and if we are too careful, we aren't open to much.

> *Laughing so hard I stopped breathing (the "Me" is the Universal Me.):*
>
> ME, CALLING OUT A NAME, TRYING TO CORRECT AN ORDER MISTAKE: *Leslie?*
> CUSTOMER: *Yes?*
> ME: *So we are sadly out of raspberry, can I—*
> CUSTOMER: *I didn't order that.*
> ME: *Are you Leslie?*
> CUSTOMER: *I ordered a—*
> ME: *Is your name Leslie.*
> CUSTOMER: *No.*

Next me, holding a pizza box and shouting: *Sue!*
   Customer walks up.
Me: *Sue?*
Customer opens the box, frowns, and sticks her finger in the pizza: *I didn't order pepperoni*
Me, with a voice devoid of any emotion: *Sue?*
Customer: *ohh no I'm (name)*
The actual Sue, materializing at my elbow: *Is that a pizza for Sue?*
Me: *Would you like some free breadsticks to eat while we remake your pizza? Another customer touched it.*
   Another Customer sheepishly mumbles sorry
Sue, who has clearly worked with the public: *you take as long as you need to, honey*
Third Me, shouting at the top of my lungs: *Iced venti vanilla latte for Jennifer*
   Male customer standing right in front of me turns to look.
Me: *Jennifer? Iced vanilla latte?*
   Customer says nothing, takes the drink, shoves straw in, takes a long sip.
Customer: *I wanted this hot. I ordered a small hot decaf skinny vanilla latte.*
Me: *Are you Jennifer?*
Customer: *No, I'm Daniel.*

December 13, 2019

People in the Jenny Craig support group write about veggies all the time and not one. Time. Have I seen it spelled like that.

December 14, 2019

Hehe!! Dress rehearsal… alto power, with one voice out and one mouth full of candy [with Ginger and Jessica]!!
Sheri B: *Hi my alto buddies!!!*
2:30 and 7:30!!! It's gonna be so gorgeous [with a reshare of Christmas with the Chorale poster].
Yes! #danceeducationforall. Before a child talks they sing. Before they write they draw. As soon

as they stand they dance. Art is fundamental to human expression. —Phylicia Rashad

Checked in attending Christmas with the Chorale 2019 at St. Barnabas Presbyterian Church: Ready for the first show!! Black Cherry x 1. Fly Girl x 2. Tiny dot of ultra gold gloss. Glossy Gloss. A lot of stuff that makes my eyes really green.

Lyn B tagged me in a picture smiling and singing, "enjoying Courtney's Christmas concert."

Me: I love this picture. Thank you so much for coming!!!

Cris A: Sorry we couldn't make it tonight! I'm sure it was great!

December 15, 2019

The Grinch stole my... (predictive text):

Me: The Grinch stole my heart out to the right of my life.

Deborah G: The Grinch stole my birthday and my nephew's graduation gift and the gift of my paper.

Josh A: The Grinch stole my money and the card is on my phone.

Peter B: The Grinch stole my phone and it was a pleasure meeting you and your family are doing well and that you are not feeling.

Erica A: The Grinch stole my phone from the other side truffle fries that were not too much of it to get a better place for it haha.

Kelly M: The Grinch stole my Christmas party.

Cara B: The Grinch stole my heart from my desk.

Jeff M: The Grinch stole my phone from the phone with my phone on the other hand so I'm going back.

December 16, 2019

Okay, that's sad: I posted a MyPoints survey that asked, "Who's your favorite Love Actually couple?" Ten percent, including myself, voted for the prime minister and Natalie. Seventy-four percent voted "I've never seen Love Actually."

COURTNEY CANNON

December 18, 2019

Checked in at Richardson Woman's Club for one last Christmassy hurrah at the mayor's dinner. Fun to feel so important. Thank you, Mayor Voelker, for inviting us.

LAURA L: That's where I got married!

December 20, 2019

Second time in two weeks... front tire just won't hold air. Found out today the wheel is corroding. Also a screw in a back tire, just for some extra fun.

SAMANTHA K: Dude I want to hug you cause you have the worst luck with tires. *hug*

[I posted a meme.] Just a yearly reminder that temperatures do not make a person sick. Bacteria and viruses do. Wash your hands, k?

December 22, 2019

This kills me: Is your stomach flat? Me: Yes, but the "L" is silent.

First concert: Neil Sparkle
Last concert: Billy Joel (bucket list!!)
Best concert: Bruno Mars or N Sync
Worst concert: Ummmm... I'd have to say LeAnn Rimes but she was only 13, and she was still stellar.
Seen the most: Neil Sparkle
Next concert: Nothing official, but boy I'd love to see Blake Shelton.
Most fun concert: I'd have to go with N Sync on this one.
Wish you could see: Elton John
Most memorable: Billy Joel, only bc it's most recent.

Love it. Hope I get part of the profits. #imwellworthanovelorten [with a Facebook quiz that resulted in, "@JKRowling Now that I'm finished with the Harry Potter series, I've decided to write a book about Courtney"].

Instead, I'm writing a novel about myself and praying I can have a quarter of the success she did. Without the horrific downfall.

> @RyanReynolds Neat. 300 pages full of swear words and sarcastic remarks.

December 24, 2019

> Christmas Eve at Phillip and Claudia's, where I felt weirdly uncomfortable and had major diarrhea... took some meds and went to Laura and Rich's, where I felt much more at ease and happy to be spending Christmas with little kids.

December 26, 2019

> [I shared a Facebook quiz: "Courtney the Scorpio. Courtney, you never asked for much. All you want is a simple life, full of love and contentment. This January is going to be a great start to an amazing..."] Here's hoping... Busquet needs to come home, that'll be a start.

I was wondering if I wrote about him at all. He almost successfully scammed me. He's most certainly the only person who's ever gotten that far. Beautiful white male in photos, his English was much better than Wayne's had been, but there were still red flags for me, including, of course, the good ol' stationed in Germany excuse. He led me on for three months, despite me saying from the beginning, "If you ever ask me for money, I'll block you." We even exchanged I love yous frequently. I never spoke to him on the phone, but his ability to send pictures that made sense for us was uncanny. (I called him Superman once, and he managed to get a really good shot looking like Superman, with the cute guy's pictures he was using.) He was good.

And then three months into it, he asked me to help him with a business deal, and a woman sent me a Cash App transaction that I then had to send to Busquet. I'd never used Cash App before, but because it wasn't costing me anything, I did it. I regretted it instantly, told him I wouldn't do it again, blocked the woman, and declined the next request. He got angry, as I expected him to, and if I can find the screenshots, I'll include them. But…ugh.

December 27–28, 31, 2019

>NYE weekend at the bar, Bonnie pregnant, no Mandy Joe! But we still had fun. Shawn's last weekend too, if I remember correctly. At the time, I felt like my heart was breaking (they were moving to Oklahoma).

December 28–29, 2019

>Crazy nights for Shawn's farewell tour, the final round. With lots of live videos.
>Very long FB survey, three notable answers:
>6. If you could move somewhere where would it be?
>Washington or Connecticut.

The only reason Washington was listed first was because Lisa was there at the time.

>11. If you could have any career what would it be?
>Writer.
>17. You have the remote, what shows are you watching?
>Gilmore Girls, ha.
>This cracks me up: "Stop hating on Texas cities. Dallas is modern. Austin is beautiful. Ft Worth is rustic. Lubbock. Waco has Magnolia. Houston has the Astros."

January 1, 2020

>Emotional roller-coaster of a weekend plus some...my sweet friend's last shows at the bar culminated in one hell of an NYE party. How we will miss you, Shawn Solo. You are so loved.

January 4, 2020

>I love this. They may not be my kids, but you can still ask me. It DOES take a village.
>[I shared a post by Shelby Beck.] "This morning while at the park I noticed a mama playing catch

with her toddler as she swayed back and forth, patting the tush of the newborn tucked tightly against her chest. A while later I glanced up to see her approach me. She shrugged her shoulders and quietly said 'I'm embarrassed to even ask, but do you have sunscreen we can use?' As if she was somehow ashamed that she forgot to pack sunscreen today.

"Dear fellow mamas, please ask if I have sunscreen. Ask if I have baby wipes, diapers, or even extra snacks. Ask me if your toddler can sit down and play with us while you find a shady bench to nurse your newborn. Hand me your phone and ask me to take a picture of you with your sweet babies— we all know mamas aren't in enough photos.

"Ask for help. Ask for love. Ask for anything. Even though we are strangers, please ask me. It's not easy being responsible for little humans but it's easier if we help each other out. We're all in this together."

January 6, 2020

I posted an FB quiz that said I was Kat Stratford from 10 Things I Hate about You: "You are highly intelligent and have a lot of self-respect. You do not conform just because something is cool. You can come off a bit harsh, but you are actually very sweet." BRO. Why are these things always so accurate?

January 7, 2020

Has anyone ever used CashApp?
RICH A: All the time. Love it.
LEE J: Is this post from 2015?
MEGAN F: I heard it is awful.

I asked because this is when Busquet asked me to help him. I trusted Rich, so I went ahead with the app.

January 9, 2020

Awkward Yeti Cartoon:

HEART, RUNNING THROUGH THE RAIN: *What a beautiful day!*
BRAIN: *Beautiful? It's cold, wet, and muddy.*
HEART: *Yep!*
BRAIN: *How is that beautiful?*
HEART: *Because I love ALL the days we get, not just the sunny ones.*

February 4, 2020

JESSALYN: *Brayden, did you fart?*
B: *Yeah, me fahhhht!*
ME: *Brayden, why do you go to the doctor?*
B: *Because me sick*
ME: *But you're not sick!*
B: *Yes me are. I sick!*
ME: *But you're not sick.*
B: *Yes. Yes me are.*
    (All the while Jessalyn is whispering "cough.")
ME: *Do you need a shot?*
B, CONTEMPLATING: *Um, no.*
ME: *Then you're not sick.*

Jessalyn whispered "cough" again, and Brayden copied her, thinking that's what she meant him to do, and she giggled.

ME: *How do you know you're sick, Brayden? How do you know you're sick?*
B: *I know.*
ME: *How? Do you have a cough?*
B: *Um, yes!*
ME: *Let me hear it!*
B: *(fakest cough ever)*
ME: *You don't sound sick.*
JESSALYN: *Okay, well it sounds like we need to get you a doctor's appointment.*

February 8–9, 2020

Skipper weekend, birthday party with the littles, then Urban Air trampoline park where I almost lost Brayden in the ball pit. That thing is scary.

March 16, 2020

> I posted a picture of me wearing my rainbow striped dress and green lipstick for St. Patrick's Day. I think this was the last time I wore makeup for COVID.

April 23, 2020

> Mya doing her homework, Brayden under the table: "Don't you dare tickle my feet, Brayden, I hate when people tickle my feet."

April 27, 2020

> Playing on the inflatable water playscape in the Skippers' backyard.

April 28, 2020

> Bonnie played Santa's Secret Teacher for the kids; the kids and me singing to the Trolls movie, which we must have watched 400 times.

April 29, 2020

> Playing limbo outside, backyard photo shoot with portrait mode.

April 30, 2020

> Playing with flour again, this time outside; adorable pic of Mya laying in Brayden's lap, his hand on her shoulder; video of all three doing a "happy Mother's Day" video for Grandma.

May 4, 2020

> Video of Mya pretending to be doing her own YouTube. She even had the asides down, as she yelled at her brother and then sneaked a word to her audience.

May 20, 2020

Singing "I Believe in Love" by the Chicks... not a bad performance at all. (For the Quarantine Karaoke group on Facebook.)

May 21, 2020

Brayden tossing his head in a circle and closing his eyes, me asking him to do it again while Jessalyn giggled uncontrollably. "And again!" I tell him, he complied, and I say, "Now what are you doing?" Him, "Rolling my EYES!"

Jessalyn and Brayden doing the ice bucket challenge (for COVID maybe?), pure greatness.

Doing the challenge where you put candy in front of your toddler and leave the room to see if they eat any while you're gone. (Brayden did really well because we forgot to turn the TV off, and Mya discovered the camera and behaved like a ham.)

May 26, 2020

Mya doing Zoom with some of her friends, looking joyful.

Jessalyn and Brayden playing "fast-food drive thru" with the Jeep.

Brayden dancing to "We Will Rock You," he winked at me.

"Are you winking?"

"Yeah. Mommy teach me how to wink."

He does it again, the cutest wink you've ever seen.

May 28, 2020

Slow-mo videos of Mya and Jessalyn blowing raspberries.

LMAO. If you've never tried this, I highly recommend it. It's hysterical.

June 1, 2020

> Most beautiful photo shoot of the kids in the backyard, playing in the sprinkler, me playing with the sunlight. Rainbows galore, there's a pic at 4:44!!

June 2, 2020

> Juno bobbing for ice cubes.
> Mya performing "Never Enough."
> FaceTiming with Mom, Cookie glaring at me from the back of the couch.

June 11, 2020

> Pool with the kids.

June 14, 2020

> Oklahoma to surprise Shawn and Mandy for their first real public performance. (COVID restrictions had lifted, but traveling had changed drastically!)

June 24, 2020

> The kids test sour candies for their YouTube.

June 30, 2020

> FaceTiming Mom, Monte looking regal from the back of the couch.

July 6, 2020

Somewhere around here was when the Skippers and I all caught COVID-19. As you can see from the lack of posts, I spent eighteen days sleeping, pretty much. I felt like I had a bad sinus infection, but the icing came when I lost both my sense of smell and my sense of taste for almost six months. I was terrified I'd never get it back again.

July 28, 2020

> Tribute to Naya Rivera with "Songbird." (Wow, days after having COVID, impressive.)

July 30, 2020

> *[I posted a picture with me, Ruby, Monte, and Cookie.] My babies, one of whom is crossing over tomorrow. He's been breaking my heart for a while now, but it's still so hard to say goodbye. Monte, you are the best little male dog this family has ever had, and you will be so missed. We love you so much.*

August 12, 2020

> *Movies with all three kids, wearing masks.*

September 18, 2020

> *Out somewhere (Legacy West with Kaitlyn most likely) with lipstick and a mask.*

October 12, 2020

> *I am 110% unsatisfied with life right now. To put it mildly.*

October 13, 2020

> *A grownup Christopher came over for dinner.*

October 19, 2020

> *Ruby barking at the crane tearing down the leasing office after the lightning strike fire.*

When the building next to mine got struck by lightning and Ruby and I both managed to sleep through the following chaos, I decided to move to Connecticut. Being alone terrified me, made me sad, and I was tired of it. So I chose to move in with my mother, halfway across the country. Dreams come true, but not at no expense.

October 23, 2020

> *Hard Night's Day at Legacy West with Kaitlyn for my 39th.*

October 24, 2020

    Dinner out with Phillip and Claudia for my birthday.

October 31, 2020

    Halloween at the dog park; Ruby wore her chicken.

September 5, 2020

    I'm reading over a diary I wrote as a kid and it's cracking me up. It's been almost 20 years, and so little has changed. I'm still dramatic and driven to love every boy in the world. Some of the entries were so "depressed," and there's a part of me who wants to shoot the kid I was, and part of me wants to hug her. Crazy how awful I found life. Every page had a new crush listed, and I was always so sure I was in love with them. #diaryofastranger #dramatica
  Joey D: That's awesome you have those. It's like pre Facebook posts.

September 6, 2020

    [I shared a post: "That broken thing you keep trying to put back together is keeping your life from that beautiful thing that's waiting to be built."] Thiiiiis, bro. #movingon

November 6, 2020

    All dressed up for a virtual choir concert (that was so hard)!

November 21, 2020

    Day 20: A holiday you love: Halloween
    Day 21: A technology: My phone. Man. I'd be lost.

November 22, 2020

  I have a notification on my Goodreads app and it's driving me crazy.
  Day 22, Something made you laugh. Gilmore Girls. Specifically Lauren Graham.

November 23, 2020

  Sometimes God is so good, it hurts. Thankful.
  Day 23: Something nice: Moving to a new state with a full-time job in pocket.
 ERIN G: What?!? A laugh but no explanation?!
 ME: Lollll I'm moving to CT to live with my mama.
 MACKIE K: That's exciting! Connecticut?! That'll be different. I understand it's beautiful!
 ME: I can't wait.
 SLY S: Sayyyy what!!!
 ABRA N: [She commented a surprised, blinking GIF.]
 BRENDA J: Courtney—I hope your move to CT and adjustment goes smoothly. Give your sweet mama a hug for me!
 ME: I certainly will. She says she loves you and always will.
 BRENDA: Big DITTO there [with a Bitmoji that said, "Sending Hugs"].

November 24, 2020

  Day 24: a book, magazine, or podcast: Seventeenth Summer by Maureen Daly. I've read it so often, it's falling apart, and I could easily read it again right now. Also, all the Harry Potters. Because, if you know, you know.

November 25, 2020

  I had the pleasure of being quarantined a second time months after I'd been sick, which afforded me the luxury of being able to pack and sell my stuff.
  Day 25: Another person. My favorite Shawn Solo. So many wonderful times and memories in so short a season. Love you forever, friend.

SHAWN P: *Love you my friend!*

November 26, 2020

Anyone ever listened to Harry Potter books on audio? Want to know if the speakers are British.
PETER B: *You have to pay extra for British accents.*
MARIA V: *No, but sounds good imo.*
Day 26: Something in nature: Turkeys. Happy Turkey Day. #GobbleGobble.

November 27, 2020

Sabrina Watson wrote, "Kinda cool to think someone somewhere is having the best day of their life today. Someone's hearing I love you for the first time today. Someone's gonna get the job of their dreams today. Someone received some kinda good news today. Tomorrow it could be ur best day so keep going."

"Our caregivers have gone on record asking you to do what you can to contain the virus. We expressed concern in public forums based on facts and our first-hand experience in the hospital. We asked you then to follow CDC guidelines: wear a mask, socially distance, stay out of mass gatherings, (watching Beverly Hills, 90210, while writing and Kelly said "gatherings" at the same time I was typing it. #clairaudient) and wash your hands... Now we have 72 people needing beds in our 60-bed hospital while the rest of the Metroplex hospitals fill up. We are asking again that you help us slow this surge." — Cindy Perrin, Texas Health

November 28, 2020

Day 28: Something that brings hope. New England. Such dreaming is happening.

November 30, 2020

Day 29: A compliment you have received: "You have a beautiful voice."

Day 30: Something you're passionate about: Singing. The end.

December 1, 2020

Do y'all think there's a difference between screaming and yelling? It's always bugged me when they're interchanged.

DEANNE G: Yes. Screaming is without anger or pain than yelling. Yelling just gets your attention.

ASHLEY B: I think there's a difference.

ME: What do you think it is?

ASHLEY: Yelling is speaking loudly. Screaming is what you do on a roller coaster. You yell at a person, you scream on a roller coaster/ in a haunted house etc. Your thoughts?

ME: I hear people tell someone all the time not to scream at them, and I literally want to be like… all he did was get louder. He wasn't screaming.

CHRISTY V: Yes. As a teacher of 37 students at one point, I would have to yell at times to get my point across to my 4 and 5 year olds who would all be talking over each other at the same time. But I would never scream at them. I feel like a scream has more emotion, where a yell is just volume.

December 2, 2020

Pic of a dragon, with [Your name backwards] the [current mood], Hoarder of [last thing you ate] and [object to your left] is your name if you were a dragon:

ME: Yentruoc the anxious, hoarder of hot fudge sundaes and dogs. I would happily hoard those things.

December 4, 2020

Pajamas and movies (for the last time!) with the kids.

NOT THE F——ING GILMORE GIRLS

December 5, 2020

> Y'all. So so so thankful and blessed. What a relief not to have to take Aurora cross-country again. I can actually accelerate!! Who can guess what I named her? #thinkdisney #alwaysdisney #connecticutbound I'm carsick from the smell though. Time for some air fresheners [with pictures of my beautiful new car].
>
> ERIN G: She's got a yellow bow, so Belle is an option… but she is blue, so I'm thinking more Moana or Elsa… but she's getting you cross-country, so Mulan and Merida would be solid choices too…
>
> ME: I LOVE your thought process. You're on the right track. But nope!!!
>
> ERIN: Am I close?
>
> JACLYNN H: Congratulations!!! She's pretty.
>
> BONNIE A: Dory
>
> ME: Would have been such a good one
>
> BONNIE: Dang. Cinderella or Cindy?
>   (Gif of the Blue Fairy from Sleeping Beauty)
>
> ME: Could have continued with the Sleeping Beauty theme!!! Lol
>
> BONNIE: Gif of Aurora and Prince Philip dancing
>
> ME: Aurora was my Subaru lol. It does not work with all my answers being randomly posted. They were supposed to go under each gif!
>
> BONNIE: Gif of the Genie
>   Gif of Alice in Wonderland
>
> ME: clooooooser lol!!!
>
> BONNIE: with which one?
>
> ME: weird, I typed it under him. Genie lol
>
> BONNIE: Gif of Jasmine
>
> ME: Bingo!!!
>
> BONNIE: It's so pretty!!!
>
> ME: I gotta get rid of this new car smell and then I'll be elated.
>
> BONNIE: Gif of Sadness
>
> ME: Sadness lol. This would be super depressing!!! Should have named her Eeyore lol.
>
> GINGER D: Dory

PETER B: *Disney or Pixar?*
ME: *Disney lol*
ANNETTE W: *Totally Dory!*
CHRISTAL K: *Congratulations*
TENESHA I: *Congratulations! I'm thinking Cinderella!*
ME: *That was in the running!*
MACKIE K: *Beautiful! Drive her safely!*
DEANNE G: *Merida!!*
KATHERINE H: *Such a cute car! How did this magic happen?*
MARCI S: *Wait, so it's Genie?!? I'm lost! Congratulations!!*
ME: *Jasmine lol. And thank you!*

Total and complete hygge. Probably 9 years of babysitting these crazy kiddos for their dad's birthday dinner night, but for at least the past three, we've done Christmas movies and pajamas and nothing. NOTHING. makes my heart happier [with pictures of me and Skipper babes].

KAREN W: *Love these pics. I MISS all of these faces sooooooooooo badly. I know you guys had a fun time—maybe I'll get to see everybody SOON (I'm dying).*

December 8, 2020

I feel this in my very soul.
A haiku about Mario Kart:
Are you kidding me
Who the fuck threw that blue shell
I will fuck you up

December 10, 2020

I posted a cartoon of Lucy Van Pelt yelling, "Although COVID-19 spreads mostly via the mouth and nose, scientists now conclude that the greatest risk comes from assholes."
VICKI E: *Nailed it*

[I posted a meme of someone thinking "Haven't seen any posts from my friend for a while. Let's che—" and seeing you had been unfriended.] I've been here...

I'll tell you what, it's been happening more and more often from people I never would have expected. God working in my life one at a time.

December 12, 2020

[I reposted Mya doing Christmas songs.] I don't even know all the words to this song. Wonder if she can still do this.
MACKIE K: *Her sweet voice!!*

I posted a meme about gender stereotypes.
CHRISTAL K: *"Man up" gets me triggered.*
ME: *Same. Man up and boys will be boys.*

CHRISTAL: *I just heard someone on tv say "act like a man."*

December 13, 2020

I posted a picture of a puppy sitting in a square of grass among snow, her owner holding a piece of plywood above her head.
SHERI B: *My chihuahuas hate snow!!*
ME: *Ruby loves it. I'm so excited for her to see real New England snow lol.*
I've started wondering lately how many people I know who prefer different pronouns than we've been using.
STACI P: *Yes. This. I just watched Gender Revolution on Disney+ and highly recommend.*

December 14, 2020

I tagged Bonnie in a picture of Dog the Bounty Hunter saying, "2020 has been hard on all of us." - Taylor Swift
KATHERINE H: *Good one!*

It's time to start the panic attacks. I'm kidding. Mostly.

DeAnne G: "You are not alone" GIF.

[I tagged Katherine H.] Tea & Sympathy needs your help! It's no secret that @teaandsympathynyc in New York is one of my favorite restaurants. It was practically an extension of my living room—I ate there at least once a week when I lived in the city, and pivotal scenes from Crazy Rich Asians and my latest novel Sex & Vanity take place at their cosy window table. But now this beloved West Village institution is hanging by a thread, like so many family-owned restaurants in New York and around this country. So please consider their yummy treats and fun gifts available online for the holidays this year (Brandy Christmas pudding, scone mix and a fabulous tea set?), and if you live in downtown NYC, Tea & Sympathy is still delivering the most delicious comforting British food right to your doorstep. I wish I could tuck into their Shepherd's Pie and sticky toffee pudding right now! https://www.teaandsympathy.com/

KATHERINE: Can't wait to take you to NYC!

ME: I can't wait either but are these the best gifts ever or what?

I posted a meme that said, "Be with someone that loves you loudly, publicly, privately, and behind your back..."

When your child is virtually learning one room away and you get a text from their teacher...

MS. HEINRICH: Hi! This is random, but Mari asked me to text you because he is stuck between the mattress and the wall and can't get out.

MOM: omg here I come.

"Yep" [with a post of a cartoon—"Haven't seen something more accurate than this lately"—and two children facing each other, one taunting the other. The bully's mother stood behind him, arms folded, her own tongue snaked through her kid's mouth].

NOT THE F——ING GILMORE GIRLS

December 15, 2020

Shared post from 2015 of Charlie comparisons: "Christmases past and present. (It makes my heart so happy to see his Suite 100 Christmas picture on the fireplace. This kid and his amazing parents.)"

December 16, 2020

Dude [with a meme: "You know why people over-share on the Internet? Because it's like screaming into the void plus validation, like if the void was like, 'Yo, I feel that too'"].

Ruby's first picture with Santa.

We had an adventure today! #pictureswithsanta #bassproshop #rubyhatesfish #rubyrose @junebugs_jive #cutestthingever #besties [with photos with Santa, Junebug, and Deanne].

Thank you God for bringing this before I get on the road. Keeping an eye out on all my stops and SO FAR, all is clear. Praying for an easy journey. I don't do well in low-visibility driving [with a weather post saying it was twenty-five degrees and blizzarding in New Haven].

December 17, 2020

Omg, CROCODILE!!!! My MAN!!!!

Omg, after four seasons, I finally got one right!! Her tone was unparalleled. #thesun #bluuuuue (It was LeAnn Rimes as the the Sun on The Masked Singer.)

   LORI M: Me too. I knew it from the very first song she sang.

   STACI P: So good!

December 18, 2020

That was a lot nicer than I wanted to be, with pic added to "Online Dating is the Worst" folder:

   GUY: Love your pretty eyes miss Courtney

   ME: Thank you.

GUY: *Courtney I love being called Sir but I am a switch, and would love for you to tie me up, can we make it happen*

ME: *No. Already told you we are clearly looking for different things. You just made that abundantly clear, despite telling me three messages ago that you're looking for more than sex. Thanks for being just another lying guy. Peace.*

JILL F: *Hahaha! Love it!*

AMY R: *Oh I've missed these posts. Men are something else.*

MACKIE K: *Block him!*

December 18, 2020

Hard Night's Day at Legacy West (for the last time!).

December 19, 2020

Couldn't have asked for a better last show. Sure do love these guys, this place, and this girl.

[I was tagged by Ashley D in a screenshot of a great reply for men.] "Hello! If you are slipping into my dms and would like to engage with me, please send $10 USD to $CocoCanCan. This is non refundable for any reason. When you have sent payment, please respond with 'I agree to send Coco $10 USD and understand that this is not refundable for any reason.'"

December 21, 2020

God, yes. Please. (Also, vaginas are stronger than balls.):

Things to stop saying to men and boys:

* Man up!
* Grow some balls
* Boys don't cry
* Stop being such a girl
* Boys will be boys
* You're such a pussy

*Mate, you're whipped!

Oh man these are awful. The alien one KILLS ME. Also, I sincerely hope my addiction comes from loneliness. Hopefully living with someone will break me of it. #talktoeachother [with photos depicting our phone addictions (the alien standing in the middle of a city, hand outstretched, glowing green, as everyone blue kept their heads down, looking at their phones, ignoring him)].

[I posted a Facebook test: "The way I draw an X determined my biggest flaw: hardheaded."] Yup.: "Courtney has a fighting spirit. She's stronger than you would think because she's faced more than you could ever imagine. Despite everything she's been through, she's beautiful inside and out, with a generous heart and a kind soul. Courtney is the sea—beautiful to watch, but dangerous to mess with. She has a heart of gold, but it won't end well if you anger her."

Another test revealed I'm -1% narcissist and 106% empath: "You work hard for your dreams, but you are unstoppable when it comes to taking care of the people you love. You are as sweet as sugar but as tough as nails. You're often under a lot of pressure, but you can bear the burden on your shoulders. You are not only an empath, you are incredibly STRONG."

December 22, 2020

I'm determined to take one trip downstairs an hour (minimum), and Ruby isn't digging it.
DeAnne G: She can come over!!
Me: Don't think she'd dig that either!! Poor babe.

December 24, 2020

My brand new beautiful Jasmine, all packed (to the brim, despite my careful calculations), Ruby in the front seat, smiling out the window.

Stopped by the kids' house for final Christmas Snaps.

> This year is weird. Christmas Eve was quiet & tomorrow I start a new adventure with my first vacation in yeeeears. Merry Merry!
>
> CHRISTIAN T: Vacation... Don't you mean permanent move?
>
> ME: Well yes but the vacation is starting it. Merry Christmas.
>
> CAROL B: Enjoy your vacation and a fresh start! Merry Christmas!
>
> ME: I'll miss you, lady. Here's hoping we can sing together again!!
>
> BRENDA J: Merry Christmas Courtney! Safe travels & prayers for a new chapter of your life. Give your Mama a hug for me!
>
> ME: I sure will
>
> KATHERINE H: You're so brave! New England awaits!
>
> JACLYNN H: Safe travels. Texas is losing an amazing lady.
>
> ME: Aww thank you, sweet friend!!
>
> JESSICA H: Aww, will miss you girl. Safe travels and keep adventuring! Solo trips are some of the best.

December 25, 2020

> First stop, a very closed Graceland.
>
> Part one was FAST and easy. Praying for the remainder to be so as well. Now we are laying on a King bed watching Elvis performing at top volume. I'm not sure there's ever been a more beautiful man. Also, I'm a little thankful the gift shop is closed today so I can't spend any money (yet).

December 26, 2020

> So long, Music City! I'm sorry I couldn't stop!

Nashville had a bomb explode on Christmas Day. I was terrified to drive through.

> Stop Two, the Tennessean, SNOW!! I'm carsick from all the winding roads. All I want is a bread basket and a Sprite lol.

KATHERINE H: *Looks cool!*
I love this view (from the hotel).
KATHERINE H: *It's so great having Ruby join you on this adventure. A piece of home, wherever you go.*

December 27, 2020

Third stop, The Omni.

Okay every city needs to get on this: "Another reason to love Portland: over one dozen 'free fridges' have sprouted up around the city! These fridges and pantries are filled with food for anyone in need, and always accepting donations. Pictured: the location at SE Grant & 9th next to Shaking The Tree Theatre. (While the white shelf is empty in this photo, I can confirm the fridge and cabinet were full.)"

Watching this Food Network special about what they all went through when COVID blew in, and it's gut-wrenching.

Frito Feet!! With pic of Ruby's hind feet sticking out from a blanket.

December 28–31, 2020

Check out my new #rainbowbrite #coloring-book. These are saving me from myself.

January 2, 2021

CSE winter challenge starts Monday! My ma is doing it with me. Anyone else?? Follow me on Insta: CocoPhoenix1313.

January 3, 2021

I copied a post that said, "Stop saying 'start a family' when you mean "have kids." A couple is still a family. A single person and her cat is a family. A couple and their plants are still a family. Three weirdly close roommates could be a family. You don't need kids to be a family."

January 8, 2021

> [I posted a picture of my new coffee tumbler from Graceland, with Elvis's beautiful mug grinning at me among the sparkles.] This man is watching me today (and every day). Happy birthday to the King!!
>
> FB Quiz: Text from Cupid: "Hey Courtney. (Hi Cupid.) Courtney, stable relationships are not for you, you'll be the single rich aunt in your family."
>
> KATHERINE H: Well that was me for a long time. Except for the rich part.

February 1, 2021

> Ruby in a giant blizzard, got almost totally covered going down the stairs.

July 10, 2021

> Outdoor sculpture museum with Katherine, Fritz, Harper, Margaret, and Mom.

September 6, 2021

> Back in the @jennycraigofficial saddle again! So excited to have some structure. A chocolate muffin, meatloaf, and chicken fettuccini Alfredo were the features today! Not to be excluded, a string cheese, a banana, an apple with TWO slices of white American cheese, and our delicious caramel vanilla ice cream. I want to be down 20 pounds by my birthday. Six weeks.

September 27, 2021

> [I posted a picture of Ruby draped across my leg, staring daggers across the couch.] Ruby has been staring at my mom like this for almost half an hour (she fed her dinner and then put the bag back without giving her seconds). She started falling asleep in mid-stare, but she resumed eye lasers soon enough.

NOT THE F———ING GILMORE GIRLS

Our show ended so I went to Hulu and looked for something we hadn't watched in a while. Started "Frasier," which we'd only watched three episodes of, and it had been at least two weeks. And the first line is "MUST this dog stare at me all the time??" #electronicspsychic #yesshemust #shesstillstaring

This was before I heard the term *clairaudient*, which was just so wonderfully perfect: having the power to hear sounds said to exist beyond the reach of ordinary experience or capacity, as the voices of the dead.

October 2, 2021

Attempted to go to the Big E, went to INSA instead, which was my first experience with a legal weed store, and MAN it was fun.

October 12, 2021

Possibly (finally) getting my tattoo for my big 4-0. My mom is having a tough time with that POSSIBILITY.

October 23, 2021

[I posted a video of the glass opal necklace Mom gave me.] "So my mom got me this opal pieces necklace and I can't figure out how to take a good picture of it because, you know, cameras don't do justice. And I can't tell if anything is happening right now because it's really bright. But I wanted to share how sparkly and flashy and very awesome it is, and a little backstory for that.

"Opal is my birthstone and I am notoriously hard on them. I shattered my opal ring at my grandma's house and lost my opal earrings, and my mother got smart and got it for me in, hopefully, an indestructible little light-bulb-looking creature, and I'm super excited about it. Ooh, I think that might do it, look, that sun's coming out. Can y'all see how sparkly and beautiful that is? (Giggled.) Plus I have glitter on my lips. (Blew kiss.)

COURTNEY CANNON

"Glitter to all of y'all. Thank you everybody for the amazing birthday wishes and yeah... back to real life as normal."

October 24, 2021

[I posted screenshots of my birthday message from Jenny IC.]

"Dearest Coco ♥ Not one day has passed since I learned about your birthday yearbook that I haven't thought about 'signing' it. I've thought of so many memories and things about you that I love, admire and appreciate about you (ie you probably have an opinion on the Oxford comma). But I am incapable of doing so many things these days, regardless of how important they are or even how much I want to do them. I hate that I didn't do it in time, but maybe you can print this out and stick it in somewhere. All my excuses aside, here goes:

"The time I spent (working) was kind of a dark time in a lot of ways, looking back. I had my new baby (blacked out) helped, and I didn't have any friends. My need to connect with someone outside my family was (thankfully!) met in my relationship with you. I was instantly comfortable around and felt like I'd known you forever. Your love of Disney music and rainbows and coloring made me so happy.

"I ran out of room so this will have to be broken up in separate messages.

"Made me happy and forget about my stressful home life. But it wasn't just your positive vibes that I loved. It was your perspective on everything. We loved (blank) and (blank) and all those babies together, we appreciated their parents together, we sometimes judged various people together, we made beautiful (blank) together.

"This is all making me realize for the zillionth time that I would love to hang out with you sometime now that my family is about to return to some semblance of normalcy. Lots of (blank) because all of our mental health is suffering and at least hospitals have beds again. Which is all to say we might turn back into real people and do things again.

"Ok, so besides the fun stuff, we also talked about hard and sad stuff, and you were a caring and insightful listener. Even though we haven't seen each other in so long, I feel like I've continued to get to know you better through your social media and it literally makes my life better. You're generous with your vulnerability, and always compassionate toward yourself and others.

"Here's an actual fact: *many times* I've seen a post of yours that was particularly vulnerable and impactful and immediately thought of that Marianne Williamson poem about not playing small. You probably know it, but if not you'll love it. The part that describes you is: "And as we let our light shine / We unconsciously give other people permission to do the same / and we are liberated from our own fear / our presence automatically liberates others."

"Ok, so I've known you've been with your mom but for some reason I thought she was here, but you're in CT?! Do you live there now? I don't know how I missed that! You're probably asleep and I should be too, so I'm gonna sign off with a birthday wish.

"I hope that today you felt all the love that so many people feel for you, whether they've expressed their love lately or not. And I hope you feel all my love and that you know how profoundly lovable you are."

October 29, 2021

I posted a TikTok of me barking at Ruby and recording her reaction. She didn't have much of one.

November 2, 2021

Took the dogs to Savin Rock beach; pics of me sitting on Mom's bed in front of the sunset quilt, looking super high but cute.

November 7, 2021

[I posted a meme.] "People ask me, 'Why are you single? You're attractive, intelligent and creative.' My reply is, 'I'm overqualified.'"

November 20, 2021

Watching "tick, tick...boom" stirred up all the feelings that "Rent" does. Crying like a baby and marveling again how short life is. Been back and forth about whether to post this, but... #nodaybuttoday

It's come to my attention recently that I am a placeholder. And by that I mean, people love me until something better (or different, anyway) comes along. It's like I'm the Buffalo nickel and everyone is attracted to the shiny new quarters. I'm not looking for sympathy or "no you're nots;" I'm just stating a fact.

I've lived my life in short chapters, and I've always been aware of that. As they say, when God closes one door, He opens a window. He's never let this extrovert be truly lonely. Moving to Connecticut was a huge, quite hard decision for many reasons, but the pull of my mother, the weather, and the politics (mostly) was stronger than my need for nothing to change. All I can say now is thank God my mother and I are making this work, because I'd be lost without her. I've met multiple men online, as usual, and they were all... duds. Still can't really bring myself to do the karaoke thing, whether it's because the germs are gross, people are gross, or because I miss what we had at the Tavern so much.

I have three or four people in my life that I can pick right back up with like no time has passed, but when you receive a yearbook and there are huge chunks of emptiness where you would have hoped to, and expected to, honestly, see messages from specific people, it's kind of an awakening. I'm a really good friend. I AM the shiny new quarter. I'm rainbows and sparkles and joy, and I want to share that. I realize everyone has their lives but if you can't take two minutes to tell someone you care about them, especially after this shithole of a couple of years, then that speaks volumes. That includes liking or commenting on social media posts. It's like I cease to exist after a certain amount of time. Texas has closed, aside from my family and a few other people. That part of my journey is done.

I hate NY resolutions, and I never make them. I try to live my life the way I want to (no one can make you happy except you), and I've realized as I've given some reflection to my life, that means being quite a bit more selfish.

I've waited a long time and thought a lot about how to write this, because the people who did participate in my birthday made my heart swell. Of course I realized immediately who didn't engage, and it hurt, but I tried to allow the good stuff to override the bad. So now I'm writing this without bitterness and without laying blame. If I've loved you, I will always love you. I will always wish you well. That's what's so great about social media. But it's time to let go.

TERRI K: You are a good and beautiful person. We've moved a lot and it's always distressing when you realize people aren't who you think they are. It's a weird time but you will find your people. And you will see who are your forever friends. I have some I don't talk to often but we always pick right back up and it's so comforting. Relax, enjoy your time with your mom and it will come. I promise. Signed an old person who has lived in 5 states and multiple cities in those states.

ME: Thank you!!!! Always good to hear real-life situations!!

ANNETTE W: I hear you. Be kind to yourself. That isn't selfish.

KT G: This is really moving. Thank you for being vulnerable and sharing this.

ME: Thank you, sweet friend.

November 23, 2021

[I posted a meme that read, "I wonder who made the decision that eyes and teeth should be separate from health care."] Lmfao. Had this exact thought enrolling for benefits two days ago.

[I posted a meme of Kevin Costner and Luke Grimes from Yellowstone that said, "I'm at that age where I could date you or your daddy."] Bro.

November 24, 2021

[I posted a video of Cookie.] Watch, even though she's so still. It gets so good. #slomodachshunds #slomo #dachshunds #dachshundsofinstagram #dogsofinstagram #cookielouise #rubyrose

November 25, 2021

Pics of homemade cinnamon rolls for #thanksgiving breakfast. Holy cannoli were these good.

November 28, 2021

[I posted a drawing of a cupcake and balloon.] Practicing without a picture to help is hard. but I'm learning! #everblendmarkers #everblend #arteza #create #creative #createeveryday #art #artist #practicemakesprogress

November 29, 2021

[I posted pictures of my Apple Watch where Siri had listened to me say, "Yeah, I wish I was just offered free food. I'm just tired of life." Siri replied, "It sounds like talking with someone might help. The National Suicide Prevention Lifeline offers free and confidential emotional support."] Thank you, Siri, but I promise it's not that serious. #suicideprevention #sirilistenshard

November 30, 2021

[I shared a silly dog instagram post.] God I love dogs.

Working on #mentalhealth today. Tired of the panic attacks. #mentalhealthawareness #loveyourself #selfcare #hygge

December 1, 2021

[I posted pictures of Ruby and Cookie under blankets.] Spending her 12th birthday loafing, as any good dog would. We didn't have cake though. #happybirthdaybaby #rubyrose #cutestthingever
    SHERI B: *Happy Birday, Ruby Rose! Here's a Tit in flight for you!*

December 2, 2021

[I posted a picture of Wendy's salad and Arteza markers.] Stepped out for lunch today. Panic attacks are coming in spades this week, and I needed to get out of the same routine. I always work through my lunch, so today, I went to do some errands. Felt amazing just to leave the store for half an hour. Back to do a little anxiety coloring. May need some Gilmore Girls on in the background. My little anxious heart is getting (has gotten!) overwhelmed. Erika and JJ started a mini-challenge yesterday, and of course I missed the announcement, so I'm starting my #cse3perfectdays today! My mom is on board too! So #applepecansalad, my go-to when I don't plan, and grocery shopping this evening!! Here we go!!
    KATHERINE H: *Oh, honey. Life is hard. LMK if I can help at all.*

#cse3perfectdays day one is a wrap! Yummy burgers and overcooked sweet potato fries and a chocolate peanut butter shake were the perfect ways to end this crappy day. #cleansimpleeats

December 3, 2021

[I shared Jamie Jackson's PSA for the upcoming holiday: "Don't come at me with your little gift bag or Christmas tin and be all 'it's not much, but...' Let me tell you something... if you think enough of

me to build, buy, make, bake, paint, craft, or grow something for me...out of 7 billion people, this one thing is just for me...that is much. Let's not forget that this year when we say 'it's not much, but...' because the thoughtfulness to think of someone else is 'much.'"] Oh man

Time for another episode of "Hardcore Reality with Coco." Keep scrolling if you don't want a double dose. Anxiety/depression is winning this week. I'll tell you, living with a mental (illness but hate that word. Disorder?) is tough. I came THIS CLOSE to calling out today (which I've done maybe a total of 3 times in 22 years). Yes I just came off a "weekend." Yes, I had Thanksgiving off and am blessed to be able to leave early some days. But my brain doesn't care. I'm bursting into tears at EVERYTHING. I've had to sit in my office with the door closed and watch coloring videos and breathe.

Normal COVID-related anxiety is abundant, as always. But add to that some physical health issues and people taking personal issue with me trying to help them, and you've got an explosive Courtney. Even showering has become a huge burden. Thankfully the weather is much different here, so I don't smell.

So. Here's the real real. I'm going to have to have surgery on my ass. I have hemorrhoids AND a fissure built up with major scar tissue. Pooping, an every day, sometimes multiple-times-a-day activity, is next to impossible. I've been dealing with it for months (and years before that but it's gotten unbearable over the last few months) and now my little brain doesn't want me to poop at all anymore. Too much pain, thanks. So I literally cry on the toilet. I wait until the very last second to make it as easy as possible. And it's still complete torture. Like birthing a baby from my butt, or so I would imagine. It's awful. And even the thought of surgery, which will likely relieve the pain, is horrifying. Will I not be able to eat for several days? Will I have to have a colostomy bag while I recover? Who knows? And no,

I refuse to Google. My doc already scared me enough by saying some peoples' buttholes just give up entirely and nothing stays inside anymore. I don't need to know what else could happen. I'm praying that (for once) something in my life goes right.

December 4, 2021

[I shared an Awkward Yeti cartoon.] Okay, Nick, get OUT of my brain!! (Or heart, as it was!).

Heart said, "I miss me. I mean, I don't feel like myself lately."

Brain replied, "We have a lot going on, Heart. It will pass."

Heart said, "And then me will come back?"

Brain answered, "I'm certain if it."

And Heart said contentedly, "Good, because the world is really missing out!"

Philly cheesesteak wraps for lunch, crispy chicken nugs for dinner. I'm digging this two servings of dinner thing. This may be the way I succeed this next challenge. #CSE3perfectdays

December 5, 2021

This #cinnaberrybreakfastbar is out of control. One for the record books, @cleansimpleeats. Look at that, over 5,000 on a quiet day. Yay!! I'm learning how to add little steps. #steppinginto2020 with @hanscleaneats [with pictures].

December 6, 2021

Chinese Sesame Chicken was yummmy. I'm loving trying all these new ones before the winter challenge. #cse #cleansimpleeats #steppinginto2022 with @hanscleaneats

Facebook test, "Who always walks by your side? Your mother: Courtney, you have inherited your mother's strength and fighting spirit. Thanks to her inspiration, you are prepared to overcome any difficulty, although you always tend to put others first, before you. Wherever you go, always remember that your mother is with you, and she is proud of the woman you've become."

Well, she's no longer walking by me, and I do wonder if she would be proud of me if she were sane. I did my best. I'm still trying to do my best, which includes writing this book, which may very well sever any chance of rekindling, but it has to be done. Honestly, I feel like I'm finally cutting through huge, painful, horned toenails or something.

December 7, 2021

> Feeling the Christmas spirit today. Took the dogs out and caught sight of my #cindylouwho hair, so naturally I had to play with #snapchat. Observations: 1, I feel happy just playing with the filters. 2, I don't think those are Christmas trees. 3, it's very hard to get a full shot of this shirt while sitting in my car. 4, the lady at my allergist called my leggings "stretchies" and I love it. Has anyone ever heard that?? 5, it's a good day. #christmaslover #christmassy #anyexcusetodressup #thebestwaytospreadchristmascheerissingingloudforalltohear
>
> Sharing these guys so y'all can smile too. #rubyrose #cookielouise #cutestthingever #dogsofinstagram #dachshundsofinstagram [with pictures]
>
> Another delicious cinna-berry breakfast square and black bean and cheese quesadillas for dinner. #CSE #cleansimpleeats #steppinginto2022 with @hanscleaneats

December 8, 2021

> [I posted a cartoon of Bugs Bunny looking ragged: "8:00 AM before your 9-5." Then Bugs sitting up bright-eyed in bed on his iPad: "7:00 AM on your day off."]
>
> So I did the math today, as my days haven't been progressing quite the way I'd like. I have to get over 7,100 a day to hit this goal!! Totally doable, of course, but quite the eye-opener as I'm sitting here coasting on my 4,000 steps. Let's hope I can start

NOT THE F——ING GILMORE GIRLS

> *tomorrow!! #10000herewecome #steppinginto2022 with @hanscleaneats*
>
> *Second snowfall of the year!!! Yay!!! #tistheseason because I live in a state with actual seasons!!!! [with pictures of Lenny's backyard]*
>
> *Sometimes this cartoon is spooky. #accurate @ theawkwardyeti*
>
> *Surgery scheduled for January 12, and the relief I felt this morning has given way to slight panic. It's gonna be a long few weeks, I fear.*
>
> HEART: *Brain, we need to find a way to be happy again. If we don't, I'm not sure how long I can go without doing something destructive.*
>
> BRAIN: *You do something self-destructive multiple times every day.*
>
> HEART: *Gasp! I need to buy some things online to help me forget what you just said!*

December 9, 2021

> *New internal alarm clock is not my favorite.*

I find two things funny here: (A) that it's only been two years that I've considered myself having an internal alarm clock and (B) that I ever hated it. I love mornings and have considered myself a proper morning person for well over ten years. Like, I crave bedtime just so I can get up. I love coffee time (I'm a chatterbox in the mornings), and I love my YouTube or music to start my day. Oh my goodness, I've missed my routine. Three more weeks and I can get back to my life!

> *#tbt to the time when LA and I were ruling the world. @la.sunflower_ [with pictures of LeighAnn and me at the Stars games].*
>
> *I keep trying to tell myself that the more work I do now, the less I'll have to do in a week or two. But when evenings are like this?? It helps heal me. #steppinginto2022 with @hanscleaneats [with pictures].*

In the pic, I'm wearing the same pajama shirt I am right now and cuddled on the couch with my dogs and blankets. And though the blankets have changed (I have no idea what happened to my electric blankets in all the moves), the dogs, thankfully, have remained the same. I'm praying for at least another two winters with these mongrels.

Opened Facebook dating on a whim, and this one was adorable rather than disgusting. I refuse to put OKC or POF back on my phone though, no matter how entertaining they are. #onlinedatingsucks; pic said, "me name xxx i me look for me partner I'm honest have big heart."

Lisa M: Wait. Facebook has dating?!

Me: yep. I was hopeful for it. It's not much better.

December 10, 2021

Just got home to my mom making chicken & dumplings and it smells heavenly and I have all the feels.

These came in the same package and made me happy (with a picture of a Rainbow Brite coloring book and rainbow pill box).

December 12, 2021

[I posted pictures of the Skippers in a beautiful log cabin, making magic with the Big Guy.] You guys. Look at these magical people. These are the most beautiful pictures. I was just talking to my mom last night about still believing in Santa, and of course these kiddos came up. I'm a grown adult and still believe in magic because…it's pure joy. And happiness. And MAGIC. Why not believe??

The world is such a harsh place, and if I can create a safe and happy environment in our own space for my kids and that includes Santa, then I pray they believe till they're old and gray. What I wouldn't do to squeeze these three and their amazing parents. Literally the only regret I have in moving is leaving them. They're continuing to grow without me. Thank God for social media.

So much to learn. But he's cute. #markers #everblendmarkers #arteza #coloredpencils #blending #art #creative #creativity #createeveryday [with a drawing of a gingerbread man holding a candy cane].

I forgot to post last night, and when I checked my steps, I was so annoyed I decided not to post at all. But then today, I walked over 100 steps every 15 minutes by setting an alarm on my watch. I already do that to make sure I drink enough, so now I can make sure I move enough. Except I'll have to do two laps around tomorrow, because once I get home, 15-minute laps will not work, and I slowed waaaay down after 4 today. Live and learn!

Comfort food in the form of pot roast tonight. Also Jenny Craig lava cake. I'm working on blooming into a sinus infection, so ow. But...it was a good day.

December 13, 2021

[I reposted a dog under a piece of plywood in the snow.] I gotta remember this for Cookie's short little legs!!!!

[I tagged Lisa M in a post from "You know you're from Texas when..."]
"Y'all. What is this magical redneck store of goodness with 9,000 gas pumps and jerky that lines the walls like pearls to Heaven's gates and looks like it came scripted straight out of a National Lampoon's movie? Dude was chopping brisket right there on the table and people were grabbing the sandwiches as fast as employees could wrap them. More baked goods in the biggest hopping bakery I've ever seen. It's like a Cracker Barrel and Walmart had a baby that made a litter of Pilot stations and those grew up and married Texas."

KEVIN C: gotta love seeing your job while you're at home. Lol
LISA M: I wish I could go!
JOHN H: Buc-ees!!!

I did it, y'all. Over 8,000. I was exhausted by 5. Building every day, and hopeful I can keep it above 8,000 for the remainder of December. I'm sure I set myself back these past two days. #steppinginto2022 with @hanscleaneats

3:36 (AM): HELLO, IT'S ME! (Marci, it'll see you in an hour!)

This was what I came to think of as the witching hour. When I have no one to worry about making noise for, I might have to figure out how to use this time wisely.

> MARCI S: Nooooooo!!!! I finally went to sleep last night—I think I was out before 10, which never happens!!! So sorry Courtney!!
> [I posted a meme that said, "Respecting Other People's Boundaries 101: Holiday Edition. If someone tells you 'No, thanks. I don't drink,' the proper response is to say 'Okay' and then respect it."] Period. (Also, "no thanks" to dessert...also okay! I don't even give an explanation, just a no thanks.)

This goes for any boundary. If you're full and someone is trying to force seconds on you, just say no. If you live in a state where marijuana is legal yet you work for the CIA, just say no. You'll live, and more importantly, so will the other person. Standing up for yourself never hurts anyone. Not doing so hurts you.

> Weeelll still a bit to conquer on my days off. But this is hella better than last week's day off, so I'll take it. #steppinginto2022 with @hanscleaneats

December 15, 2021

> I'm waiting for it to happen in my new hometown. Come on, Hallmark. You're letting me down. #newenglandliving [with a meme that said, "Please remember, Christmas is not about buying expensive gifts. It's about going home to your small town and falling in love with Ryan Reynolds"].
> I updated my PP to me as a kid, cheesing in front of a Christmas tree:
> I was an awkward preteen, as most are. Braces, glasses, and a weight problem. Thankfully I never got bullied; I was much too outgoing and friendly for that. But looking through these pictures today has been interesting.
> First off, look at those legs!! Secondly, never started really gaining until my parents got divorced. (The first ones. The second ones came with all new issues.) And thirdly, I have clearly always had an

obsession with food. But I am learning more every day, and enjoying it too. And still enjoying food.

Wednesday will be my "off day" from steps. I am very far from my goal still, but my back and hips suggested more sitting than walking today. (Remaining steps: 108,389. Days left: 16. 6,774 steps per day. Is that possible????? That's exciting!!!)

AMOS H: You were a cutie.

KENDRA R: You were/are precious.

ME: You're so sweet. Back atcha.

Yessssss [with a picture of a white cat sitting in a window, a reflection of a cloud beneath him.] Took a pic of the cat lookin out the window and accidentally turned him into some sort of god.

December 16, 2021

I really love to make people laugh.

SHERI: ...and you do!!

Okay, y'all, we are getting somewhere!! Reached 7,000 before 3 today!!!! I'm learning. #steppinginto2022 with @hanscleaneats

December 17, 2021

This kills me under normal circumstances, but right now it's so much more touching. Y'all. I saw a panhandler counting a huge wad of cash yesterday (it looked like he had just been handed a miracle by the expression on his face) and I wanted to cry. I was so scared someone was going to jump out and mug him. Both my mom and I have been intimate with some of these situations; it's horrifying [with a post of twenty-four heartbreaking rules parents had to make for their children when they were poor].

My allergies are kicking my ass, and today my energy waned before I got out of bed. I'm thrilled I got to 5,000. #steppinginto2022 with @hanscleaneats

December 18, 2021

Another slowish day. Rain and a horrible headache made me sleepy. I'll make up for it tomorrow; I've got a busy day!

December 19, 2021

Fuuuuuuuuck I feel this so hard [with a picture that had a green scribble on one side labeled My Anxiety and a green scribble decked out like a wreath labeled My Anxiety in December].

Y'all know I gotta play with new filters. A few hundred more steps today. I'll do another few thousand tomorrow. Shooting for 9K!! I'm not doing the math again until a week out. Trying my best!!! #steppinginto2022 with @hanscleaneats

December 20, 2021

I'm on Santa's Naughty List because…" predictive text game…
- ME: I'm on Santa's Naughty List because I'm going on the phone call tomorrow.
- MIRANDA P: I'm on Santa's Naughty List because I have never been to the store.
- ME: Somehow I bet that's not true!
- BRITTANY C: I'm on Santa's naughty list because of the way I read this post.
- ME: Yes!
- DEBORAH G: I'm on Santa's naughty list because I don't have a lot to say but I'm so sorry.
- BONNIE A: I'm on Santa's Naughty List because of my family birthday party so I'm sorry to be so sad but I'm so glad I got it lol.
- BETTY W: I'm on Santa's Naughty List because of the video I got to watch on your site.
- SHERI B: I'm on Santa's Naughty List because I'm going on the phone number so sorry to bother but I will have it in your mail tomorrow morning.

SANDER W: *I'm on Santa's Naughty List because of the weather and the rain and the snow and the other thing I can do.*
KENDRALYN R: *I'm on Santa's Naughty List because I'm so tired. This is true.*
HEATHER H: *I'm on Santa's Naughty List because of my family.*
ME: *Jack or Josh? Hehehehe.*
ANGELA W: *I'm on Santa's Naughty List because of my life with my friends #theonlyreason.*
JEFF M: *I'm on Santa's Naughty List because I don't want you in my room anymore and I'm just trying not to be rude.*
DEANNE G: *I'm on Santa's Naughty List because I'm a little confused.*
CAROL B: *I'm on Santa's Naughty List because I'm going to have a little bit of a fun night and I'll let you know when I'm done.*
Watching "Endangered Species" and they're on vacay in Kenya.
MOM: *I'd love to do something like that.*
ME: *Me too, but the traveling would kill me.*
MOM: *Oh, true, me too.*
ME: *If I ever do a real trip like that, it'll be to Bora Bora. (Show her some Pinterest pics of said place.)*
(Characters see hyenas and get super excited.)
ME, SILENTLY: *Now hyenas are really ugly, if I never saw one in real life, I'd be okay.*
(Guy on tv: There are no hyenas in Bora Bora.)
MOM, AFTER I TOLD HER WHAT I'D BEEN THINKING: *Now that's a true Witchy Woman moment.*

December 20, 2021

For our (main) Christmas treat, I splurged on @fatandweirdcookie for Mom and me. Let me tell you, we have only split one so far, and I would willingly hand over the same amount of money just to have this one again. Aptly named "Santa's Sauce," it's a cocoa cookie with a melty marshmallow center, and it's insanely incredible. Limiting ourselves to one may be tough. But I'm determined not to backslide this week. Stepped it up a little better today. Still feeling quite behind. Maybe I can work through my rest day this week.

December 21, 2021

I'll always have hope, no matter how many men bite the dust.

"One day someone will walk into your life and get it right where everyone else got it wrong. One day you won't have to wait for a call or a text back. One day you won't be the only one giving your all. One day you'll finally meet someone who wants to help you grow in life. One day you'll finally meet someone who isn't afraid to give 'love' another chance. One day you'll finally meet someone you can trust with everything. One day you'll have your best friend, your biggest supporter and your teammate all wrapped up into one person."

Tonight's @fatandweirdcookie is #thebrad. Sadly couldn't taste much oatmeal, so it was like an overhyped chocolate chip cookie. But it was still delish. Can't get it together on my days off, so I'm going to have to start adding an actual workout video or step it up on my work days. Did do the math again though, and I need just over 7,600 a day. Totally doable. #steppinginto2022 with @hanscleaneats

December 22, 2021

"Everyone thinks they're an expert on schools because they were once a student. But thinking you know how to teach kindergarten because you were a kindergartner is like thinking you could direct a movie because you once watched Star Wars. Teaching is an art and a science. It requires specialized education and years of practice. Listen to teachers."

Okay, kicked Wednesday Lazy Day's butt!! What's more than getting enough steps, I closed all three rings!!! #applewatch #steppinginto2022 with @hanscleaneats Tonight's @fatandweirdcookie was #blackbeauty, a cocoa cookie with white chocolate chips, Oreo chunks, and Oreo cream filling. Yummmm. Also made #cleansimpleeats pizza.

December 24, 2021

It may all melt off this afternoon, but we have a white Christmas Eve!!!!! Joy!!!! [with a picture of little paw prints in snow]
SAMANTHA K: It's 80 degrees here. You miss Texas?
ME: Not for that reason!!
Pic of our little tree with presents around it, all decorated by me. It's little, but it's ours. Missing my Dallas fam tonight, but this was a perfect Christmas Eve. Merry Christmas to all, and to all a good night!

December 24, 2021, 4:44 PM

Ruby flying like Superman from my bed to the couch, with her blanket in her mouth. My Angel Super Dog.

December 25, 2021

It was a good Christmas [with a Snap that read, "Merry Christmas from Jolly McSparklenose"].

December 26, 2021

Yay!!!!!! I'm DOING IT!!!! Look at these rings!! (53 mins of exercise when two weeks ago, that ring wasn't moving at all!!) I'm so excited to have gotten over 10k again. Helped to lessen the gap between me and 202,200, and it made me so happy. I want to build that habit permanently!!! #steppinginto2022 with @hanscleaneats

December 28, 2021

Pic of my uncle Frank from 35 years ago, having colored a Rainbow Brite picture in completely wrong colors. Pic of a current Rainbow Brite coloring book, colored by me in completely wrong colors, trying to break free from my comfort zone. "Thanks for the inspo, uncle Frank."

FRANK U: My pleasure.

Man, this @fatandweirdcookie was amazing. #animalcookie. Kicked my workout's butt by 11AM and still only got to 7,650 today!!

December 29, 2021

Another fairly successful day off: okay on steps but closed all three rings again!!!!! Allergies kicking my butt though. Waiting for a good snow. #steppinginto2022 with @hanscleaneats

December 31, 2021

NYE comes again, with no end to this weirdness in sight. We've slowly begun to adapt. How I pray we can make this "new normal" permanent. Despite missing the ease with which I used to go in public places.

Things I've learned since Hannah created this challenge and I've been much more conscious of my steps:

A busy work day does not equate steps, but it does make the "move ring" close much faster.

Getting lots of steps doesn't necessarily mean I've gotten much exercise.

The more I move, the more I want to move. I couldn't sit still until about 10:30 tonight.

Good challenge. Monday starts the #cleansimpleeats #winterchallenge. I've enrolled in two challenges in which I'm betting on myself to lose the weight. #healthywage is cool!! Starting off slow, but if I win, I'm planning on rolling half of my winnings into a new bet. Money has always been the best motivator for me. And so, at 11:18 EST, I bid you good night. And happy new year. We've got this.

Okayyyyy! "As everyone starts posting their 2021 highlights please know that if the only thing you did this year was simply survive that is something to be proud of. You're still here. You did it. I'm proud of you."

January 1, 2022

Why did I wake up this morning surprised by some of my pain? #newyearsamebody
LISA M: Best thing for it is to get up and get moving!
ME: Haha I'm keeping on... sweating currently from dancing while stocking.
Y'all, I put on makeup today. Just a teeny bit, and I rubbed my eyes six hundred times, but the lips!!!! #metallicmagic #lipsense and I am obsessed. Can't wait to try it over another color!! And see it in the sun lol.

January 3, 2022

Sharing my "before" pics in the actual "before" because for some reason, I feel like I've got this this year. I hate even numbers. 2022 can suck it. But 22 is my mom's lucky number, and I'm living with her so...
Grocery shopping early failed as usual. Forgot to take beef out to thaw. Didn't have ONE ingredient in MULTIPLE dishes. So we opted for loaded baked potatoes, carefully measured and macro-balanced as well as I could without a degree. Delicious and nutritious!!
Forgot to take a pic of my chocolate peanut butter brownie shake. But I'm sure you can tell I liked it!!
Off to a good start! Bloodwork tomorrow in preparation for my surgery, and then planning on a lot of coloring and bullet-journaling for 36 hours or so.

January 7, 2022

Dogs in snow: #wakingtoawinterwonderland
This. This is why I moved here. Aside from my mama.
CRISTA: Gorgeous! How much did you get?
ME: 13 inches!!
ASHLEY P: Isn't snow the best?!?!!! Also, I have many memories of spending "snow days" at your

> house (and busting our butts on the ice in the alley)
>
> ME: Literally. Even when it's all over my floor, I love it. And so funny that you said this, I'm about to do a sweep for everyone's detailed memories!!!

I posted mirror pictures in skinny jeans. Finally at my official lowest since… Not even sure when. 1 more pound, and I'll see a number I haven't seen in years.

That graph, y'all. (It looked like a roller coaster, literally.) My body doesn't play with the fluctuations, I'll tell ya.

Wanted to show this one spot of mad itchy eczema, but then I enjoyed how my brand new skinny jeans are looking. My collar bones are beginning to peek out again. Gotta do a body scan too.

Forgot pics of my delish aloha chicken kabobs and my amazing double chocolate banana bread, but it was another good day. #cleansimpleeats

> CRISTA L: Proud of you girl!
>
> ILSE D: I'm so freaking proud of you!
>
> ZOË L: Courtney, yay!!!!!! So happy for you! What a way to start this year!
>
> AMOS H: Congratulations keep up the good and hard work.
>
> LISA M: Fantastic work!!!
>
> DEANNE G: Go Court Go!
>
> CAROL B: Yayy yoooouuuu! Inside and out!
>
> GINGER D: Woohoo!! Looking good!
>
> ANDREA P: Way to go! Keep it up!

January 8, 2022

Happy birthday to this insanely sexy man. If he's the only love of my life (aside from Ruby), at least there are pictures like this [with another sizzling picture of the King of Rock and Roll].

January 9, 2022

"Coco will be there. #ifyouknowyouknow." [This was my caption for a meme of He-Man (I think) on a sparkly rainbow background that said, "The CDC recommends you wake in the morning and you step outside and you take a deep breath and you get real high and you scream at the top of your lungs WHAT'S GOING ON."]

January 12, 2022

[I posted pictures of me in surgical gear and mask, IV in hand.] 6:15(AM) call, was in recovery by 8. Still groggy, but twilight anesthesia meant no funny waking video. Y'all. My mom had to stop the car for me to throw up. Never had that happen before, even with general. Motion sickness rears its horrible head. #runsinthefam Sitting in the car while my mom picks up the necessary supplies for recovery, including a pretty intense pain pill! If you're the praying type, please pray for no constipation. I'm terrified. Also, the enema ahead of time may have actually been one of the more painful things I've experienced in my life, and I've torn my cornea and broken bones. So thankful to be on the other side of this. Praying for full and speedy recovery. #fissurectomy #fissuressuck #surgeryday My mother had to give me the enema. I was in so much pain, I couldn't conceive of putting something up my butt. So I had to lay on my stomach and let her do it. I shrieked, at 4 in the morning, and my poor landlords thought someone died. It was horrifying in multiple ways, but I kept telling myself she'd seen my butt many times before.) Does this have any typos? I'm being really careful, but I'm heavily sedated.

January 16, 2022

On the phone with Grandma for a memory from her...

ME: Is there any memory you would be willing to share that I might be able to use at some point? (Said as slowly and loudly as possible.)
G-MA: Any what?

ME: Any memory. You know just any rando—like sitting at home around the radio you know, with all your—

G-MA: One of the memories is gonna shock you if I tell you...

ME: Okay!

G-MA: The first time that my husband kissed me.

ME: Ooh, I'd love to hear this one!

G-MA: Okay, I was married to your father, husband number one (she thought I was my mother) and we were not getting along, and he was telling me all the things he was doing which were not mentionable. And I rebelled, I said I don't wanna hear any of that. And along came husband number two and he kissed me on the dance floor. And it shocked the daylights out of me.

ME: Aww. What year was that?

G-MA: What what?

ME: What year? How old were you, do you remember?

G-MA: Probably in my late twenties, early thirties.

ME: Okay! That's a good one!

January 16, 2022

Talking to mom about a different word for "dinner" so we could discuss it without the dogs getting all excited, Ruby heard "supper" but I determined Cookie was starting to go deaf; two hours later, they got excited again because it was really dinner time!

January 17, 2022

Ruby had severe "chompies," like she had food stuck in her teeth.

February 14, 2022

Cookie growling at the portrait of Ruby in the Sky I got Mom for Valentine's Day (and she hated.

This may have been where she started getting sick and I didn't pick up on the signs yet.).

March 6, 2022

> *Went to see Waitress at the Schubert, with masks.*

March 25, 2022

> *Teaching Ruby to hand me her blanket so she could jump without it in her mouth.*

April 2, 2022

> *Selfie, my eyes looked wild.*

April 3, 2022

> *"Home Edit" on my iPad; I was beginning to retreat into myself.*

April 13, 2022

> *Awkward Yeti cartoon:*
> *BRAIN: Chores are finally DONE.*
> *HEART: Wow! This feels GREAT!*
> *BRAIN: Now imagine how great it will feel to get them done EVERY week!*
> *HEART: EVERY WEEK?! WAIT. This was another one of your WORK SCAMS?! (turned waste bin over on Brain's head) NEVER AGAIN!*
> *BRAIN: sigh.*

April 13, 2022, 12:22 PM

> *Kisses from Ruby, my Angel Dog.*

> *Cookie rolling on couch, Mom's voice sounds depressed and slow, my laugh sounds high-pitched and manic.*

April 29, 2022

> *[I posted a Snap:] Coco in the sky with diamonds (or dollars). [In the picture, I am grinning as dollars fall from the heavens.]*

May 5, 2022

>All dressed up for interview with Laura and Jean, my Jenny Craig Market Directors, for the center director position in Manchester. I knew that job was mine.
>[I am using the same Snap filter, raining dollars, but in my car this time, singing "Lollipop" by Mika and totally confident that job was mine.]

May 9, 2022

>Mom recorded me holding Cookie like a baby and singing "Don't Rain on My Parade."

May 12, 2022

>My nose twitching madly, like a bunny rabbit. I had never experienced a tick like that before.

May 13, 2022

>Argument with Mom, in which we'd decided to spend a night in the Omni Hotel for a treat. She was so angry that I'd offered to walk to save us $20 for parking.
>MOM: Courtney, we both wanted to do this. It's ridiculous that in your, in my opinion, that in your endeavor to save us money, you're having to walk two miles. That's what it is. I don't get that. I don't get that.
>ME: Okay, then I'll spend the $23.
>MOM: I know, you've said that several times, you've also said several times "but I want to walk." What do I...what do I want to do for you? How can I help you?
>ME, CRYING: It seems like I'm not helping you.
>MOM: Well, at the moment you weren't. That's okay. At the moment, I wasn't asking you to help me. I had asked you to help me half an hour ago.
>ME: I did.
>MOM: No, you gave me generalities, you did not give me specifics and that wasn't what I...

NOT THE F——ING GILMORE GIRLS

ME: *But it is generalities at a hotel!*

MOM: *No, honey, no it's not. You look all that up and you budget it, you figure it out, you know in advance what you need to have in cash and what you need to have—what you can pay for with credit.*

ME: *Check-ins and check-out times are the same.*

MOM: *Not always. Sorry. But they're not.*

ME: *I already looked up dog fees.*

MOM: *Maybe at Omni they are. Dog fees we haven't even yet sat down and continued to talk about. I couldn't see it on there when I went to look. I did tell you I would go look up all of the stuff, I did go look it up, I just wanted to watch the end of the movie. But you're very upset with me for something and I don't get what. I don't get what.*

ME, THINKING FOR A MOMENT: *I don't think I'm upset with you. I literally had to just think about it, and I was like, "I don't think I was mad?" (Manic giggle and shrug as I struggled not to start crying again.) And yet you kept getting so mad. (Started crying again.) I didn't do any... I don't know what I did? (pause, pause) Except for offer to try to save us money. And if that's not that big of a deal, then I'll just park my car there! I mean it's not that big of a deal!*

MOM, QUIETLY: *I don't even know why you're crying now.*

ME: *Because that's what I do.*

MOM: *Which shuts down the other person completely.*

Me, nodding and rolling my eyes as I raise my eyebrows and I shut off the camera, thinking so does the silent treatment, which is what you do.

May 14, 2022

Cuddling a client's baby, the exact therapy I needed.

May 23, 2022

The dogs were eating... sparked a conversation about dachshunds being named Hoover, which I'd heard multiple times before:

MOM: No, they're not. You tell me one dachshund, other than me telling you, named Hoover in the next three minutes.

ME: K, hold on.

(Pause)

MOM: Oh you're just going to google Hoover dachshund and you have the whole world at your (looks for the word) fingertips.

I laughed uncomfortably.

MOM: So you're going to be able to. But no, I've never heard...

She trailed off.

Naturally, of course, if she had never heard of one, it meant they didn't exist.

May 26, 2022

Ruby had to eat lamb, and she watched Cookie through the entire thing before deciding to dive in, and even then, she picked something out and spit it on the floor.

Ruby smacking in my face; Mom, sounding angry, "I can't believe she won. I'm moving to England."

Me, "Ruby, was that good or gross?"

Mom, as I'm cutting off the camera, "do you know who Marjorie..."

June 1, 2022

Playing tennis in the backyard with Ruby.
Pardee Rose Garden.
Snap Concert, "Will You Still Love Me Tomorrow;" "Criminal;" "Let's Give 'Em Something to Talk About."
Dog park, clearly trying to stay out of the house.

June 2, 2022

    I posted a blue Snap that said, "Mood. A whole mood."

June 4, 2022

    Went to Milford with Mom to see Cassie at work at Archie Moore's.

June 6, 2022

    Dressed for my first day "at the office," as Jenny Craig Manchester's newest center director.

June 14, 2022

    I posted a Snap of me as a bull, breathing green smoke. Even shaking my head hurt. WTF did I do?? Lots of others, including video:
    So I did something to my neck and can't move my head or my arms which is an awesome way to start a new week. Um so I'm playing on SnapChat because that's about all I can do. And watching "So You Think You Can Dance" cause I'll finally have enough wherewithal to focus on it. I don't even know if I said that word right. Yeah.

June 16, 2022

    The Awkward Yeti:
BRAIN: *What if we fail?*
HEART: *What if we don't?*
BRAIN: *What if we aren't good enough?*
HEART: *What if we* ARE.
BRAIN: *What if we can't get what we* WANT?

HEART: *What if we get something* BETTER?
    Butterfly comes to rest on Brain.
HEART: *Keep going! I can do this* ALL DAY!

June 22, 2022

    Torturing Ruby by flipping her ears inside out, but she won't shake her head to fix them, then doing the same thing to her sister and Cookie doesn't care either. I said, "I feel like it would be like your toes overlapping. Don't you hate it when your toes overlap?"

Pic of a snake asking a raccoon why he's sitting all slumped over, reading his book on the floor. Raccoon said, "my heart just feels a little heavy today."

So Snake slid under him, grabbed the book with his tail, and lifted Raccoon up to sitting.

June 23, 2022

Snapped a Brandi Carlile lyric: "Sometimes seeming happy can be self-destructive even when you're sane. Only insane." And then another, "Here I am, I'm so young. I know I've been bitter, I've been jaded, I'm alone. Every day, I bite my tongue. If you only knew my mind was full of razors to cut you like a knife if only sung. But this is my song."

Snap filter as a drag queen, "Don't tell me I can't sing this song / tell me that I've got it wrong / cause this is where I belong."

June 24, 2022

Awkward Yeti
BRAIN: *Are we good enough?*
HEART: *Good enough for what?*
BRAIN: *Good enough to be loved, good enough to follow our dreams, good enough to be happy with ourself...*
HEART: *BRAIN. YES. It's always YES.*
BRAIN: *It can't ALWAYS be—*
HEART: *YES TIMES INFINITY ALWAYS YES.*

June 25, 2022

[I posted tons of Snaps.] Turning a blue day into a spa day. #fuckthesupremecourt

June 27, 2022

Awkward Yeti!

BRAIN: *Come on, Heart, there are a million things we need to do!*

HEART: *We* NEED *a* BREAK*! How can we expect to take care of things for* OTHER *people if we can't even take care of our* OWN NEEDS*?*

BRAIN: *Fine. What do you* NEED*?*

HEART: *To retire to the mountains and never return!*

June 29, 2022

[*I shared a meme that said, "I don't post for likes. I post because I have ADHD, and if I don't tell someone every thought that comes into my mind, I'll die."*] SHHHHIIIIIT, *who was listening to my inner monologue this morning???? Wow. (Crying on my way to work bc, anxiety, I was thinking "who's not sick of listening to me IRL??" Literally racking my brain for someone to talk to. And then...*SOCIAL MEDIA. *Y'all don't wanna read, scroll on through. But boy it helps to lessen the brain-load.)*

June 30, 2022

I had 4 people tell me I should start a YouTube channel this week. #foodforthought What would you watch, if anything?

MARIA V: *TikTok over YouTube. YouTube is stripping payments away big time.*

ME: *I didn't even know that was a thing. I'm so lost with social media sometimes.*

June 30, 2022, 4:44 PM

Dogs doing their "dinner song and dance"; my darling Angel dogs.

July 1, 2022

Cookie is in bed with me, I'm grinning but can't be happy.

I posted a meme that said "I don't feel like sparkling today" with a sad star next to it.

> In bed with a scared Ruby, who was crying at the fireworks.

July 2, 2022

> Snap car concert: "Let me love you and I will love you until you learn to love yourself. Let me love you, and all your troubles, don't be afraid, oh I can help!"

July 4, 2022

> [I posted a picture of me, Shawn, Mandy, Bonnie, and Jon at live-band karaoke a few years before.] This picture makes me smile for many reasons. Here I am in the middle of my favorite people (as I often was if I could help it) and my bright AF keys and wallet are in the middle of all the drinks. Post-fireworks, I think, though I don't remember actually seeing them. So many amazing memories with these guys, but one of my favs will always be this. Karaoke is always fun; live-band karaoke was another rush entirely. Miss you guys and loving you all from the east coast.

July 8, 2022

> The Elvis movie with Mom...
> Okay, so that was fantastic. Baz Luhrmann is a genius. Austin Butler is a GENIUS. (Flatten my eyes and raise eyebrows.) Genius. And Tom Hanks has been a genius all my life! Love him, go see the movie, uh, be prepared to cry if you're an Elvis lover.

July 11, 2022

> Awkward Yeti:
> BRAIN: I'm trying my best, but it's still not enough.
> HEART: Enough for WHO?
> BRAIN: For YOU!
> HEART: Yeah I want a lot of impossible things, immediately.
> Pause, pause...

NOT THE F——ING GILMORE GIRLS

Heart: Buuut! You're doing great!

Comparison shots between October 2020 and now, about 55 pounds down: Holy shit. It may be slow. But you can't tell me it doesn't work. Come follow me for support and motivation for what works for you.

July 16, 2022

Sitting in Katherine and Fritz's backyard, fan blowing my hair: Beautiful summer night in New England. #iheartnewengland

I posted Snaps with Kath and my mother, an attempt to be normal.

The Skunk...

We were outside later than normal one night, and I didn't have my phone. But I had a strange sensation, and I went on high alert. There was someone else in the backyard with us, a huge, hulking black guy I couldn't see clearly. Ruby barked, alarmed, and I shrieked at the dogs, trying to convince them to stay away. We all knew the instant it was too late, and we all ran inside anyway. The smell was horrific. There is not a strong enough word to describe it. If you know, I salute you. If you don't, I highly recommend you never find out.

July 17, 2022

I'm at work. Look how frizzy my hair is. This new stuff is awesome. It makes it fluffy and clean and awesome... um just wanted to get on and tell y'all today's song challenge is a song that mentions birthdays! Other than the Beatles' "Birthday!" I wanna hear y'all's thoughts. I already know which one I'm gonna pick but I need new birthday songs.

July 29, 2022

Cookie standing outside Mom's cracked bedroom door, I eek it open for her and giggled.

August 2, 2022

Morning snuggles with Cookie, morning torture for Ruby.

August 4, 2022

Tickling Cookie, Mom is telling me, "I told Susan about Margaret saying that her new doctor, doctor F, whoever he was, was um, throwing psychotropic ideas towards Margaret?"
Me, "What kind of ideas?"
"Remember the mushroom conversation? Mushrooms are psychotropics. And um, so I was telling Susan, I got all excited cause I thought 'can I share these with you?'"

August 13, 2022

[I posted a meme.] "Oh, what a shame. It's storming. *makes tea* I had so many errands to run. *lights candle* So much laundry to fold. *Grabs fuzzy blanket* So many groceries to buy. *burrows* So much cleaning to do. *opens book* What a shame."

August 14, 2022

Awkward Yeti:
BRAIN, SITTING IN THE GRASS: Good things come to those who wait, HEART.
HEART, pouting with arms crossed behind BRAIN. HEART disappears out of frame.
HEART REAPPEARS, BAGS IN HAND: I couldn't wait, so I bought some good things!
Mom decided that she couldn't talk to me about anything ever because I asked her not to talk about being murdered in her bed at 8 PM. She got angry because I "never listened to her"; I was crying because it gets exhausting listening to your mother tell you you're her main stressor.

August 15, 2022

    I posted a meme of two figures, one rainbow with flowers blooming out of their head, one not. "You've changed." "We're supposed to."

    [I posted a meme.] "Picture it. It's late October. A cold front just blew in. It's chilly and breezy. The air is crisp. You're home in comfy clothes, baking cookies and watching scary movies. #ihatesummer"

August 16, 2022

    [I posted a Snap with a possum on top of my head.] "What happens when you don't feel like smiling?" … "Make yourself."

    [I posted a meme.] "Can't wait for that cool morning when the heat has to be turned on & I'm all cozied up in a blanket with my coffee."

    "When you say things like that… What did you just say?" I asked, tears clogging my voice.

    "I don't know," Mom answered smugly, putting her giant leather bag on the floor and sitting down. "Ask me again."

    "You said if I put you in the hospital"—she hummed affirmatively—"I will lose your relationship."

    "You will!" she affirmed again.

    "Mmmkay, so that's a threat."

    "It's not a threat!"

    "Mother."

    "Courtney, you don't understand!"

    "I do. I do understand. I've been through this several times…"

    She stood up, grabbed her satchel, and said, "I'm not talking anymore."

    When she got home from her outing, we continued to argue, this time about money. She kept trying to tell me I was going to be paying the $1,200 by myself, and I said, "No, I can't do that. We are splitting finances."

So she got angry and said, "Then we need to move, and I'll find a one-bedroom by myself. You're my issue, sweetheart, and we need to solve the issue."

Devastated, I started talking to the audience rather than her, "She said that she was going to leave and that she would be fine on her own."

I said, "I'm not gonna be fine on my own."

She said, "That's a choice you're making."

And I said that was not a choice I was making. I was trying to get her healthy and get her some help, and she blamed me for it. I inhaled a deep, shaky breath, the tears leaking out of both eyes. I didn't know what to do because...she didn't know she was sick. She admitted it twice, that she was hypomanic, and she thought that was normal, that she needed to live with it. But it is not normal. It had been twenty months—well, eighteen months—of fucking awesome living!

I recorded her making her own video, talking to her phone as if it was her therapist.

"I am so, so grateful for a lot of things, like maybe I can have my own little life back again."

I said, "Oh my God."

She looked up as if she had forgotten I was there.

"I'm not hoping for that," she said, shaking her hand at me.

I burst into tears and said, "No, you are!"

"Okay," she backtracked, "I'm hoping the stress will end, okay? I'm hoping the counseling will work, because I want to live with her. I adore her. That is not the issue. I can no longer continue the communication that Courtney and I don't have."

One guess if I ever got her to therapy with me.

Aside from the silent treatment, the most frustrating part about trying to talk to Mom was her tendency to put her fingers in her ears like a toddler.

NOT THE F——ING GILMORE GIRLS

August 17, 2022

In the morning, she told me she'd leave the house we were in. She loved that I was happy and safe, and I wouldn't have to get a cosigner. And she hated the neighbors and hated that they knew her business, so she wanted to leave. But she kept saying if I didn't find a therapist, she would move out.

I calmly told Mom to go ahead. (I had decided from here on out to record every conversation we had as "proof." I was tired of being gaslighted.)

MOM: Can you think of anything that might be connected to my Wells Fargo card that might have happened today for $45? 'Cause Wells Fargo's saying…they're declining it as fake. So, um, this is the description of where it's from? Dascpt.com? I was hoping it was the department of Connecticut because I tried last night to get a driver's license and couldn't. But it's not. So I'm just making sure that you don't know of anything that might have gone through.

ME: I do not.

MOM: Then I'm okay with them declining it. That's all.

"I just had…the most helpful consultation I think I probably could have had today. Um, not many clients on board today, and I was kind of hoping to make a lot of phone calls today and kind of just be by myself, and it's worked out well. And I'm calm, happy, despite my life being a wreck right now. And talking to this sweet woman twenty minutes ago was a huge blessing. Turned out, she was a therapist and kind of understood a lot of what I had to say. And I hope I gave her as much help as she inadvertently gave me because it's tough to deal with mental illness when (I nodded knowingly.)… It's tough. Don't know what else to say than that."

I posted a video of "Hot in Here" by Nelly accompanying a video of me at the doctor's office, twisting for angles in the mirror.

Another video with Mom:

ME: *Okay, so she told me that her boss, Jeff Carson, is on hold...*

Mom started to shake her head but bit her tongue.

ME: *Standby to be a witness for her at therapy.*

Mom nodded vigorously.

MOM: *I did.*

ME: *Because why?*

MOM: *Because I need someone who recognizes if I'm in a manic or hypomanic stage, neither of which does he think I am, and he will def... and he has had plenty of experience with bipolar.*

ME: *You know why he doesn't think you are?*

Mom rolled her eyes and leaned closer.

MOM, SARCASTICALLY: *Why?*

ME: *Because he hasn't talked to anybody else. So he's seen this side of you—*

Mom, raising her hands to her heart, nodded.

MOM: *Right. Right. And so he's my witness.*

ME: *For three and a half months.*

MOM: *Right. So he's my witness...that everyone I talk to other than you...*

ME: *So when you split up from Joe—*

MOM, PALMS IN THE AIR: *Could I talk?*

ME: *You started being sick.*

Mom turned in a huff to the computer.

ME: *And it's gone downhill from there and has gotten really out of hand this...today...this week...this week. And so now this poor man who you're working for, um, and I thought would be a really awesome fit for you and I hope still—*

MOM, EXCITEDLY: *He is. It's so wonderful. It's so wonderful!*

ME: *I really hope...I really hope you can stay there, because I think it's gonna be great.*

MOM: *I will, hon. I have no problems staying there.*

She waved her hands in the air.

ME: *But, Mom?*

MOM: *Yes, sir. Ma'am.*

ME: You are hypermanic, not hypo. Hypermanic. Overmanic.

She laughed.

MOM: I'm hypomanic.

ME: That means low.

MOM: I know.

ME: No, you're hypermanic.

Mom stood up quickly. I thought it was in anger, and she was either going to throw something at me or hit me, but it clicked what she meant, and I immediately said, "Okay, okay, no, I'm sorry, I'm sorry. I get what you're saying. I'm sorry. I get it. Hypo is below a crack-up."

MOM, CALMER: Exactly.

ME: Okay, so you're hypomanic.

MOM: That is what I offered to the doctors.

She sat on my bed, still standing above me.

MOM: Maybe I will admit I could be hypomanic when I went and pulled up the diagnoses and what is required. First of all, hypomania does not need to be hospitalized. And second of all, I'm not even hypomanic, if you go through all the items. (She mimed highlighting.) As in...

ME: Then you're a step below hypomanic.

MOM: Can I finish?

ME: Sure.

MOM: Are you sleeping enough? Yes, twelve hours. I take my meds at eight the best I can, wake up at seven. Okay, eleven hours, as best I can. Um, and always. Never miss a medicine. Okay? (She ticked her fingers.) I'm sleeping. I'm eating. I'm going to work. I'm gracious and kind to everybody else in my life.

ME: Else.

MOM: Yes, there you go. Actually, the hypomanic, I'm gonna have to actually say I'm not even that. But I was willing to say that at the doctor...

ME: But you're a step below that...

MOM: To get out of the hospital. That's all.

Me: Exactly. So you're willing to talk yourself out of it instead of taking a couple days to maybe get some relaxation meds in you and chill out and realize how sick you are, because it's just gonna keep climbing. And like I said twenty minutes ago, I'm scared you're gonna end up standing on the street corner.

Mom: That's not going to happen. I've given you every—

Me: Do you want me to get Lenny down here right now?

Mom: Why?

Me: So we can figure out our living situation.

Mom: Sure. I'd be happy to move out. Happy to. (She raised her hands again.)

Me: Oh, you will. You'll move out.

Mom: That's fiiiiiine, honey. I want...I don't want to be in this silly neighborhood before, now that you've told everyone. (She gestured at me grandly as if brushing something under a rug.)

Me: Where...where do you think you're gonna go?

Mom: I will hopefully find a one-bedroom apartment somewhere in West Haven. Jeff will help me with that too. (She nodded sagely, one hand on her knee, one hand on the corner of my bed, poised for flight.)

Me: Mmmkay. Oh my Lord.

Mom: Yeah. I don't need a cosign. You do, sweetheart, so I will leave you this...

Me: I'm so concerned how close—oh, I...I'm not leaving!

Mom: And that's fine. I told you that this morning. I huffed a laugh through my nose.

Mom: Did you film that one?

Me: Probably.

Mom: Okay, good. That was one of the first things I said to you, that I realized you needed to stay in this house so you don't have to cosign...get cosigned. Not me. (She pointed at herself and shook her head as if I didn't know who "me" was.)

ME: Right.

MOM: So I can move.

ME: Riiiiight. How you gonna afford it?

MOM: The way I've afforded it for however many years I've been affording it.

ME: Except for you're sick and working twenty hours a week...

MOM: I'm not. And I do.

ME: So you're gonna go get an $1,800 apartment somewhere...

MOM: I'm not gonna go get an $1,800 apartment, honey. If I have to live somewhere like Lloyd Circle again, I will. I will get a cheap apartment because that's what works!

ME: So you're willing to live an hour away from West Haven somewhere...

MOM: No, I want to move to West Haven.

ME: To get a ghetto little house somewhere and be miserable. No, actually, probably pretty happy in your quiet little hamlet again even though most of the time you enjoy being with me.

MOM: I always enjoy being with you, until we're talking about finances.

ME: Right now, I don't think you do.

ME: So she's choosing that and...

MOM: I'm not choosing that. I want therapy to work, honey!

ME: I don't know what else to say. I'm just...I'm just done.

MOM: I want therapy to work!

In the evening, after battling her all day again, I told her if she went outside to air her business one more time, I was going to start answering the neighbors when they asked if she was okay. She gave me permission to tell whomever I wanted, including Jimmy, including Katherine, and including the neighbors, which was possibly the clearest indication ever that she was sick.

August 18, 2022

I posted a TikTok with "Pumpin Blood" as the song, getting my blood drawn. She can't get a vein, so she switched arms, then switched to my hand. She's digging in there, man. Digging. Where's my blood? Is it a sign I've cried too much that my blood won't come out? Follow me if your life feels like this sometimes, #criedoutdriedout

"So, sweetest phlebotomist on the planet has poked and prodded both my arms...with no luck. Um, and gave me a bottle of water to go chug, and I had my Gatorade and I chugged that. And now I'm out here walkin around tryin to get my blood pumpin because I'm a zombie and there's no blood in there. Back up... hopefully in 5 minutes, we'll see."

Switched back to my arm...and bingo.

Then back outside. "Whatever she just made me do worked. But then, bless her little heart, my blood started running out halfway through the fourth tube, which, four fucking tubes? Four? Four tubes of blood, I looked shocked into the sky, but she said that three and a half should be enough, so here's hoping. Let's get some answers."

Cut again to outside the ER, where I'd come to pick up my mother, visibly shaken and tears clogging my voice. "Just had a panic attack in the waiting room of the ER. Can't do it, can't do it, can't do it!

Panic attack induced by horribly barfing guy in ER, topped off by my mother saying exactly what I knew she'd say when she saw me: "I can't be in the car with you."

I wish I could google search my own mind and just type in stuff like "what are my favorite movies" or "what was the name of the place with the really good egg rolls."

[I posted a picture of a black dog looking horrified.] My emotional support dog after I tell him all my problems.

August 19, 2022

[I posted a meme in rainbow letters.] "What we don't need in the midst of struggle is shame for being human. —Brene Brown"

Mom in her bedroom, Michael Jackson blaring, me going, "Hey." She responded but so quietly I couldn't hear.

Me: *I didn't know we weren't talking.*

She said something about the dogs, who she wanted to separate to eat from then on out because they had gotten in a fight over the food.

"She bit her in the face because she went for her food. It sucks, but it's a dog thing."

Then she said something about feeling comfortable feeding her. So I said, "Do you mind getting the food ready at the same time and then splitting them off?"

And she said, "No, I don't mind at all."

And I said, "Okay, well, isn't it dinnertime?"

"No, not for me."

"But for them…"

It was thirteen minutes after, and my scheduled military mother would not normally let that happen.

"Oh yes. Shut the door."

August 20, 2022

"Court, you opened my closed bedroom door and despite how I asked or demanded you stop talking and leave me alone, and you wouldn't step away or close the door. You are 5'10" and easily 60 pounds more than me. I pushed gently but firmly and you still wouldn't close the door. As I was pushing you so I could close the door, you reached around and pinched me hard enough to bruise. Then yesterday, after I showed you the bruise you talked to, I believe Jimmy while sitting next to me and said to him you now doubt what I said back in 2001 that Jimmy gave me a black eye…"

[I posted a meme.] "One awesome thing about Eeyore is that even though he is basically clinically depressed, he still gets invited to participate in adventures and shenanigans with his friends. And they never expect him to pretend to feel happy, they just love him anyway, and they never leave him behind or ask him to change." He's always my favorite character. What a winner.

At 6:36, she's sat on the couch and said, "Oh my God," with her hands over her face, "it was real! He's been sending me musical messages!" (A strange revelation to have when Clapton is singing about shooting the law.) She sounded joyful and looked over at me, who was already filming, "And you can tape me. He HAS been doing it." She continued rocking, her hands over her face. "Oh my God," she whispered, and then, "Oh, my God," a little louder. "I'm not nuts," she said on a relieved sigh. "I'm really. Not. Nuts."

I yawned in the background, and she turned to look at me again. "That's what the blue light was about," she said, gesturing toward the sky. "That's why Lily..." she trailed off, into her own brain again, and covered her face. (I'm so glad you have your ear pods on.) That's why she cried. He turned and sat in front of me and put the blue light on. Oh my God, man. I've gotta email him. I'm doing it."

Mom was sitting at her computer, rocking manically to "Cherry, Cherry."

> ME: Mom, are you trying to talk to me? Do you need to text me something? Mom? Hello? Hello? Motherrrrr. You keep turning around like you need to tell me something. If you need to use the phone, you can! HELLOOOOO! MOM. For the love of Jesus, could you just acknowledge that I exist?"

Suddenly she turned around, grinning, and got out of her chair, snapping off-beat. "What is going on?" I asked.

"We're soulmates," she said, continuing to snap.

Me, wearily, "Who? Who is soulmates?" She ignored me again, which killed me, and I screamed, "MOTHERRRRR. WHO. ARE YOU TALKING ABOUT??" I took a breath and said, "If I go back and watch these films and you're talking about Neil Sparkle and being soulmates (I butchered the word), I'm gonna call an ambulance. So you need to turn around and talk to me. Mom. I'm not gonna chase you down the street like Jimmy and I had to do when he was 17. So if you don't turn around and talk to me, I'm gonna call the cops. I'm giving you about 20 seconds warning. This timer says 1:22. I will give you until 1:42 to turn around and say something to me. And this is being filmed. And I'll get Lenny and Cindy down here as witnesses if you need me to. You have six seconds. Mom. Are you cracking up? Mother? Are you cracking up? Okay!"

A few moments later I got up and went behind her as she typed manically, an absolutely insane email to whom I could only assume was Neil himself. "Oh my God, it's so real," she sobbed.

"Mom," I said, startled. "Okay." I decided to go along with it.

Whatever conclusions she was coming to (I stopped recording the computer; it was too hard to read), she was blowing her own mind. The exact same thing that had happened twenty years earlier.

Finally she turned around and said, "Promise me you will let me send this letter. Promise me you will let me send this letter, no matter if the cops come. Promise me that, okay?"

My voice flat, I said, "The person on the other side of this letter doesn't affect me. You can send the letter if it's important to you."

She went back to her letter and ignoring me, and I tentatively asked if I needed to call the cops.

"No, please don't. I promise you."

"What is going on right now?" I asked, her excitement starting to catch on to me.

"I've had a little bit of a breakthrough, not a breakup or a breakout or anything... I've realized something."

"How bout a breakdown?" I asked.

"No. I'm just not able to explain it to you yet. You can film me, are you filming me? Please don't call the cops. Please let me send this letter."

"Agreed."

At the end of the email, she turned and asked me to film again, "Neil, my darlin', I figured it out. So what I propose is that you meet me at Mary's Place and, I have to listen to it again to remember the words about Beth and Cyn that I played for Beth on the car ride up to drive her home. Oh my God, you're gonna have to back it up, I'm very shaky. But anyway, I would like my daughter to listen to the words and hear what I hear, cause I'll explain it to her. And by the way, I still think you beat Paul Simon with Taproot Manuscript. (She flinched, as if breaking bad news.) His came later than yours. Thanks. Okay here goes."

She turned back to her computer, and I asked, "Should I stop it or..."

"No, I'd prefer you filmed it. (Okay. Okay!) This is historic, Courtney, I promise you it is."

She began "Mary's Place" by Springsteen. "This is Bruce's song to me," she said.

"Bruce Springsteen?" I asked, alarmed, hoping she wasn't about to ruin him for me.

She started telling a story, and I asked again, "Wait, that's Bruce Springsteen singing?" She'd never gone outside Neil that I knew of.

She talked over me, ignoring me, "You did offer me a doctor, somehow, maybe it was in my mind (she put two clusters of fingers against each temple, looking like Patrick Stewart in X-Men.) But you did offer me a doctor when you had me come up to... There were those firemen that just died."

Lost, I asked if she was talking to me or "them."

"I thought you were filming me."

"I am filming you."

She wanted me to switch the song to the tv so I could read the lyrics. "This is pretty miraculous, what you're witnessing right now, my love."

"Okay," I said, willing to play.

"This is miraculous. (She splashed her water onto her shirt and looked down, plucking at her shirt.) I'm sorry, I'm trying to lose weight, I'm on the divorce diet, you know how that goes. Um and 'Shiloh,' 'Shiloh' is what broke the code for me tonight. Playing 'Shiloh' is what broke the code. Okay, let's watch this. I need you to listen to the lyrics. And I'll explain what I'm hearing. I am psychic. And this is gonna prove it. And Neil, it's about time that we agree that this is happening. And thank you for sending the number one fan, I don't remember who she was, but oh my God, that night was wonderful, wasn't it? You played with me, you invited that wonderful little lady shaking like a leaf…" she got distracted and resituated on me.

"Courtney of all people, she recognizes how psychic I am. (She's wringing her hands in her lap.) It's a proof. Like when my father broke his hip and … we will talk about it later."

We started "Mary's Place" over again, and she sang along, apologizing for her "awful singing." She then proceeded to hear something completely in her own head. Finally, about halfway through, she turned and said, "We can still do this when my mother's alive."

"Ohhhh, I see, you think it's Marie-Ruth's. Okay."

She continued regaling me with memories, not all Neil-related, speaking to Neil and his dead musicians. Then suddenly she said I was psychic too. I asked her to repeat herself, then said, "I am psychic, yes, but how did I help you with this one?" I giggled as she ignored my question and went hunting for another song. "I mean, I'll take the accolades, I love accolades, I just don't know what I did to deserve them."

She then had me name all her favorite songs, not just Neil. She stayed up "late" watching Gilmore Girls with me.

August 21, 2022

[A video of us walking outside, early in the morning.] "It's Sunday, and it's our day off, and we're walking at..." I checked my watch. "Okay, it's already 7:20, so it's a little later than I thought it was gonna be. And we're walkin..."

I moved the camera to show Mom, who put her hand on my shoulder and said, "You're walking with catch-22."

I continued, "Walking, getting our exercise. We stretched. Hopefully, this is a new habit. Some healthy habits being built, yay."

A moment later, in a new video, I recorded our shadows walking, and I said, "Ready? Come on, let's go."

Mom yawned hugely.

Mom asked, "What are you thinking of?"

"Just making my reel for later. My TikTok."

Mom's shadow put its arm around my much larger shadow, and I said "Look how long I look" right as she said, "My Wendy."

Uncomfortable, I said it again, "Why do I look so long?"

"I don't know, but can I hear the music?"

After our walk, she waxed poetic about the night she went crazy on Highedge, saying Brenda was "an angel, an absolute angel," saving her life.

"It hurt her to have to be dragging me through mental illness. And it's kind of the same way I feel about you. I think you're absolutely an Angel. I can't keep burdening you with my...thought process. That's what I'm scared about, 'cause you get really frustrated if you can't hear me. And I get really frustrated cause I feel like I'm not being listened to."

She went on.

"I had a huge breakthrough in understanding things yesterday, honey. And it took all the pressure away from me. And maybe it's 'cause I prayed so hard to God. I prayed so hard for someone to listen to me. I've been praying and praying. I used to rock in my bed. Do you remember that? Oh, I still do, don't I? I learned that self-soothing helps me…"

"I really do believe in God. I had to explain all this to Edie, who's been my 'Kentucky Woman.' I had to. Okay? I think it might take a couple of weeks before I hear anything back from her. But for some reason, 2-22 is trying to say to 'Kentucky Woman,' 'I'll meet you at "Mary's Place."' Did you film it?"

"Yes. So you think Neil wrote 'Kentucky Woman,' Bruce wrote 'Mary's Place,' and 2-22 is your birthday…"

"Oh my God, you're getting it," she whispered.

"For what purpose?"

"Can I not say that to you yet? What I really believe?"

"Oh, okay. Is that one of the things you wanted to wait on? If that's one of the things in the email, okay. Now wait, what do you think's gonna change that means we don't need therapy after all?"

"Because I think you're listening to me now even if it's crazy-sounding."

"But I always listen to you, Mom," I whined, beating my head against the wall. "Okay. We're gonna agree on that today."

9:15 AM:

MOM: I need you to be the historian, Court. I need you to write the book about me. I need you to understand me. So, again, any questions you have as you think about them, as we're watching TV or whatever, write 'em down. And I'll tell you my side of whatever happened. Anything at all. Okay?

ME: Okay!

MOM: Is that fair?

ME: Sure?

MOM: *I'm not asking you to believe me, but have I ever lied to you that you know of?*
ME: *No. That's the thing is, I believe you. Jimmy has been known to lie, he's a liar/joker, I don't even know what to call him anymore, but...I know that there's also two sides to every story. You've proven that to me these past few weeks every time you say my perceptions matter. Well, of course they matter.*

She's nodding, and interjected, "And that includes being sick, hon."

"I believe you."

"Well, you do now."

"Your perceptions matter, but my perceptions matter too."

Mom is buttering her English muffin. "Of course they do" (this after giving me the silent treatment the evening before). "But not—not—not allowing you to hospitalize me for instance."

ME: *Well, and I didn't try to hospitalize you...*

I paused and started over.

"That's not true. Well, I called the ambulance knowing they'd take you to the hospital; I was thinking you'd probably have to spend one night, they asked for two."

MOM: *You know what I was thinking?*

"What?"

"That the police and the ambulance would get here, they would talk to me, not you, as the patient, me, and see that I wasn't out of my mind. And that's what I was banking on. And I asked you, I truly..."

She took a deep breath and looked skyward, then mumbled "We're making headway" before turning back to me. "I truly ask you... Um...I don't know what I ask you. We're almost making headway."

She flaps her hands at me. "Can we watch this?"

And then moments later, I must have said something about posting on social media, because she gave me permission, which is super out of character.

"I swear to you that we can film anything. You can film anything at any point, and I'm not gonna be embarrassed or shy or stupid. I may have to sometimes sit over here and rock out to the songs. I'm not going nuts..."

ME: That's fine. I promise I would never share those on social media anyway.

She laughed as she took a bite of English muffin.

There was laughter in my voice as I said, "I mean, I know you wouldn't really want that. Sharing it with, you know, somebody that needs to see it, might, but...social media doesn't need to see that."

We spent the rest of the day allowing her to ramble as much as she wanted. I stayed as high as I could to cope, but mostly, it was really fun—exhausting but fun.

Mostly, she kept telling me, "This is how I think the TV is talking to me. Have fun with it."

And I needed a new way to explain to her, "It's when it stops being fun and you start thinking the TV is actually talking to you that I get worried."

At the end of Calamity Jane, she mentioned again that things would be good in two weeks. I asked her (again) why she thought they were bad right now.

"I think they're wonderful since last night. I think we both got a lot of weight off of our hearts and brains. You don't realize what kind of breakthrough I had yesterday. Such a huge recognition of how much you love me, how much you care, and how hard it has been to hear harsh words from me. To you. I realize that, sweetie. I know that. I feel like I've been hammering at your door for a long time. And all of a sudden I feel like"—she froze—"we're having a breakthrough. She's listening to me. So I think maybe two more weeks, two weeks notice. And then we can enjoy each other more."

She shook her whole body in a no.

"It's not me being weird or psychic, I promise."

I never did know what came at the end of those two weeks for her. She swore up and down she'd have an answer from Edie or Neil or someone.

While watching Enchanted, she started crying. "Stay with me, Mom, a little bit longer," she begged, then breathed deeply and calmed down. "Oh, I'm so sorry, Court."

"That's okay," I assured her, having been known to cry at a few weird places in Disney movies myself.

"She walked on my gr…"

She stopped herself on a sob. "My heart." "Do you feel like you need to call her?"

She gasped. "No, it's too early her time. But yes. I'll wait. Then I can go see Mom."

"Wait, you're gonna go…see her?"

"I feel like I need to. I swear to you, I need to see my mom before she dies, and I don't know how soon that's gonna happen." She took in another sobby breath. "And I need to hold her and tell her I love her, because nobody seems to believe I do, including her."

Despite wanting to roll my eyes at that, I arranged a FaceTime with Grandma.

When I resumed the movie, she thanked Grandma for praying today. My staunchly atheist mother suddenly believed her word from Grandma was thanks to prayer.

6:34 PM: We watched the credits of a movie we'd just finished, and Mom kept up a running commentary.

"Jimmy Romano. Thanks, Ray. Amy Wells…Amy Boland, do you now know? Scott—Scott in Powder. Thank you, Sean Patrick Flannery. We both think he's gorgeous."

She stopped, so I turned the camera on her, and she was rocking, brushing imaginary something off her fingertips.

"Hey, can I ask you a question, babe?"

"Sure." I was totally game since her mood was good.

"Do you remember when Neil picked us out of the crowd on your seventeenth birthday, and it sort of seemed like he was pointing to us?"

I must have been staring too long, because she continued.

"I know that was me being me, but didn't it sort of seem like it?"

"I don't remember it," I finally said. "That's what I was. I don't remember that."

"You don't remember the concert?" she asked, incredulous.

"Well, yeah, I remember going to see him in a limousine, I think."

That earned a "Mm-hmm" from her.

"But no, I don't remember specifics about the concert."

"Oh my God, that was so good. You were a little bit...hypnotized at the time."

Did she mean by her or by Neil?

"The scales had not yet been removed. But, oh my God, that's a hard one to do."

"The what hadn't been removed?" I asked, a laugh stuck in my diaphragm.

"Scales," she said, looking me straight in the eye.

"What does that mean?" I asked.

She mumbled something incoherent and smug, then took a sip of water.

"Oh, is that part of what you figured out last night?" I guessed, and she mm-hmmed me again. "Okay," I murmured quietly.

"And thank you for recording it," she said, shaking her head.

August 22, 2022

I introduced her to a few of my favorite songs that helped me when I'm down. She heard them in much different ways than I do.

Meme that said, "If you feel like you need to record conversations to prove you are not crazy, a liar, or delusional… you are in an unhealthy relationship, most likely with a narcissist."

[I posted a meme with Winnie sitting at a table, fork and knife in hand, honey pot in front of him.] "Reminder that Winnie the Pooh wore a crop top w/ no panties and ate his fave food and loved himself and u can too."

August 23, 2022

[I posted a TikTok of the dogs.] Good morning to all our fellow dog parents!!

We watched FRIENDS and Mom told me which character was my colors. It was Tuesday morning, and I asked if she was sure she didn't want to send Jeff, her brand new boss, a video saying she was okay, but she needed some time off. (I'd been suggesting the same thing for 36 hours; she'd started off not wanting to take time off at all and ended up completely ghosting him.)

August 24, 2022

She started off angry that day, yelling at me. "If you say it one more time that I'm sick, I am leaving!"

Of course, this was after two days of her not sleeping and into her third day of ghosting her boss.

"Do you want to watch some videos?"

"No," she snarled as I walked into the kitchen. She turned to look at me, her eyes afire. "I want you not to say I'm sick. That's what I want. Don't say I'm sick again."

Her finger was in the air, punctuating every growl.

"Don't. Say. It. 'Cause I'll leave."

"You've managed to say it this last couple of days, which I thought was meaning we were getting healthy." Tears were thick in my voice.

"Uh-huh," she interjected sweetly.

"You were excited to talk to Dr Lavern today. You are not healthy right now, and I'm sorry if that pisses you off. And you're more than welcome to leave because you shared your location with me. I'll know where you are and if you're fine."

She turned her back again and said "No, I'll take my location off" with a flippant hand gesture that was likely meant to be the bird.

"Please don't," I begged, not sure I could handle her going off grid again.

"Watch what happens," she threatened as I continued to say, "Please don't do this to me."

"Don't say to me one. More. Fucking. Time that I'm sick!" she screamed at the ceiling, knowingly looking upward as if she hoped our landlords could hear her. "That's all I'm begging you! I've been soft-mollycoddling you on the couch. I've been asking what I can cook for you..."

"Do you know you told me last night...do you know what you told me last night?" I sniffed. "'Thank you for taking care of me this past few weeks.'"

"Because you have!"

"I know I have, because you've been sick."

"I haven't been sick since I've been home from the hospital."

"That's not true. All right, I'm done with this."

A few moments later, I said, "I just want to make sure you realize you're going to lose your job."

"I know that. I already told you that. I know that."

"And you know this is a done deal, that you're healthy today, in your words, and you're not going to go to work."

A couple hours later, she calmed down enough to tell me she knew we were okay.

"God has us," she assured me. "You look so sleepy."

"Well, I believe that too, but..." I laughed in disbelief.

"But what, babe? Use your words."

"I just don't know what made you decide so all of a sudden."

"What, about God?"

"No, that...you're so sure we're gonna be okay and all that."

"Because I believe in God," she said firmly. "That was my breakthrough the other day. It was like an epiphany. God is around me. All the time. All the time. And I know that. And I put my head up off your lap four days ago now? And said I did it. I figured it out. So I wrote Edie a letter. And I want you to read that letter. But you're not ready for it yet. It's a beautiful noise, but you're not ready for it yet. Shut the fuck up. I might have to put my legs behind my head."

I had literally just asked her to start doing yoga with me because it was good for relaxation. She told me she wasn't supposed to because of her back.

"Why?" I asked.

"Because I need to stretch."

"I thought you weren't supposed to."

"Oh, I'm a little better now."

Stubborn ass.

A few minutes later, she exploded in laughter that almost turned into tears.

"You okay?"

"Mm-hmm. I gotta giggle every once in a while. I'm excited. I feel like someone's coming."

"Someone's coming?"

"Um, Dinah and her horses."

I thought for a moment, but I couldn't make it make sense.

"I don't know what that means," I admitted, unable to hold back a laugh.

"Didn't you sing that song the other day? 'She'll be coming 'round the mountain when she comes.' That's what I was talking about."

Suddenly, she began playing with her face, making faces like a four-year-old. Her mania was palpable, and she sat forward, letting her hair fall into her face, pulling it over like a curtain.

She finally pushed it back, examined her hands, and said, "I've got clammy hands. It's like we're in a haunted house. I just don't figure it out, except for tonight. I think. Okay, I won't explode Earth, I promise."

"Did you say you won't explode Earth?"

"I did, sorta. Don't listen to me. I'm jabberwocky."

Unable to sit still, she paced the living room as You've Got Mail played. She cried a bit and wouldn't respond when I asked her what was wrong, what she was worrying about. But finally she sat down again.

"I can see myself happy," she said quietly, crying pretty hard. "I don't want to see myself unless it's what I really am. It's so weird."

She sobbed, rubbing her face.

"I have to come down and understand this better."

She sat there shaking her head, struggling against the tears.

"I don't know," she said out loud. "Could I go crazy from it? Would it be too weird? No, I don't think so."

"Could you go crazy from what?"

"I'm talking to the TV right now. I'm sorry," she amended. "The TV is talking to me."

"Yeah, but you could go crazy from that."

My voice flat, I asked her to stop the movie and asked if she realized what she had just said. When she said no, I repeated it.

"You said, I'm sorry to someone whose name I didn't catch, and 'I did not mean to kill myself. I just hate the voices in my head.'"

"That is what I said," she confirmed.

"What does that mean?"

"Um, I don't know. I'd have to play with the words a little bit?"

She stared at me for a beat.

I said, "That's the second time in two days you've said something about killing yourself."

"Oh," she said, unfazed. "Okay, I'm going to watch."

She unpaused the movie.

"No, can you hold on a second?" I demanded, scared.

I then continued trying to talk to her, and she covered her ears like a child.

"I'm not ready to talk right now. I'm going to watch a dream."

12:22 PM: Mom sat there watching TV, lost in her thoughts and laughing so hard she was crying, then suddenly closed her eyes and looked as if she was praying. She then whispered what sounded like "Stones" and began to bob her head, tossing it like a horse. Next, she began making faces, crossing her eyes, twitching her lips like Elvis, clearly amusing herself when Tom Hanks and Meg Ryan weren't. She smiled secretly and then laughed, miming a zipper.

"It's a broken mouth."

She then whispered, "Pentatonix?"

A moment later, she said she was tired.

"Tired of what?"

"Being sick."

"Do you want to go to the hospital?" I asked as gently as I could, hopeful.

"Why would I want to go to the hospital?"

"So you can rest and relax and get the right meds."

"You're not even beginning to tell me that I'm sick, right?" she asked, her lips thinning out.

"You just said you were sick."

She scoffed and got off the couch.

"You promised me," she said angrily, shaking her finger at me. "I did not say I was sick, and you promised me."

"I didn't promise anything," I said as she opened the front door. "Mom, where are you going?"

You could hear the laugh in my voice, even through the stress.

"Mom, you don't have any pants on."

Thankfully, she came back in of her own accord, but she did ask me if I called the fire department.

I swear she sounded hopeful. Some part of her must have felt horrible.

Listening to Springsteen's "Glory Days," she began to talk again.

"Anthony, did you reset it? I'm still in prison. Grandfather's clock. You were cuckoo as a closet bird. I tried to tell you to shut it up. And all you could tell me was I was insane."

She changed the song to the Carpenters. Instead of talking, she began miming birds appearing, a strange smile on her face. Then she sang the line, "On the day that you were born, the angels got together. And decided to create a dream come true. So they twinkled stardust in your eyes…"

She trailed off as the lyrics failed her, but when Karen sang "Eyes so blue," she said, "They're green," confirming my idea that she'd been singing to me.

"I don't know," she said eventually again.

"You don't know what?"

"What's stressing me out."

"But I thought we were going to talk to the therapist and…"

She lifted her iPad and said, "I gotta have something different. I'll kill her. I'll kill her if she says it one more time. I'm gonna kick her so hard…"

She shook her finger at my legs hanging over the couch.

"I'll rip her leg off, if she says it one more time."

"Me?" I asked.

"Yep."

"Says what one more time?"

"Anything."

"Oh," I peeped.

"About therapy or therapists or anything. Medicine or any of that."

"Okay. I'm sorry."

"Huh?"

"I said okay, I'm sorry."

At 2:15, there was some kind of wellness check where they made sure we both agreed to go to medi-

ation and therapy. Mom ended it—"I'm done. Good night"—as if she was queen of the world.

She skipped her doctor's appointment that she'd been promising to attend. She refused to get on her computer, saying if the doc had wanted to keep the appointment, she would have found her (lying in her bed).

At 3:45, she said, "Courtney, you're being too bloody stubborn."

"About what?"

"Pretending to me that you feel fine. You're sick. And I'm tired of this. You have sat here on this chair, thinking I'm sick, for four days. Get up and go to work. I'm just tired of your moodiness. I'm fucking tired of it. I have had it with your moodiness."

"I have video evidence that says otherwise," I said flatly.

"I don't even know what you're talking about, but it doesn't matter, Courtney. You're moodier than shit."

"You're right, it doesn't. You're right, now I am sad again. It has been a roller coaster of a few days."

"I don't know what you're talking about."

"I have video evidence."

"Show them to me."

"No, I'm good," I said, scared she'd delete them.

"I'd like to see them."

"No."

"You keep offering. How come you won't show it to me when I say okay, show me?"

"Because I need a break now."

"I showed you Edie's letter to you. I have shown you everything. I've talked to Esther. I've talked to Gail. I've talked to everybody I can talk to, and I can't get through to you."

She sat forward to get as close to my face as she could while we were sitting next to each other.

"You just won't listen to me, you son of a bitch. I'm tired of it. I am tired of it, Courtney, and I'm about to institutionalize you. You're forty fucking years old," she screamed at me, and Ruby, who was between us, raised her head to my mother's face. She sat back. "Get off your high horse."

Just when you thought she was done...

"Fucking asshole. I'm so tired of it, Courtney. Miss Prima Donna thinking I'm the one that's sick. And you've sat here for four days, not moving, not talking to me."

She stood up off the couch to come stand in front of me, pulling on my toes like she did when I was a kid, but with malice.

"No matter what I say, just refusing to talk to me."

She put her hands on her hips and glared at me. I stayed calm, at the end of my rope.

"You're just giving me the proof that I need, so please keep going."

"Okay." She kneeled down and put her elbow on the end of my recliner. "I am begging you on my hands and knees to snap out of this."

"I was out of it," I whined, "for two days that I thought we were doing well, and I thought you were going to come out of it, and then today you snapped at me again. Just snapped into..."

The anger on her face was enough to melt gold.

"I snapped... I have offered..." she said incredulously, and then she began angrily slapping my feet and legs. Her teeth were gritted as she stood up, smacking me as hard as she could.

"Okay, okay," I said, pulling my legs in, my lap desk and iPad flying, "that's my proof."

I called the cops, and they basically scoffed it off to a domestic dispute.

August 25, 2022

[I posted a meme of Tom the Cat hugging himself, tears flowing freely.] "Me comforting myself while going through a hard time because I don't want to worry my friends and family about my own problems."

"So it's possibly been some of the stressfulest... months of my life, um, and this crazy-looking burger has been calling my name for the entire summer. And it's gonna be the last week on the menu. And it looks disgusting and it better taste freaking awesome because this is weird." I made faces as I scraped something off. "I left the lettuce off of it because who likes lettuce on a hamburger? I just think that's so weird, it gets all hot and gross. Anyway. Bottoms up!" I picked up the burger. "Yay, Sonic! Got a big ol' diet Ocean Water too. No sugar." I grinned, then bit the burger. I chewed for a minute, nodding, my eyebrows knitting together. "Weird," I confirmed, then shook my head. "Not worth the hype."

When I got home from work, there were broken Oxo containers in the kitchen and raw sugar and other things strewn across the floor and counter. Already exhausted, I sighed and set to work cleaning it up, crying quietly, while Mom came in and out to help while dancing in the living room.

Later that evening, Ruby stood very close to me, concerned. Mom, blurred out so far, reached over to poke my arm.

"Go," she said. "Go, sweetie. Get out of here!"

Ruby turned to glare at her and scooted closer to me.

"Do I have to yell?"

I answered sullenly, sounding like I was eating something, "I don't know. Maybe that will convince the cops that you're fucking insane."

"Okay, let's do it. Call the cops. Can we do it again?"

"No. I tried last night. It didn't work."

"Right. Call them again."

"No, I'm good." I said firmly.

She was quiet while Ruby stared at me, her nose as close to my face as it could be.

"Courtney," she said finally, venom dripping from her tone, "I hate you."

Whatever I was eating caught on the sob in my throat as I croaked out, "I'm sorry."

"I hate you with every atom of my body," she went on, sounding so cold she made my skin crawl.

"I'm very sorry to hear that," I said and started to cry for real, the food since swallowed.

"I hate you so much. I hate you, I hate you, I hate you, and I hate you," she said as I sobbed, Ruby again getting super close to me.

She sat back, pleased with herself, as I cried, "Why? Why do you hate me for trying to help you?"

She flipped open her Dorothy Dunnett book but then said, "'Cause I have tried your entire life..."

A minute later, she was back in my face.

"You wanna film this? Is that what the camera's on for? Why is the flashlight on?"

"Because I'm filming you," I said calmly.

"Okay."

She put her hand up to cover the lens.

"I love you. So much. So why are you filming me?"

"Because I just filmed you saying something entirely different two seconds ago," I said and started to bawl again.

But half an hour later, she asked to be on camera again.

"I think you need to film me"—she squatted down in front of me, pausing as if thinking up her reason—"telling Neil Sparkle I love him."

"I think I did that the other night," I said flatly.

"You filmed me telling Neil Sparkle I loved him?" she asked, looking both confused and hopeful.

"Mm-hmm."

"I don't think so. Show me. Show me."

"I'd rather not right now."

"I would like you to look it up."

"Please. Please?"

"Okay, then tonight you can film it. Would you like to film it?"

"It's eight o'clock."

"Oh my goodness, we're seventeen minutes before eight," she said sarcastically, tilting her head at me like a cocker spaniel.

"I don't understand why you're acting like a... Sorry. You're being sarcastic right now. Do you want me to film you saying something or not?"

"Yes. I want you to film me telling Neil Sparkle I love him."

"I just did."

She looked startled and confused again.

"Well, I haven't been to the play yet, but I think he loves her."

(She was talking about A Beautiful Noise on Broadway.)

"Who?"

"Neil Sparkle."

"He loves who?"

"Me."

"No. You're wrong."

"No, I don't think I was."

"Okay. I'm sorry. It's gonna break your heart again."

"Go ahead and film me. It's okay."

"I am. I'm filming you. I've been filming you."

"You're filming already? Okay, press the button and make sure it's on video," my boomer mother said, instructing me to use my iPhone.

She stood up, adjusted her nightgown, and said, "Okay, I'll do it here."

She put her left foot on the end of my recliner and leaned on her knee.

"Neil Sparkle," she started seriously, "would you marry me?"

She stared at me as if I was supposed to provide the answer.

"I don't understand if you're being funny or you want me to send this to somebody."

"Pretty much the norm," she responded cryptically.

"I don't know who you are right now, though, so that's hard for me to decipher."

"I know. I keep doing personality profiles, isn't it, or multiple personalities or something like that?"

She sat back on my bed and lifted her foot, which had Cookie's collar latched around the ankle.

"Snake pit or something like that?"

"Borderline schizophrenia? Which you were diagnosed with when I was twenty?"

"Yeah. Actually, I was diagnosed with that by fifteen, when Susan told Mom I was bipolar. She said, 'Send her up to my bed, and I'll let her rock in Seattle for a while.'"

"Uh-huh," I sighed. "Are you ready to get help yet?"

"Yeah."

"You're ready to go to a hospital?"

"You bet."

"You're ready to go to a hospital tonight."

"Yes, ma'am."

"Why are you so ready?"

"Because you're telling me I need to be evaluated," she said like it was the most obvious thing in the world.

"No, I'm telling you you need to stay in a hospital."

"Can I stay there on the couch?" she asked, pointing to her spot.

"No," I said, wanting my room to myself.

"Why?"

"Because you have a life to live?"

"I try every day. Do you? I don't see it happening."

"I'm going to work every day..."

"You come home after a hard day's work, and I've got requests for dinner and...cereal... My God, you have been working hard today, haven't you?"

"Oh, we're done."

I cut the camera off.

Her gears shifted again. She was back in my face, her chin resting angelically on her hands.

"Tell the joke," I told her sullenly.

"Was it funny?"

"I didn't hear anything," I said (because she hadn't said anything yet).

"I know you didn't."

"K. Then can you get out of my personal space?"

"It was a pretty funny story. But once again, even though I told you the story, you don't hear it. You wanna watch Neil Sparkle ask me at the play that Katherine is inviting me to. Do you think he might ask her to dance? I think he would."

She reared back, getting excited.

"I mean, it's a possibility, isn't it? She chased him all across America. What do you think? Will you go with us to the play? I think he might ask her. I really do. I mean, she's told us so many stories about him. Wouldn't that be cool? Wouldn't that be cool?"

It was so strange to hear her say "she" when she was talking about herself. I think that was the first time I ever truly understood the schizophrenia part.

She assaulted me again, off camera this time, but I remember I screamed that time. I called the cops again; my mother was ready and patient. She was being so kind to me as she prepared to go to the hospital, and as I watched the videos to write this, I thought she must be so relieved in some ways but also so scared and disgusted and angry.

August 26, 2022

The pups are with me in bed and I'm feeding them breakfast; I'm having blueberry pie with whipped cream. [I posted footage of the dogs and their rough week, asking for people to show us love and spread some joy.]

August 29, 2022

Comparison photos from CSE challenge, I was anxious about the angles and sure 8.8 pounds didn't look like much.

August 30, 2022

> [I posted a meme from Mike Mitchell.] "If you want to know how the week is going, I just took a pillowcase out of the dryer, put it over my head thinking it was a t-shirt to wear to bed, spent 15 seconds inside it searching for the neck hole, and then mumbled 'what is this, pants.'"

> [I posted a meme from lil spinach freak.] "Yes toxic relationships are hard, but do you know what else is hard? Your first healthy relationship after a toxic one. No one talks about how hard it is to unlearn all the toxic behaviors you adapted as coping mechanisms. How hard it is to convince yourself that you're safe now."

I'm sorry, dear Papa Bear.

August 31, 2022

> "I'm not really sure what's going on here, but I kind of dig it, I just listened to That Guy With Hair's Official Video and now it's stuck in my head! And my mashed potato brain is going to get all fried... into french fries!" I smiled and froze, squinting my eyes. "Yeah that's about as creative as I can get."
>
> It's been a month, y'all. Like. But tomorrow is a new one. I'm thinking of giving myself a break from the scale for a few weeks, just as a test. I'm not one to get hung up on the number until I'm in a contest where I need to be at 232 by December. Seven pounds never took so long.
>
> My mood, my living situation, and my job have been such a whirlwind this month, I've sort of quit thinking about the food part. Which is both a huge accomplishment and a huge problem lol. Being mind-less about my eating is what has always gotten me in trouble. So for September, I'm committing to daily posts again. Perhaps minus the scale.
>
> I'm kind of in an odd state of mind right now. My chemicals are all in line, we crushed our goals in my new center (first month as manager offi-

cially!!), and I'm losing weight fairly regularly. But my mom isn't home and healthy, and that puts a kind of stress on me I never imagined feeling again.

September 1, 2022

I posted a video on TikTok: "Who is your Disney twin?" I pushed the button and spoke. "Okay, I'm going to do this month's"—I giggled as the filter started—"challenge a little different this week. Oh, what the hell. That is not appropriate," I complained when the spinner stopped on Beast. I held a piece of paper up backward in the camera. "Thirty-day book challenge. Y'all, I need help, 'cause I am not reading enough. I need you guys to tell me the best book you read last year, something that you think I should read as soon as possible. Help me!" I trilled on a smile.

September 2, 2022

I added a sticker to the top of the screen that shouted "Attention, please!" and put my hand over my face. "So this one's fun." I giggled, then dropped my hand, pouting my lips dramatically when the filter appeared. I batted my newly huge, newly lashed eyes and simpered, "Do I look like a Disney character?" Bat, bat, bat, bat. "Anyway, today's book challenge is a book that you've read three times or more." I tilted my head, admiring my face from every angle. "That one's easy for me 'cause I love to repeat things."

September 3, 2022

I posted a meme: "Someone once asked me, 'Why do you love music so much?' I replied, 'Because it's the only thing that stays when everything and everyone is gone.'"

September 4, 2022

Ruby sat in my lap early in the morning, looking sick or scared; I was pouting at the camera. Then I subjected her to Snaps. I then found a TikTok filter that morphed my face into someone else's. I used Kelly Clarkson's gorgeous mug and wrote, "My darling doppelgänger. This worked pretty well!"

In another one, Ruby stared adoringly at me. The captions scrolled across her face: "She's finally caught on that I'm the one doing dinner this week. She's been staring at me for about half an hour." Then I asked her if I could help her with something, and her ears perked up.

Later that evening, we watched Grey's Anatomy, and I filmed the scene when Derek got shot. "Bingeworthy" was written in script across the screen, along with, "This scene will never fail to make me cry. Follow me if you love TV characters like they're family."

September 6, 2022

I colored a mandala. Ruby and Cookie snoozed, attached to whatever part of me they could touch. My little caretakers, pressed firmly against me. Follow me if you don't know what it means to care for yourself. #mentalhealthawareness #endthestigma

September 8, 2022

[I retweeted a meme from @KeanuReeves.] "If you have been broken, but still have the courage to be gentle to other loving beings, then you're a badass with the heart of an angel."

September 9, 2022

A Jenny client brought her standard dachshunds in to see me. They were huge and sausagey and exactly what my heart needed.

I posted a meme: "Reminder: You can start over at anytime. Your day is not ruined. Your world is not over. You do not have to be the same person you were five minutes ago. Take a deep breath and start over again."

September 10, 2022

I posted an Awkward Yeti cartoon:
BRAIN: Want to pick a new book to read?
HEART: Yes yes yes!
BRAIN: Okay. Here's a mountain of new books we bought but never read.
HEART: Those aren't NEW new! Those are OLD new!
BRAIN: They are new to us!
HEART: I can't hear you over the sound of us buying more books!

September 13, 2022

I made a time-lapse of practicing my blending, shading, and handwriting on the word hopeful.

September 14, 2022

[I started to film, my eyebrows raised, eyes wide.]
"Okay, so I'm trying to convey what..."
I blinked, as if trying to create tears.
"I don't think I'm going to be able to do it and show at the same time!"
Linnea, in the background, said, "How are they gonna see it?"
"Well, I'm trying to get some information for my mom. So if I'm looking straight ahead at whatever this is"—I used my right hand to gesture—"the shapes are over here," I said, moving my hand to the left as if I could touch something.
My voice got louder, sounding slightly panicky.
"So I can see myself just fine [in the camera]."
Linnea interjected again, this time closer.
"Okay..."

"But if I put... I'm recording. I'm sorry. Hold on. I mean, you can talk. I don't care. But...come here for a second! Put your hand right here for me."

I pointed at my own left arm, which was holding the phone. Her hand appeared, and I continued.

"Nope, I can see it. Put it right here," I instructed, tapping a little farther down my arm.

She did, and I said, "Nope, I can see you just fine. Weird! I can still see the flutter, but I can see you just fine."

I opened my eyes wider as if something occurred to me, made an annoyed noise, cocked my head, and shut off the camera. The next moment, I was sat in front of my computer, looking at the screen with the phone propped to my left.

"Okay, so it's...if I'm looking at my computer, it's right here," I said, using my right hand to grab something out of my field of vision, "like I can grab it out of the air..."

I used my left hand to move into my field of vision and gestured with my right hand.

"Yep, see, I can't see my fingers right here."

I stared.

"It's a squiggle."

I moved my right hand over the top of it as if to try to break it up. I blinked, fully annoyed.

"That is utterly bizarre. All right," I said, blinking hard and turning toward the camera. "I think we've had enough computer work for the day."

September 15, 2022

It's been one helluva few months. I've slacked on the food posts because I've been concentrating on swimming. But I'm getting better every day that my mother gets better, and I am here for you. Ask me anything. Tell me anything. Unless you're planning harm, I'm a vault.

September 16, 2022

I used a filter that made my eyes big and round and my nose long and swingy like an eggplant. As I tossed my head and grinned, I sang, "I'd put myself first...and make the rules as I go!"

September 17, 2022

I posted a video using one of my favorite filters, the purple fairy. "I would just like to say, don't be surprised if you see six hundred videos of me wearing this, because if I can't figure out how to be this for Halloween?" I paused and examined myself gleefully, then added, "I need to be this for Halloween." Sure enough, later, I did "My Song" with the purple fairy on, then a quick clip eating a ham and Swiss baguette, then later a longer clip eating an egg salad sandwich.

I took several clips of the dogs whining for dinner. In the final one, I asked Cookie if she was ready for dinner, and she actually nodded.

September 19, 2022

I posted a meme: "I was going to start dieting, but Halloween is here, then Thanksgiving and Christmas candy. Before you know it, it's BBQ season again and I'm not about to turn down a cheeseburger."

September 24, 2022

"So I just had a really interesting lesson in patience, which I of course get tested in every day!" I started cheerfully, squinting in the afternoon sun. "Um, a forty-five-mile drive home, you guys know the drill. Getting gas every four days right now? And there's a gas station right next to my Jenny that I love and is cheap, and there were a bunch of fire trucks blocking it off today. Instead of waiting to see if I could wait or get around or anything like that, I went in the opposite direction even though it was literally walking distance from me, and my car was very low already.

"So I went on to the highway. It told me it was about two miles, got there. Of course it was closed down. Went to another one, two miles again, and finally, thank God, it was $2.99, as y'all can see from this beautiful video. And I learned a lesson in patience because"—I flicked my fingers and started rustling some papers—"uh, don't remember."

I cut off the camera, then picked it back up when I remembered.

"Sometimes, it pays off. Literally. It pays to be patient, y'all. Every time."

Later that evening, I treated myself to a journey down baby memory lane, making screen recordings of the live versions of my photos, earning hidden giggles from Anderson, amused awe from Brayden, and much more.

September 26, 2022

I posted a video in the car: "So I just went to pick up Advil from"—I looked over my shoulder as if to see the store—"wherever I just was. Um, my whole body hurts today."

I adjusted my sunglasses, uncomfortable.

"It's not an easy day. Standing hurts. Sitting hurts. The only thing that doesn't hurt is lying down. So I treated myself to this fun little gum."

I held up a canister of Trident Vibes Sour Patch Kids.

"Trident Vibes."

I giggled and removed my sunglasses.

"I thought it would be fun to see if it was sour."

I made a face, opening the gum.

"Now to be fair, I did just drink my water, which has a little kick to it, which was sour."

I caught myself in camera and tilted my head.

"What do y'all think of this…crazy hair?"

I held up a piece of the square blue gum, popped it in my mouth, and started to chew. Almost immediately, my face contracted, and I knitted my eyebrows together.

"Yep," I said between smacks. "That's sour."

I continued chewing, clearly struggling.

"Oh my God," I managed, trying not to swallow the gum. "Okay, Sour Patch Kids were never that sour. Were they?"

I rubbed my forehead, looking slightly amused.

"Adult version" chew-chew, "of giving your kids" chew-chew, "Warheads for the first time," I finally said in a rush, my hand coming up to my chin to catch the spit.

Next stop on the sugar train was Chick-fil-A.

"Okay, I don't do Chick-fil-A very often anymore, but they've been advertising this autumn spice milkshake, and it's freaking phenomenal and worth most of the calories. I don't know about every calorie, but most of the calories."

September 27, 2022

[I posted a TikTok duet with a man: "Five things you didn't realize you are doing with high-functioning anxiety: (1) You have a good, kind heart, but you people-please too much. (2) Any mistake you make, you beat yourself up for it. (3) You obsess over some of the smallest things that most people don't even notice. (4) In every situation, you obsess over picking out the worst-case scenario. (5) You know how capable you are, but you don't believe in yourself."] This guy knows. Believe in yourself. No matter what. You got this.

September 28, 2022

Walking outside in the sunshine after work, you could hear the excitement in my voice.

"It is a beautiful day...autumn. For all intents and purposes, I live in a place that has autumn!"

I unlocked my car and slung my huge purse inside.

"New England livin', baby. Anyway, I'm in a really good mood, and I just wanted to spread the love and say I hope today is fantastic for all of y'all too. Love you, guys."

And I signed off with a blown kiss.

A few minutes later, in my purple fairy costume, I said, "I just wanted to say hi and that I love you. In my purple fairy costume. Waiting at the red light. I'm here if you need to talk. Love you."

And another blown kiss.

Moments later, in the same purple fairy, I blared some music, then turned the volume down and said, "Thought y'all would enjoy that. Y'all, guess what I just had to do! Put the heater on. In my car. With the windows open. In fall. In Connecticut. Because I don't live in Texas anymore."

September 29, 2022

I posted a meme: "It's okay if you thought you were over it, but it hits you all over again. It's okay to fall apart even after you thought you had it under control. You are not weak. Healing is messy. There is no timeline for healing."

Later, in the silly purple fairy, I said, "So part of the craziness that is involved with my body that we are trying to figure out has to do with...what I think are probably blood sugar issues? Um, depending on eating."

I shrugged and sniffled, sounding completely stuffed up.

"I mean, y'all, how fun is this stinkin filter?"

I giggled and sniffed again, then continued.

"Um, I was super hungry and decided to get my favorite Jenny Craig snack, which is our new popcorn."

I held up the open package as proof.

"Delicious and yummy. And does not take fairy wings very well," I said and put it back down. "Um, and about halfway through it," I hemmed and hawed, growing weirdly awkward, "that weird sensation came that you are either going to"—I lowered my voice and gestured—"throw up or sneeze? And I wasn't sure which. And thankfully it was just a sneeze and not anything extra but definitely lost my appetite, so don't know what that was!"

When I got home from work, I had an odd feeling that I should stay in my car. I obeyed the feeling for the rest of the song but then got out. Standing on the other side of my car was a wolf of a Siberian husky looking at me warily. I knew she lived in one of the houses. I just couldn't remember which. I called Mom outside, who must have been angry with me, because I remember being nervous to call for her. The dog approached her but would let neither of us catch her.

Eventually, Mom was able to read her collar, and I called the phone number. The owner was at work but was so happy to hear we knew where her dog was. She got her mother out there, and we ended up chasing the dog down the street, along with another neighbor of ours. If you've never chased a husky, I don't recommend you try. I knew it was fruitless, but my heart was so desperate to help someone.

September 30, 2022

"Y'all, check it out," I instructed, a gray fleece scarf draped around my neck but nothing else other than my three-fourth-length sleeved shirt, sending a puff of breath into the air. "Aww!" Another puff. "You can see it!" One more puff, as if I had never seen my breath before. "It's cold."

October 1, 2022

Sitting on the couch with Mom, listening to "Rise Up" by Andra Day. I scratched Ruby and she chomped at me, then I sang along a little, scratching her some more, trying to invoke another chomp. Mom participated in her scratching, trying to get some kind of a response, then called her a lazy butt. "You really are," I added, disappointed. She flipped to her back, adorably, and I scratched her chest once more, earning a good snap. "There ya go, that was a good one!" I praised her, giving her one more rub, then she grabbed onto my hand with mouth and paws.

NOT THE F——ING GILMORE GIRLS

October 4, 2022

I posted a meme of a rainbow galaxy, over which was written, "My favorite conspiracy theory is that everything is gonna be okay."

October 5, 2022

I made a video as I lay in bed. "So I went to the doctor for a C-spine X-ray. If there is something seriously wrong with my neck and it's taken us this long to figure it out? Interesting. So now I'm at home, lying down and watching The Halloween Bake-Off. Yay for sick days. I also think I might have lip gloss ring from my mask."
I nodded and brought the camera closer to examine.
"Pretty sure."

October 13, 2022

I posted a meme of a sunset that said, "Have a panic attack. You've earned it."

October 14–20, 2022

I posted mostly Ruby and Cookie videos while we got the house packed up.

October 21, 2022

I posted a whole slew of Awkward Yeti cartoons, each more accurate than the last:
YETI: I'm so tired. (He turns to address Brain.) Please stop thinking about every possible future scenario in our life.
BRAIN: Don't be ridiculous. I haven't thought of every possible scenario. But don't worry. I won't rest until I do!

October 23, 2022

I posted birthday Snaps, including one that said, "Prediction for me: find a soulmate."

October 26, 2022

Sitting in my car, I made a TikTok: "This is gonna be a whole story. Come follow me if you don't know what it's like to take care of yourself.

"So I'm outside Walgreens, waiting for my vaccine or booster, whatever you want to call it these days. The sun's right in my eyes, but I don't want to put my sunglasses on because..." I sat up straighter. "There, that's better! Now y'all can see my glitter."

I paused, pursing my lips and cocking my head.

"Um," I said again, and you can hear the raspiness, "I've been pretty sick for a long time, and it's getting glaringly more apparent every day that goes by how sick and for how long. Getting some answers, getting some...help? And yet I'm sitting here thinking, man, do I even know how to feel good? And that's the part of this that made me think, 'I'm gonna jump on TikTok,' because...we all deserve to feel good. All the time. That's not that true. Not all of us. Most of us."

October 28, 2022

Sitting in my mother's computer chair, Ruby is in my lap. I scratched her and whispered, "This is what happens." Ruby kissed me a few times and jumped down. Later that night, the dogs watched Mom closely as she took bites of her hot dog.

October 31, 2022

Halloween Filter concert: "Rocketman," "Rhiannon," "Fortunate Son," "Open Arms," "End of the Innocence," "Sister Golden Hair," "Fat-Bottom Girls," "We've Got Tonight," "Crazy," "Pink," "All-American Girl," "Desiree," "Dreaming of You," "Bye Bye," "My Song," "Kind of a Drag," "Dancing Queen," and "It's Over," by Roy Orbison. Which, if you haven't seen "Black and White Night," a tribute to him, I highly. HIGHLY. Suggest remedying that immediately.

November 1, 2022

    I posted more karaoke Snaps. Man, music is healing. "My Church," by Maren Morris.

November 6, 2022

    All moved into the new two-bedroom, Ruby wearing her thunder shirt, I asked her what she thought of the place. She looked at me as Mom asked, "Do you know where the hangers are?"

November 9, 2022

    I made a TikTok of my hands, which had visible sores from either scratching or twisting them. Lyrics played as my hands danced. "But all my friends they don't know / what it's like, what it's like / they don't understand why / I can't sleep through the night. I've been told I could take something to fix it / damn it, I wish it was that simple."

November 10, 2022

    I held my left hand up and brought it back down, smiling.
    "Hi," I said, remembering to greet everyone before proceeding and putting my hand back up.
    With my right hand, I touched the spot I thought it would be and said, "I'm not sure you're going to be able to see it. So there's a lump right here. That's like..."
    I pulled my finger back.
    "It feels like..."
    I moved my pointer one more time, and the lump protruded.
    "Eh, there it is. You see it? Eh...eh...eh."
    I fake gagged.
    "It's like the size of a pea. Any ideas? 'Cause it is not on this side," I explained, pointing to my other hand. "And it freaks me out, and it hurts a little bit when I push."

November 14, 2022

Lots of delicious-looking food with "Billie Eilish" playing as the song. It said, "We are back in full swing. Next goal, 15 pounds off by Christmas. Who's with me??"

I colored in my Stoner Princess coloring book, still trying to find peace even after a week of being in the two-bedroom.

November 15, 2022

"Follow me if this makes you smile," captioned the video of my day, "Pure Imagination" playing as I spoke. "Hello. It is finally cold and beautiful. Look at that blue sky. New England. Cold. Got my stars shirt on, my glitter lips on, and"—I pause to pull my shirt up and show my belt—"my rainbow belt. It's a good day."

Cut to the inside of a store.

"So we came to this really awesome Dollar General while we're doing laundry at a Laundromat! And...look what I found!"

I held up my booty, excited.

"An Axe-smelling air freshener. Oh my God, and Dreamworld-flavored Coke."

I nodded sagely.

"Can't wait to taste my dreams."

Cut to back inside my car, where I opened the Coke.

"Okay, here we go. Dreamworld-flavored."

I took a swig. I didn't look pleased, and I nodded.

"It's about what my dreams have tasted like in the past."

November 15, 2022

"It's snowing. It's snowing. It's snowing, snowing, snowing," I sang outside in a video, watching the snow fall.

November 20, 2022

> I made a TikTok of Snaps and dogs. It was an anxious kind of day, but I overcame by making myself laugh. How do you cope with stress?

November 21, 2022

> Grr 3 AM wake up comes even without blue-light before bed. Okay: insomnia 4,899,071, Courtney, 3.
> KATIE V: Ayyye! I'm up too! Everyone's still asleep but I'm up for whatever reason.
> I reposted Brandon B: "You are not the darkness you endured. You are the light that refused to surrender." The more people I get to know via this social media blackhole, the better. I met Brandon when he photographed my choir a few years ago. Never spoke a single word to him and yet I knew he'd be important in my life. Y'all. Reach out. You are not alone. Don't let that light flicker out.

To add even more color to my life, Brandon became a published author, which was my dream. It has been so fun to watch his journey. Look up *The Wonderland Saga* by Brandon T Bernard! He's awesome.

November 22, 2022, 4:44 PM

> I made a TikTok of the dogs being silly for dinner. At Angel time again!!! God, they're precious.

November 23, 2022

> It's the 3 AM witching hour, but today I'm starving. Not fun.
> I posted a picture of the game Perfection. I mean...fuck:
> The older gens that are like, "You can't *all* have anxiety and depression," are the same ones that gave us a game called Perfection in which, if you weren't perfect in a limited amount of time, the board literally blew up in your face."

November 24, 2022

Yes, it's the 3 AM Witching Hour. I'm drinking a Fresca. (Unrelated.)

Over at Katherine's with the dogs for Thanksgiving; Ruby is enthralled by Blossom, who doesn't even budge when Ruby sticks her face in her bed. I wore my FRIENDS Thanksgiving shirt and sat in the living room and played with filters.

November 27, 2022

I went live on FB: So we're trying something new. Facebook recommended it so let's see how that works. But apparently I am eligible for monetization if things get followed. So yay! Uh this is picking up. We're going to eventually do some kind of live question and answer kind of thing when I get the base for it. But, Hi Kathy, that's not happening yet. The more the word spreads, the more I can get that out there.

If you like what I have to say, if you think I'm cute, if you think I'm funny, anything like that, share, spread the word, um, legitimately just want to help as many people as I can. And in my little hamlet in Connecticut, it's quiet. So social media, here I come. Um, yeah. It's Sunday, I'm not usually at work on Sunday, so that'll probably be my live hour, but Tuesday might work too? I'm gonna keep talking until I don't even know when because I want to get this out there.

So bottom line, I'm a weight loss coach, I work for Jenny Craig, but I know a lot about a lot. And I'd love to help you get to your goals. Follow me, share me, I'll run some specials once that gets rolling. Give me a call, send me a message, I'm here. Talk to y'all soon. Bye.

I'm intrigued by this "professional" mode on Facebook. Share me please!!

I updated my cover photo to comparison shots of weight loss.

HEATHER H: Way to go!!

CAROLE K: *[She commented a GIF that says "Well done."]*
TENESHA I: *Yes Girl!!*
JEN I: *Holy moly!!! Outstanding*
KENDRA R: *You look amazing! You can see all the inflammation gone from your face and just overall you look like you feel so much better.*
KAYLA M: *Amazing!! Congrats, my friend!!*

[I posted a video reel of food.] Today's Noom lesson...is what made me want to start this "niche" on my feed. I will not be posting these often. Please message me for a link!!

November 28, 2022

I mean, this isn't getting annoying at all. Fuck. *(Is it a self-fulfilling prophecy now??)*

I went live on FB, talking about coffee, fasting, and weight loss. You guys, come do this with me!! My friend Kayla, another health and wellness coach, is leading a fun step challenge!! Hashtag-city!!

I posted food videos. It was an "extra chocolate sauce" kind of night. Ask me for the secret. Come follow me if you love food and want to lose weight. Come follow me if you need a laugh. Come follow me if you need support. I'm here to listen.

November 28, 2022

I posted a meme: "I dream of never being called resilient again in my life. I'm exhausted by strength. I want support. I want softness. I want ease. I want to be amongst kin. Not patted on the back for how well I take a hit. Or how many."

"All right, so these one slash two slash three alarm...fires?"

I snorted a laugh. "I don't know what was about to come out of my mouth. Wake-up calls are getting really old."

I paused to contemplate. "I think we're into the second week now? Of every night? So I'm kind of a zombie. I feel like I have cotton balls"—I gestured toward my forehead, also struggling to breathe, as I was walking around the center—"in here in my head. It's very strange. So in the three o'clock slump hour"—I hissed air in—"I eat breakfast really late a lot, so I didn't eat till, like, 1, 1:30, something like that? Not on purpose. I was pretty hungry by then."

I shrugged.

"So now I'm running around here, trying to get my blood pumpin' as fast and as furious as I can with an injured foot."

Huge sigh.

"Trying to get my energy up, talking to you good people."

November 29, 2022

Bro. It was 12:30 the last time I looked. (Slept early today!!) This is getting silly.

I made a TikTok duet with a guy using "Made You Look" for a transition video. At the top, I wrote, "4:30. This is after 12:30. 1:30. 2:37. And 3:30. W. T. A. F." And then a moment later, I wrote, "This insomniac has had a rough two weeks."

So I've been drooling over the Meghan Trainor TikToks since the wee hours. I'm doing it.

I went live on Facebook for ten minutes to practice the "Made You Look" dance.

November 30, 2022

Live on Facebook for 1:22 to talk about food, #allthehashtags. Follow me if you need a friend, follow me if you need a hug, follow me if you love to laugh, follow me if you love food but want to lose weight, follow me if you're bored. Share the love. I'm here for you.

"I did this without a filter and then I got on here and there was this one."

Beautiful. It looked like I was standing in the falling snow.

"So I had to do it. Um, so I just finished lunch, which is my mac and cheese at Jenny Craig, which is phenomenal. And it has broccoli and carrots, and I was so full after the noodle portion that I only ate two bites of broccoli, which is not something I want y'all to practice, 'cause you need those calories."

I shook my finger at the camera. "But I also want you to listen to your body. And what I did today, at 2:30 in the afternoon, 'cause dinner is gonna be in a couple of hours, is listen to my body. And my client this morning told me that... at... Oh my gosh...Alcoholics Anonymous, Narcotics Anonymous," I said under my breath. "Overeaters Anonymous! She used to learn that they say one (I'm not going to be able to do it!), one is too much."

I paused, thought briefly, and grinned.

"One is too much. The whole box is not enough."

I giggled and repeated it one more time without stumbling.

"One is too much. The whole box is not enough. So let's take Little Debbies. If you bit into one of those Christmas tree cakes that are just so..." I squinted my eyes, raised my fist, and thought hard, continuing, "Calling your name, 'cause gosh knows they're calling mine."

"Take one bite. Take the time to think about if it was good enough. Take the time to think if you really want more. You'll figure it out!"

December 1, 2022

I tagged Nikki C.: I had a client tell me she was a "big fan" (of mine) today, and I'm still glowing. Spread the love, y'all. Please.

NIKKI: You spread sunshine wherever you go, Courtney!!!! Thank you for being you!

"Hi, y'all! I'm sitting here sending my emails, listening to my music, and it's a Christmas song from Glee that I love, and of course my body had to move! So I started twistin' 'cause I'm doing my emails! So I thought, this is a great idea for y'all who can't necessarily get up a lot, whether it's feet problems, which I have, or a sitting desk job, which I have, or...any other thing! You can still move. You can still get your heartbeat up"—I accentuated those points with my right index finger—"any way you want.

"Oh, my Lord, my nails need to be done! So that being said, all I'm doing, let's see if I can do this"—I propped the phone up and backed away from the desk to show my full body—"is sitting in my chair, in my candy cane knees, and twistin'...to the beat. Now I told y'all in the last video, always keep your"—I pointed to my belly button—"what is this called? Belly button."

I exhaled a laugh in disbelief, annoyed that I had blanked on the word.

"Pulled into your spine. And it'll engage your core."

I resumed twisting.

"Get that heart rate up any way you can. Y'all can do this."

December 2, 2022

I told myself a loooong time ago that I'd get up and move every time I heard this song (with a video of me dancing to "Cupid Shuffle"). I made a video of me kissing Cookie, who then escaped me. My huggabug. Done when she's done.

Who has funny Santa-kid pictures I can use for TikTok?? (Looking at you, toddler-moms!)
ERIN G: Poor EL looking traumatized in two years' pics.
ANGELA W: Not a toddler anymore but still funny. He still wants nothing to do with Santa lol.
ME: yup these are the ones I'm looking for!!!!! Most priceless if I was present for the actual viewing.
ANGELA: Santa's face is the best lol.
ELENA T: Cutie pic.
ME: Omg her sweet face!!!!
CHRISTY V: My poor babies, but it sure is an adorable picture!

I updated my cover photo to Mya and Brayden playing in the leaves, Santa behind them, the word joy written above them.

KENDRALYN R: *Her hair OMG*

ME: *My sweet little troll doll is turning into a true rock star!!*

KENDRALYN: *I love it! I've always loved her hair color and knew it would be beautiful.*

December 7, 2022

I posted a word search where the first four words you saw were your mantra for 2023. I saw power, alignment, self-care, and love. (I'm choosing to hear "power" as superpower, not anything negative!!). What does your 2023 look like, my friends?

"Trending on TikTok? Yes please!! #allthedoghashtags" Ruby and Cookie to Taylor Swift's "Anti-Hero."

December 8, 2022

My babe and snuggle bug [with a cartoon that said "Love is…that extra bit of blanket in the middle of night" and a woman putting a blanket over her dog].

December 11, 2022

"So I'm sitting here watching Holiday Baking Championship, trying to figure out these filters. Ooh, there it goes."

My face began to burn away.

"And wondering if I were to decorate my room with Christmas lights, which I want to do, because that's how my aunt has her dining room, and it's beautiful, if…"

My face reappeared.

"Hi! That would mean they wouldn't be as special to me during the Christmas season. This filter is weird. Hi."

I started to disappear again, giggling.

"And there I go again. My question is, for people who love decorations, does it take away the specialty when you leave them up all year? Or does it just make it that much more fun to walk into your bedroom slash house slash wherever? Every day!"

December 13, 2022

"So I'm awake at five whatever-it-is, which isn't all that abnormal. The really abnormal part is how good I've been with my eating and my exercise for…a month? Trying to get ten pounds down by the end of this challenge? And…stress? Because the scale is not budging the way I need it to. It's going like this. Deet, deet, deet, deet."

I angled my hand and directed it upward.

"Despite being next to perfect. Like, this has been a freaking awesome couple of weeks with food. I'm beyond frustrated, and I know what I would tell my clients, and it's not doing me any good! So I'm taking to social media. Yep. It's gonna be a rough…seven days."

December 16, 2022

I posted a video of me dancing alone in my room to "Catching My Breath" by Kelly Clarkson. I stripped to bra and shorts and switched to trying to do the dance for "Made You Look." My idea must have been for a transition video, but I never got there.

December 18, 2022

Ah, the fateful night Mom scarred Cookie for life. I can't come near the poor pup with clippers or scissors before she's turning tail. Mom, in a fit of manic excitement, cut Cookie's toenail clear off, and I couldn't stop it bleeding. Cookie was shaking and chattering, and I thought I was going to have to take her to the ER, but I bandaged her and held her foot as tightly as we could. She lay on me like a baby, as pitiful as could be.

When I had made sure she was okay, I retreated to my bedroom, freaked out beyond belief, and changed into a pretty blue teddy. I put my sparkling fairy lights on and added a wintry filter, then said, "So I have this really cute couple of lingerie thingies that I've been saving for either a boudoir shoot or saving for somebody special." I wrinkle my face uncomfortably. "And then I realized tonight that I already have somebody special. Me. I don't know what I've been saving them for or what I've been waiting for, but I'm good enough to use the stuff that I save for somebody good to see. I'm good enough."

December 19, 2022

A filter started spinning that said, "In 2023, I will..." It landed on "Meet the one." "Hmm," I said, "interesting, sitting here getting all nostalgic in my brand-new bedroom, watching my baking shows, thinking, 'Hmm, wouldn't it be nice having someone to share this with?' Maybe by next year! Next Christmas, I mean, 'cause that says 2023. Yay!"

Welp. I'm real hungry. 17 hours left in a 26-hour fast. Think I can do it?

KATHERINE H: Yes. Go to bed.
PETE P: Of course. You got this!
KATIE V: You've got it if you want it but also maybe a snack if you're hungry!
CRISTA L: You can do it!
KENDRA R: All the water.
SHERI B: Yep!
GARY G: You can do it!
ME: 4 more hours

December 20, 2022

I used a filter of a comforter and sleep mask, making it appear as if I was snuggled in bed. "This is literally my day today. I'm so sleepy, and I don't know why. But here I am, watching my movies on my day off."

December 21, 2022

I duetted Alicia Keys on "Santa Baby" on TikTok.

I used a filter that said, "More of this in 2023." "So here's a fun one," I said and started it spinning. It stopped on "More inappropriate yodeling." I giggled and complied.

Later, I saved a meme, probably crying while I read it: "One day someone will walk into your life and get it right where everyone else got it wrong. One day you won't have to wait for a call or a text back. One day you won't be the only one giving it your all. One day you'll finally meet someone who wants to help you grow in life. One day you'll finally meet someone who isn't afraid to give 'love' another chance. One day you'll finally meet someone you can trust with everything. One day you'll finally meet someone you can trust with everything. One day you'll have your best friend, your biggest supporter and your teammate all wrapped up into one person."

December 22, 2022

The filter said, "Why am I still single?" The sound said, "I'm up for adoption. Does anyone want to come home to this?" I looked confused when the filter stopped on "A disappointing birthday party," as if I had forgotten what the original question was.

In the next one, it was a karmic sound, and the screen listed ten zodiac signs, Scorpio included, and said, "On December 24, 2022, there will be a massive change in your life, a one-time offer, and your deepest wish will come true. Don't skip this sound. Save it. Use it. Karma is real and exists."

December 23, 2022

Some crazy rash popped up on my legs. At work in my elf gear, I did "Delight" for karaoke. After work, we went to INSA. (Another sign Mom was manic: she was willing to put five hundred dollars of pot on her credit cards I had been working really hard to pay off.) I tried caramel apple crumble cannabis-infused ice cream.

Late in the evening, I sat in my car, tears shining in my eyes as text scrolled, "Sitting in the car listening to the song 'Rainbow' by Kasey Musgraves, which I've always loved, when a text from a literal angel comes through, and I'm reminded once again how amazing God is. And thankful. Merry Christmas to one and all."

December 24, 2022

I tried to make some more Meghan Trainor content as I was getting dressed for Christmas Eve at Katherine and Fritz's. I looked beautiful in a gold dress (I took a TikTok that said I felt like a filter of myself!), and there's even a slew of pictures of me and Mom smiling together. But I feel, for some reason, that we drove separately that night.

My final video of the evening, I'm glowing as I said, "It was a good night. And now I'm in the holiday portal." Ornaments and snowflakes fell as I tilted the phone. "Cute. Merry Christmas, everybody. Tomorrow, I am home. No plans. Kinda chillin'. My mom is making cinnamon rolls. It's gonna be a pajamas and karaoke and Hallmark movies kinda day. Everybody have an awesome Christmas if that's what you celebrate."

December 25, 2022

It's Christmas morning and I'm sitting by our tree with the dogs. Pretty much a normal morning occurrence and yet it's so much more fun bc it's Christmas. It's a beautiful time to be kind, no matter what you believe. Thanks to some wonderful aunts, we even had presents to open.

Later, I watched Elf for the first time. "The best way to spread Christmas cheer is singing loud for all to hear."

At 12:45, looking at my mother's closed bedroom door, I whispered, "I just cried through Elf because it resonated so deeply." I was so stuffed up from crying, it was hard to talk.

"I'm watching it by myself because my mom's in her bedroom. Soooo I just want you guys to learn to be the partner...that your partner needs you to be. Whether that's a friend, a lover, a mother, a father, whoever your partner, your ride-or-die is. Learn how to love them, learn how you can support them... if they're supporting you? Learn how you can support them. Merry Christmas."

To lift my heart, I put on Willy Wonka and the Chocolate Factory and made TikToks singing to the music. By 5:00 PM, I was in my bed, watching Gilmore Girls.

My mom just called me arrogant for believing she might learn something in therapy. How's your Christmas going?

Lu B: I literally went through this with my mom. Finally got her to go!!! Good luck!

December 26, 2022

At 3:31 am (so close to that angel number!), I made a video. Ruby settling into her new rose blankety, a present from our wonderful aunt. Ruby loves soft, comforting things, a habit she learned (was forced upon her?) from me, who can't be without comfort items. My mom says I've "humanized" her. I will never be sorry for that. She is my baby.

I hope everybody had a good Christmas. Um, mine was not great but I was thoroughly blessed and I would like to pay it forward a little bit! This has been a dream of mine for as long as I've been on social media, to somehow eventually be able to do this one day, including tipping my waiters! If I can get to 500 followers by Friday, I think that's New Year's Eve, no Saturday is New Year's Eve, um I will do a giveaway and if you want to be a part of it, share, like, and comment what you would like to see the prize be. It's gonna be self-care of some sort; food or massage or something like that. Comment what you want; we'll do the drawing on Saturday.

In the later hours, I did a karaoke video for "Commitment" by LeAnn Rimes, which I'd only just learned, followed by "Human Touch" by the Boss.

December 28, 2022

I was planning on doing an every day drawing challenge and hoping to get my niece to do it with me. I knew by involving her, I would be more likely to stick to it myself.

Later, I put on a Harley Quinn filter and asked, "I'm curious if there's anybody who's had COVID and is now, almost three years later, experiencing things going wrong with their body they've never had before, like bad nausea. This girl has thrown up, like, four times in her whole life. Not digging the new trend and curious if anybody's definitely, for sure gotten 'Oh, that's COVID' because my body ain't the same anymore, I'll tell you what. It's not fun."

Later, I texted Mom the video of the every day drawing challenge.

MOM: *That looks like fun! Really! What a great idea. Was this yours or Grace's idea? I don't suppose I could join?*

Since that was precisely my hope, I said, "Of course you can. I'd love that. My idea. I've been carrying these around for months, waiting for January. I'm gonna make TikTok videos daily [for when we all complete it anyway!], so I'll do short, sped-up clips of hands drawing and then pics of the finished sketch. She's excited, Audrey is excited, I'm thrilled, hehe."

MOM: *No need for videoing me at all. I'll be a silent participant if that's ok.*

ME: *Well, that won't be as fun for me, but you do you*

MOM: *I never thought of it from your point of view, to be honest. I just don't want to horn in on your thing with Grace esp w the way Audrey feels about me. If you think Audrey won't*

mind, add me in. But I think she will. Please please tell me this did not anger you.
ME: No it didn't anger me Mom!! Sorry, my phone stays on DND when at work. I already told Audrey you're gonna do it with us and she "loved" it. If you want me to work on repairing the relationship there, I will. But I'm excited to be repairing my relationship with her first.
MOM: I am thrilled that you two are trying. That's what I meant about not horning in. We can talk later ok?

December 30, 2022

3:56 AM: Must be the season of the witch.

December 31, 2022

A filter said, "Guys ghost me when they find out," and I pointed as "I really mean just friends" popped up on the screen.

December 31, 2022

3:36 AM: Another witching hour calling.
I'm in bed. At 8:30. On NYE. Where are my people?? I'm not letting the fact that I'm in the same position on New Year's Eve as I would normally be... get me down. Cause I've said it for a while, and I'll say it again, 2023 is my year. 23 is my lucky number, the 23rd is my birthday (granted my 42nd birthday, which doesn't seem very lucky but I'll take it!). We got this this year. For all of y'all who want to come along for the ride, please do. The more believers, the more achievers, the more supporters, share the love. Come follow me. And have a happy, blessed, safe, prosperous, everything you believe, everything you wish for, new year! 2023!

January 1, 2023

Moved my body at work to "Mama Wanna Mambo" and sang some "Human Touch."

I was home before two, punching the air to "(I Can't Get No) Satisfaction." By 2:30, I was in tears.

"That was not fun," I mouthed to the camera as Zac Brown sang in the background. "Not a good way to start the new year."

I shook my head in disbelief for a few moments, trying to be quiet. By 4:30, I was back in the living room, watching something on the TV with Mom; by 6:40, I had drawn my first every day drawing challenge, a shoe. I enjoyed seeing the differences in my and Grace's interpretations.

I'm posting this several places hoping to get more than 12 recs!!

"12 Months to Read 12 Books."

AUDREY M: *Recommendations from Grace: Backlash, Mockingbird, Counting by 7s, Fish in a Tree*

HEATHER H: *Not sure your reading style but I really liked Verity and Tomorrow and Tomorrow and Tomorrow. Also enjoyed Lessons in Chemistry. All very different. I may steal this.*

DEANNE G: *The Silent Sister*

ASHLEY B: *The Serpent and the Wings of Night. I'm nowhere near done reading it. But so far I'm intrigued. It's about a human that lives in a world of vampires. She is the adopted daughter of the king of the vampires. Apparently a love story is coming out of this too.*

ANNETTE W: *Wool.*

JULIANA R: *The House in the Cerulean Sea by TJ Klune or The One Hundred Years of Lenni and Margot by Marianne Cronin or What Happened to the Bennetts by Lisa Scottoline.*

DEBORAH G: *The Bodyguard by Katherine Center. I just discovered her and read all of her books this year. This is her latest book but I recommend all of them. I love her writing style and she's from Texas so it's prominent in her books!*

January 2, 2023

I used footage that Jimmy sent me from his Christmas party, tasting a horrible beer with Walt in his arms. The faces Jimmy made while taste-testing were hilarious, but it was his reaction to his reactions that were the funniest, not to mention his best friend's and our father's reactions.

Later, alone in my room, I took a before video for the next weight loss challenge. Then we conquered the day 2 drawing challenge, a lamp.

Janaury 3, 2023

Couch karaoke with Bruno Mars and Meghan Trainor. We made "baked banana bread oatmeal" and tried to watch my choir concert from four years earlier. She didn't last long for that (I didn't expect her to). So I went about the third drawing, a purse or a bag.

January 4, 2023

I made a TikTok applying LipSense, desperately trying to feel like myself again. On the day's drawing, a mug or a cup, I finally succeeded in seeing shadows and was able to make the mug look 3D (a white mug on white paper). It was hard!

January 5, 2023

"Y'all know what's weird? Body pain."

I laughed.

"I can't figure out if it's couch, bed, computer chair, old, fat. Who knows? But it hurts. Right now, it's my hip, so I'm trying to get in the habit of stretching more often. So when it starts to hurt, I stand up out of my chair, my little office chair, and crouch"—I lifted my eyebrows—"in a dress. Thankfully, I have tights on. But stretch the hips. I don't think y'all can see much, but I just butterfly! Plié! Butterfly is in sitting position. And stretch. Eeh. It hurts. But it hurts so good."

I just had a funny reaction from a client who found out that I "need" a weight loss coach too... slash support. Um, it made me laugh because lawyers need lawyers, doctors need doctors...therapists need therapists! Trash-men need trash-men! Everybody needs somebody. Even everybody who everybody thinks is on top of the world. Bill Gates. Elon Musk, he has a therapist. Or if he doesn't, he should. Weight loss is not taboo. Taking care of yourself is not taboo. Be healthy. Be happy.

During a conversation with a friend tonight, I had a conversation with myself about something that I would tell her later, and said "the reason I feel like I can make it work with anybody (I smiled) man, woman, ugly, skinny, fat, poor, rich, anything is because of how much I love myself. Which was kind of a weird epiphany. I make myself laugh a lot. I think I'm really funny. I think I'm awesome. And I want somebody else to experience that and complete me and do life with me. Excited. It's gonna be fun."

January 6, 2023

I drew a guitar while we watched a movie called 1BR, "which of course means one-bedroom, on Peacock, I think, and it was"—I made a face, not sure how to put it—"a dystopian version of what I'm trying to achieve in creepy horror world parallel universe. But it was really weird, because I've pretty much quoted it to somebody or another over the last few weeks. It's creepy."

I lower my voice so my mother couldn't hear me.

"I'm a TV psychic."

Ten months later, I'll learn the word *clairaudient*, which I'm obsessed with.

So it's 8:00 on Friday. I'm watching Grease on my tiny little TV in my closed-off bedroom, which is still such a novelty to me after almost two years of living in my mother's living room. Um, see my little fairy lights and everything? And my beautiful dog? Couldn't be any cuter. And 3 miles from work. Pretty much the best. Ummm...this is about self-care, weight loss, taking care of yourself...all the good stuff. Follow me cause I love to talk and I'm here to listen.

January 7, 2023

I drew a picture of a candle jar, then retreated to my room to TikTok using a red light from my new ring light.

"Hi. 'Tis me. It's absolutely my favorite time of night. Everybody's gone to bed. It's only eight, but it's the number one reason I want an amazing bed, because it's kind of my happy place sometimes. Got my..." I turned the camera to see the TV. "Hmm, nothing on there yet. Jerry Maguire tonight on my TV, my little pup, my nightly cocktail"—I held up a piece of chocolate—"which is almost gone, and I'm sad, but there's another flavor to be found. Um... it was kind of a weird day. But we stayed on plan. We'll see what tomorrow brings. Y'all have a good night."

In green for another one.

"Are you green with envy that you're not here with me tonight? The question is, what are you doing tonight? It's Saturday. Um, in the past, I'd probably be at my karaoke bar, which I miss a lot, but mostly the people in it. Um...one day, I'll find one close to here, but I'm sure the people won't compare. Still in search of my crew, my Connecticut crew."

Finally, in blue.

"Last silly showing-off-the-ring-light one. I haven't been on TikTok all day because it was a crazy, busy workday, thankfully. And then I got here and still didn't get on because I was trying to be with my mom. But now I'm on, and it's fun. And I miss it, and I still haven't gotten on to see how many followers I'm at. But it was at 493 this morning or yesterday, whatever the last time I was on, and I'm really really excited to see if I've gotten to 500 because I really wanna do a giveaway. It's not gonna be much, but hopefully, it'll be something great for the winner. Um, yeah, fingers crossed."

January 8, 2023

"What do you do when your mom is in a mood, doesn't wanna watch anything on YouTube that she likes..." I look at the camera, at a loss. "I don't know. This is what I do!" I was cuddled up on the couch with my dogs, blankets, and markers.

"2:22 PM! We made it to five hundred! I'm so excited. It's Sunday, so that of course means as many videos as I can and"—I looked sideways at the camera, smiling through a filter—"sparkling! So I'm relaxing my neck. Um, yeah, I hope everybody's having a good day. Thanks for the follows! I'm super excited. Uh, as soon as we double that, I can go live, which is gonna be really fun. So self-care drawing coming up! Three ways to enter. Share this video, comment... Hold on. Share this video, comment, and follow me if you haven't already, and more to come!"

I drew my rainbow ring for the day's challenge, then movies and filters.

"It was not a fun day. Thankful I somehow managed to set my wallpaper to change my pictures." I scrolled through a bunch of screenshots with Ruby as the star.

"Also thankful for Fat and Weird Cookies. I really wanted to eat all of them."

January 9, 2023, 3:32 AM

Watching Gilmore Girls for the "Season of the Witch" hour again.

I screenshotted a conversation between me and my aunt:

ME: Final end to yesterday, dear aunt. So mom has spent most of the day in her room, weirdly and martyrishly. I was on the phone with a friend at 5:30 and ended the call to go watch tv with Mom just so she didn't "think I was mad." At 7:10, I mentioned something about

Jimmy and she goes "Courtney do you talk to him about what goes on between us?" And bc I can't lie, I said "yes but I don't know what you think goes on between us." She got up and went to her room and I said do I need to stop the TV? And she shut her door and goes "good night Courtney." Guess what you selfish, stubborn ass, I talk to Audrey, Susan, and Katherine about you too. So after a lot of reflection and talking with many people, I've decided it's time for me to step away. I will be separating myself from her as she's done to us in the past. She's unbearable while she's "recovering," and I'm going to run out of Xanax. As long as she has her roof and some food, that's all I'm concerned with. I'd really really like someone else to approach her about bankruptcy so I can free up her disability check, but I can handle it even if that doesn't happen, so...

AUNTIE S: This sounds like a good idea, for you to step back. I think sometimes Cyn may forget she's your mom and so it's your story too, maybe even more than hers. So good for you, withdraw a bit. (sorry if the green heart has a meaning I'm not aware of, I just thought it was pretty.)

Today's drawing, ironically, was organized chaos, where I drew a Christmas tree of lights. At work, I put on a sparkly blue filter.

"I just did this filter with 'Baby Got Back' just because I thought it was fun. But I really like it, so I'm using it again. It was another rough night of sleeping for me. Three o'clock witching hour...I was bright and awake, but there was no witching to be done just yet that I know of for sure, though I did hope and pray and think and wish and sprinkle good vibes everywhere. So I hope somebody feels it somewhere, the good witching, because there's bad ones too. And I will never mean that. For anybody." I smiled sadly. "I hope it's a good Monday for y'all."

Later that night, in bed with a red filter, I said, "Makes certain parts of my face look strangely red. Anyway, um, I'm curious how many people know what it's like to live with somebody with mental illness. Um..." I tilted my head, clearly uncomfortable. "I don't talk about it very often because my mother is a very private person, and when she's healthy, she doesn't want anybody to know her business. But my aunt put it to me really well tonight that even though it's her story, I'm her daughter, and it's my story too. Um, even maybe more so, which was pretty eye-opening to me because there are sisters and brothers and other people—oh my—involved."

I smirked harshly, anger evident in my eyes.

With another filter, after I'd cried a little, I said, "I'm sitting here cuddled up with my YouTube Disney channel shows that I've been in love with these past couple of days and envisioning my dream Disney vacation and crying because... my happiness relies on other people's. And as happy as this stuff makes me, I want somebody to share it with."

I shrug and laugh a little hysterically.

"That's all there is to it."

January 10, 2023, 2:48 AM

[The music played over my voice until I could understand I had been watching more Disney YouTube, that one featuring Harry Potter World.] "It's times like this I wish I could go live, because I'd love to know if there was a reason I'm getting up this early in the morning. Every morning. For weeeekkkks. And weeks and weeks. At least it doesn't seem to be affecting my every day life too much. Oh well."

When I woke up for real (after ten), I made an apple crisp that I'd been dreaming about for weeks. With cranberries that my mother "hates" bc she's being an asshole. (That sounded crueler than it was intentioned.) Drinking my water. Talking to my God and my Dog(s). Centering myself. I've done this before. I can do it again. I am important. I am more than her daughter. However, in the meantime, if you're a praying person, I could use them.

Later, listening to Charlie Puth, I wrote "I don't know if this will even work because of song rights or whatever. But I felt this particular part was super important today and I couldn't get it to line up. Excuse my voice bc I didn't expect to leave it." The lyrics were "No matter where you go / you know you're not alone / I'm only one call (or message. Or TikTok. Or Snap. Or... scrolled across the screen as I sang) away / I'll be there to save the day. Superman's got nothing on me (I winked) / I'm only one call away. And when you're weak, I'll be strong / I'm gonna keep holding on / Now don't you worry, I won't be long / Darling, when you feel like hope is gone, just run into my arms!"

iTunes was on it for the "fuck you" songs today, which I played pretty loudly. First was "You Need to Calm Down," then "Hot and Cold," for which I wrote "who can relate? (I'm tired of it)."

"You're a 10, but..." spun by and landed with an attack on "you catch feelings too easily."

Later that evening, I put on freckles and said, "I just had the pleasure of jumping on my first live thanks to my friend Melissa, and that was really fun. I still don't know quite what was going on, but I gave some presents and some roses and some dogs (Hallmark movie commercial just said dogs at the same time I typed it. #clairaudient) or something strange, and I hope I helped him. And I gained fourteen people...fourteen new friends! And I followed them all back. This is gonna be very fun. Um, so thanks for doing that, DadBod! That was cool. I'm excited."

Ah, this man has become a good friend, oddly. I've never met him in person, and yet I know his magic. My first time in a grow live, this man's energy was second to none. If you're a TikTok fan, look him up: Dadbod146.

NOT THE F——ING GILMORE GIRLS

January 11, 2023

"One wacky piece of information: no witching hour for me last night! Hope everyone else is safe. After being in bed most of yesterday and hiding a lot about Saturday too. I've been in my bed a lot lately. But I'm taking care of me so."

I switched to outside, walking around. "Um, walking around. It is gorgeous outside, cold and gorgeous, just how I like it, although it's only January. I mean, it's already January, and we've only had snow once, I think. That's a bummer. Gimme my snow."

I drew my hand, which was the challenge for the day before (ten days in, and I had already skipped). Then I played with a filter of a dandelion that said, "The wind says..." Then when I blew the flower, it said, "Good news is coming!" I'll take that. I just put deposit down on my first adult furniture which is pretty exciting. Aside from the couch I bought with babysitting money when I was like 22. But that was...a disastrous couch anyway, so this one... no, no couch, bed, and dresser. Gorgeous and I'm so excited and they're my forever pieces. Forever. For-eh-VER. (Mimicking The Sandlot.)

January 12, 2023

At 3:00 AM, as usual, I played with several silly filters. I finally talked about a pizza I had ordered the other day from a new place next to us called Checkers. "Y'all may have seen some of my pictures, but it was called like, 3 AM Diner Pizza. And it was beef and bacon and pickles and mustard and ketchup instead of sauce and don't remember what else, but it was so good... oh, French fries were on top of it. And it was so good, and I've been kind of daydreaming about it for a while now but being awake at 3 AM in the morning without much dinner last night, I'm actually so hungry." I swallowed heavily to demonstrate. "I need this pizza now." I giggled.

"I need something now. I'm hungry. Somebody feed me. Feed me, Seymour."

At 10:44, I put on a black lace mask filter and said, "I've been thinking about how to send this to you for a long time because…it's weird. Dealing with my mother as an adult is a whole new game, and I just want to tell you thank you for dealing with her for nine years. However long? 'Cause I'm into my second, and I'm gonna go crazy. So I didn't know how you did it, but thank you. Thank you for taking care of us. Thank you for continuing to take care of us. It's a hard road. Love you. Have a good Thursday. And tomorrow is Friday the Thirteenth, yay! More luck!"

A few minutes later, I made another video, this one a hot mess of lyrics, captions, and layover text. The song was T Swift's "Midnight Rain," and I spoke.

"My brain isn't even working, y'all. Like, this is so… What is happening with my hair?"

(Overlay: Taylor's lyrics hit. Hard. Sometimes. Can you listen to her and read me? I talk a lot, y'all!)

"Don't know what that is either. This is night… forty something? Forty days and forty nights of waking up at three o'clock-ish."

I blathered on about how frequently I woke up and how long I stayed awake.

(Overlay: Sometimes, you just have to talk. Keeping stuff inside is toxic. Go outside and scream "Fuck you!" really loudly. It helps.)

"Finally, I fell back asleep after hearing my mother take the dog out, who has bad diarrhea right now because she's sad and sick and overwhelmed like me. (Uggggh, Hallmark channel ad said "diarrhea" at the same time I typed it. #clairaudient) Thankfully, it's not manifesting in me in any health issues, because God knows I need less of that while I'm dealing with the mental health issues. So there's that. Good morning. Happy Wednesday."

(Overlay: Happy Thursday.)

"Wait, whatever today is."

Later on at home, I was in bed, crying.

"You know those moments when you don't have anybody to talk to?"

(Edit to add, "You don't want to burden anyone any more than you already have?") "That's why I come to TikTok."

I lay there for a moment, breathing, the tears slowing down.

"It's tough."

Taylor's "Calm Down" ceased playing over my voice, and I sniffed.

"Why did this make me feel better immediately? Thanks for listening!"

After bedtime, I was much calmer.

"So after the mild panic attack upon coming home and my mother being my mother and the only victim, as usual, um, I took a Xanax and went to bed, and I think that was about 2:30. So I think I slept for, like, four hours, and I'm so tired, I'm slurring. So I'm gonna take my regular nighttime meds and hope I sleep through the night."

(Overlay: I am strong, and I am an eternal optimist. I can handle your heart. Talk to me.)

"Because...I'm tired. My brain's tired. My... brain is tired. My body couldn't care less, honestly. I hope you guys have a magical Thursday. Good night!"

A few moments later, I was back in my blue freckle filter.

"This filter is life right now. I didn't put a whole lot of..."

I paused and laughed. "That's not true. I had a lot of faith that I would get viral or whatever on TikTok. Um, I know nothing about it still. I'm doing a pretty decent job with my videos. I think they're pretty funny. Um, but my followers are growing with leaps and bounds, and I can't express enough gratitude. I'm so excited because I literally can just jump on and cry"—I blew air through my lips like a horse—"like this afternoon, to a phone, and I feel better. And isn't that kind of magical right now when we're all alone in this world?"

January 13, 2023

 Another one I quite don't get the point of. It's weird. Happy Friday, good morning! I slept through the night, with the help of the Xanax, but I'll take it. Feel a lot less foggy today, although definitely not 100% better. Uhh hope you guys have a fantastic day and don't get too motion sick from this filter!

 I used a filter that looked like a Post-it note was stuck to my head, and I wrote, "Orthopedic doc...again." I started the filter, and it landed on "You're on the right track. Stop worrying." I wrote, "My God has me. But this has been a hard...life. Don't worry. Be happy. Easier said than done, eh?"

 Okay, most blessing of a doc appointment ever. Um, I could tell the women behind the counter were Friday-the-13th-crazy as we tend to get, and when I exited, one of the grumpier ones had white nails, and I just like, "I love your nails!" and she goes, "thank you," and her whole body relaxed. And so I took it one step further, or two steps, and said, "and your earrings and your hair, you're really adorable." And she looked up and she goes, "What??" And so I repeated, "And your earrings and your hair, you're really adorable!" You should have seen her face...through her mask. She giggled and lit up and said "oh my God, you are so cute," and turned around to the other lady and said, "Lori's so cute too. We are all cute." And it just...it lifted her. Which of course lifted me because, phew, it's been a couple of days. Have a good Friday.

 At work, I did karaoke with "Something Just Like This," "why does every song make so much sense??" written across the screen. Later, I caught up on the "every day" drawing challenge. And then I did "I Kissed A Girl."

 In bed, I played with a "palm-reader" filter, cheating the system and doing it over and over.

Holy cow, another clairaudient moment. I was watching *A Fabled Holiday*, which is already echoing too close to my life, and someone said "Over and over" at the same time I wrote it. I cannot make this stuff up. But back to the past!

> The song was "Bejeweled," which is likely why I wanted to keep playing... first card said "Your heart line is short. Your love is hiding secrets from you." I said, "duh," and tried to start the filter again.
>
> "One more time," I said, and held up my palm. The filter didn't start, and I said "aw," paused it, and said, "Now one more time." Again, my hand stayed blank, and I yelped, "For real?"
>
> Finally I made it work, and this one said "Your wisdom line is short. Your strength is your heart, not your brain." I put my hand down. "Damn true."
>
> I lifted my hand again, "Be careful not to fall in love too easily." I closed my fist and shook my head. "I always do!"
>
> And finally, "You better save up now," over which I wrote "time or money??"

January 14, 2023

> I lip-synched to "Stronger" by Sara Evans. Music. If it doesn't help heal you, you're not doing it right. It cracks me up how I use my hands in these videos. I hope I don't do this IRL.
>
> As I left work, it started to snow. I opened my phone and said, "Guess what! It's snowing! Y'all probably can't even see it. I'm gonna turn the phone. Hehe, and it's not even a filter. But it probably won't stick. We'll see. Buh-bye. Oh, I forgot to tell you one thing. I have to drive in it because it's like regular weather here."
>
> I lowered my voice confidentially.
>
> "Although people still can't drive in it because it's like rain. No one can drive in the rain either."
>
> Since it was snowing, I spent some more time catching up on drawing. I made a sped-up TikTok and wrote, "Why does even the fun stuff feel like a chore when you're depressed?" Then I played with filters, had oatmeal for dinner, and spent a cozy

afternoon watching movies. It was Ruby's thirteenth Gotcha Day anniversary, so I drew her too.

    Here's my little witching at 9:48 because this is the second night that I've slept through the night, and it felt really good. I had some energy back today (Golo commercial talking about getting energy back) and we're calling it the third night in a row. Third time's a charm. So I'm wishing all my insomniacs out there, all of my people who suffer from depression or anxiety or bipolar or...God bless, all of the other freaking illnesses that are out there right now... I wish you peace. And a soothing night of...peace? Sometimes that's all you can pray for, right? Because it hurts. Life just hurts. Love you guys, good night.

January 15, 2023

    I had a very sick dog today (Cookie), so we snuggled and took care of ourselves. I also had a super bad headache. I had taken about sixteen Advil since it started. Later, I got in another fight with Mom. I wrote "I'm still shaking" with a tense face. "I can't stand when I'm being genuinely nice and someone takes offense. But my own mother? She's supposed to be my partner. How does she not know me better than this?

    "I'm a little bit lost for words right now, which does not happen to me very often. Um...my mother just screamed at me that she 'cannot be under my control like this anymore.' She has two job appointments this week after months of me begging her not to get a job, that I'll support her, that I'll take care of her, that I'll let her lounge around the fucking house and do nothing. Excuse the snotty facial expressions every so often. When she gets like this, I find myself reverting back to my teenage self real fast. And pay the bills, because that is my hope and my goal for my life, for my entire life—to be able to take care of her. I'm at a place now that I can, and she wants to do this shit?"

    I shook my head in disbelief.

NOT THE F——ING GILMORE GIRLS

"Actually speechless. Literally speechless."

Talia just told Anderson she was speechless in *A Fabled Holiday*. To continue, she said, "I am a writer. This I know. It is my calling. It is in my bones. It is in my heart. I'm not questioning that. I am a writer." #clairfuckingaudient

> *I made a quick TikTok to "I'm Petty," which I signed with my eyebrows cocked as the singer rapped it.*
>
> *I posted a meme that said, "Your light is gonna irritate a lot of unhealed people."*
>
> *In the evening, I made another panicking video: Well, I'm definitely not calming down. I just wonder if there's anybody out there that takes care of a parent or a grown child or a grandparent or anybody. I don't know what I'm doing wrong to make her think she's under my control. She has a car. She has food. She has a roof. Nobody's stopping her from leaving. She has a phone. I'm...I'm...I'm not controlling her.*

January 16, 2023

> *4:12 AM, I had to take two Xanax to get to sleep, not to mention my regular nighttime aids. And here I am at 3:45 in the morning because my mother told me I control her. So my sleeping through the night for the last three nights has gone to the birds or the dogs or whatever the phrase is. I do believe TikTok needs a flash, but I like this app. I mean, filter. I'm definitely still sleepy, but my brain is going four hundred miles a minute.*
>
> *How do I stay up? That's my issue, I think. I feel just ready to go for the day now. Five and a half hours of sleep. No medication hangover. Lots of anger at my mom still in the pit of my stomach, so maybe that's what's fueling me, but...4:30, baby. Rise and shine!*
>
> *I passed back out for another couple of hours, finally getting up at nine. I felt fine so far, but by seven, I was in my room, dancing to "Shake It Off" by Florence and the Machine. "Today was a harder-than-normal day. Big, life-altering decision*

was made today. I made it with a clear, calm head, and I slept on it. It still felt horrible. I don't think anyone likes being the bearer of bad news, and I delivered a killing blow. But I saved myself, and right now, that's what I have to celebrate. The smile on my face during these lyrics is genuine. But so is the shrug at the end. We will see what tomorrow brings."

To end the evening, I wrote: You think you've risen from the ashes, but you keep getting burned. I've never understood so clearly why my name for everything is Phoenix Lover. And then shared a post by Alys Cerda:

"There is a TikTok I saw of an 80-year-old woman who said when she was 8 years old, she was trying out makeup for the first time. When her mom saw her put on blush she told her she looked like a clown. 72 years later—to this day—she hears her mom's voice saying that to her when she puts on blush. She ended the TikTok with how the words parents say to us haunt us forever. When you reflect on your childhood, it's the things that were said to you that shaped your image of yourself and also shaped how you speak to yourself. If you are a parent or plan on becoming one, don't become your child's negative voice for their entire life. They'll face enough negativity and bullying in the world, they don't need a personal bully at home."

January 17, 2023

"So despite being a day off, it's been a quiet day for me. Um, I've slept a lot. I didn't sleep much last night again, and now I'm making up for it. And I have a sinus headache and a neck"—I stretched my neck and made a face—"sinus headache. But I've gotten through the day. It's 7:30. Um, I downloaded a calendar to make myself laugh and happy and have a reason to celebrate daily, and it's National Calendar Day or National...Day Calendar. And today is National Bootleggers Day and National Hot Buttered Rum Day."

This came out in the captions as "Hot Butter Drum" and made me laugh.

"So I suggest... no, no bootlegging please. I suggest making a hot buttered rum. If you're a Harry Potter fan, make it a butterbeer, because yum."

January 18, 2023

I woke up and turned on TikTok, blinking into the camera at the brightness of the light.

"Good morning," I whispered. "I'm just twenty-seven... twenty-seven followers away from being able to go live. I'm just... blown away! Now I did a lot of work for the gifting thing yesterday and grew on a couple of really awesome people's lives. They were fun. I wanna go live so badly. It's Wednesday, which means we're probably pretty slow at work. Um... I'd love to go live and help people decide how to take care of themselves this year. Twenty-seven more followers, y'all. Twenty-seven."

At work, I put on the dandelion filter again now that I had learned how to blow. "The wind says..." popped up on the screen, and I said "Well..." and blew.

"Wishes do come true," I stated faithfully, gesturing across the screen right before the words "Your wish will come true" appeared from the dandelion.

I gasped, astonished.

"Okay, that was weird."

I pointed at the words still lingering.

"Does it... that was weird."

I regained my composure and continued.

"But hey, that's even better. So fact of the matter is, I'm over a thousand. I can go live soon, which means weight loss questions and answers specific to Jenny Craig for a while. Um, as you can see, that's where I work, and I'm super excited for the changes that are coming down for our company. I can't wait to get you guys on board. Clean Simple Eats, which I love and adore, and intermittent fasting, that's how I'm losing... Oh, and Noom. Duh, a big

one. Um, any of those options and of course self-care. That's what I'm here about."

I managed to find a trending filter I hadn't used even though it bugged my eyes.

"Today was a good day," I said, smiling. "I had nine hundred and something followers when I woke up, jumped on a grow party, grew to a thousand in time to go live for my lunch break, which was just fun. And I would love to do every day, uh, kind of a question-and-answer Jenny Craig thing, so we'll see if that works out. Um, the self-care... Oh my God, I'm so sleepy, y'all. It's only 8:45. I hope I can sleep through the night. Um, self-care slash mental health giveaways, drawings, whatever, will still happen as often as I can."

January 19, 2023

"2:22 AM: So I'm up with a very sick dog. I was this close to sleeping through the night. I can feel it by the way I'm talkin'! Her sister has been sick for the better part of a week. I don't know if she ever threw up, but major"—I gestured, unable to say the word diarrhea at two in the morning—"liquid poop, and Cookie doesn't do that. Ruby, on the other hand, has put me through the ringer with stomach issues. I am not...I'm not in the right mindset for this right now. I do not need a sick dog. So here I am on TikTok because I don't need a sick dog."

I did a tribute video to David Crosby, who died earlier that day: "Southern Cross," which had become one of my favorite songs.

I saved an Awkward Yeti cartoon that had Brain asking, "Do you think happiness is an illusion?" and Heart replying, "I hope so! I love magic!"

"So in a new and fun twist, it's 11:33, and I haven't gone to sleep despite smoking, despite a muscle relaxer that is doctor prescribed, despite a Xanax"—it came across in captions as "his annex"—"that is also doctor prescribed. I think it might be time to visit a sleeping pill, and I don't like that.

Oh, but you know what? I didn't take my gummies. Maybe that's what I'm missing.

"So now I'm watching Gilmore Girls and talking to you fine people and still marveling about getting kicked out of my live for hateful behavior. God bless. Can you imagine? That's the last thing I'm about."

I smiled sadly, thinking of all the people who had called me a bitch in my life.

"Um, everybody, have a good night. Friday tomorrow. I hope that means a lot of delightful things for you."

January 20, 2023

"After midnight, when I went to sleep last night, I still didn't sleep through the night... I woke up bright and early! 4:45, 5 o'clock, something like that. Went back to sleep. Woke up with my bed soaked as usual, so I think that's how I'm losing this weight right now. I'm not drinking enough water. I never do when I get stressed out or sick or anything, but...I think I'm sweating it out, for whatever reason, at night. And the scale is constantly moving right now, which could be attributed to stress, or..."—I rolled my eyes and used my fingers to quote—"the divorce diet, as my mother calls it. But I'm still trying to eat to take care of myself. So something I'm doing is working...finally. Um, we'll see."

"Okay, I'm officially asking the social media world for help. Um, my mother is bipolar. She has been cycling for about a year, and this is gonna be the third time, and I'm afraid the third time is gonna kill her. So what do I do? Because she won't listen to any of us. She won't listen to anybody. She thinks she's on top of the world right now, which mentally she is. Sort of. Uh, she just removed me as an authorized user from the phone account that I pay for, so I don't know what that's gonna do to the automatic payment in four days, so I might lose phone access for a little while! So when you start messing with my life, what do I do but get in there and"—I rub my chin nervously, embarrassed to admit it—"pause all her Internet devices at home? Which could conceivably cause her to get so angry that she shows up at my work. So we'll see how that goes. Good luck."

When I got home from work, something had me so angry that I went to her closed (and locked) bedroom door and yelled, "Open the goddamn door. Please!"

Quietly from within, she said, "Courtney, you're begging me now like I've begged you for a year and a half. No."

Anger made my voice rise.

"What would you do if I kicked you out of this apartment, Mom? What would you do?"

"Kick me out, Courtney. Please do! Kick me out!"

My voice broke. "I don't want to. I made a vow to you."

"I made a vow to you," she retorted.

"But you're not honoring your part of that goddamn vow." My anger was out of my control when I started saying that word.

"You're not honoring it," she shrieked back at me several times while I pleaded "Listen, listen" to the audience. "What am I doing that's not honoring it?"

I flipped the camera around and stopped addressing Mom.

"I really need to know that. What am I doing? Because"—I started counting on my fingers—"I paid all the bills. I'm taking care of our dogs. I've tried to keep her in food. I've been a little slack at that because neither of us have had an appetite. Um, I'm at the end."

I can hear her saying something in her bedroom, and I freeze, trying to make it out. It sounded like, "I have people behind me, thank God." "She has people behind her that she was making up, so that meant there was bipolar involved..."

Rewatching this, I think she must have meant metaphorically behind her, where I might have thought she meant literally by the expression on my face.

"Why won't she believe me when I start to see the signs? And why won't she listen to any of us when we know what we're talking about? This third one's gonna kill her. This third one is gonna kill me. Um, I'm afraid it's gonna kill our dogs."

I looked down at the concerned pups at my feet. Then I heard laughter from inside her bedroom.

"She's laughing. She's manic as shit. When is she gonna fucking learn? When is she gonna learn?"

A couple of minutes later, Mom said, "I'm not gonna beg you..."

"I have...I have never once said I didn't wanna live with you."

She laughed. "Last night, you told me living with me was a nightmare."

"I did say that," I admitted, "'cause it is right now. You're a fucking nightmare."

"I am not a nightmare, Courtney. You are," she said calmly.

"Right, because I'm the only one who's ever done anything wrong in her forty-nine years of living."

How old was I?

"Thirty-nine," I corrected. "My mother is never once at fault for anything that's happened over these twenty-two years."

"I'm always at fault, Courtney, and I always come back and say—"

"No, you don't," I interrupted hardly, as her inability to apologize for anything was the biggest point of contention with all her children. "That's bullshit, 'cause if that was true, you'd apologize for anything that's happened over these last eight months."

"So would you have."

"Hmm." I made a sound like a buzzer. "But I'm not sorry!"

"And I have! I told you what I was sorry for, Courtney."

"I'm not sorry, though. I handled everything really well."

"That's the problem. That's the problem, honey."

I snickered. I hated it when she called me pet names when she was mad at me; it was so condescending.

"Right. That's the problem, Mom, is you think I owe you an apology for taking care of you."

"No, not for taking care of me."

"Well, that's what I did. And that's what I'm continuing to do. And like I told your sisters last night?"

She interrupted me. "You couldn't even get me toilet paper, Courtney, much less food. I'm done!"

"When did you ask for toilet paper, Mother? We have a Costco-sized box of toilet paper."

"I'm. Done."

"Kiss my lily-white ass. My mother."

January 22, 2023

"9:47 on my Sunday day off, and I've already lived through two temper tantrums. Um, my aunt's coming over at 10:30 if everything goes as planned. Not really a plan of action in place, but"—I shrugged—"I'm at my end. I literally am at a loss for what else to do for this woman, so...yeah. We've got one very concerned dachshund."

Cookie yawned. I laughed.

"As you can see. And then this one..."

Ruby had her head hung, looking miserable.

"Hey, can you say hi to your fans? She's still real sick. We've got grumbly stomach. We've got somebody who won't eat, which is not okay. This one"—I touched Cookie—"on the other hand, tried to finish the blond one's breakfast. So she's feeling fine."

I danced in my bedroom for a while, in need for everyone to know I was doing the best I could to remain true to me, that she would not conquer me this time. Then I spent some time on the phone with T-Mobile, trying to get control of my phone again while my mother was in the same vicinity. Cookie spent the afternoon square in my lap. Later, my mother ventured out of her room, and I dared to ask her how to get my phone back. Naturally, her insane logic drove me to the brink of insanity. I watched a couple of episodes of Nashville to calm down and made a TikTok where I was bawling: "If you don't believe in the magic of music, watch Nashville. Powerful."

I ended the night in my bedroom, looking through old photos in which I looked happy, and I noticed a trend that involved babies, lipstick, and dogs. I put together a reel to make myself smile.

January 23, 2023

It's only 8:58 and I already need a nap. But since I don't have to be at work till noon, I think I'm gonna take one! Yay for insomnia. But yay for having the house to myself this morning because my mother apparently got a job. We'll see how that goes.

So, I have an injured right shoulder. Haven't had shoulder yet. Elbow, always, wrist always. Shoulder's concerning. Am I tapping too much? Am I sleeping on it wrong? I don't want to lose function in my entire right arm.

January 24, 2023

3:55 AM: I'm watching YouTube as I usually do with insomnia, but my dreaming brain wanted to go to the grocery store and create myself a "fun little Harry Potter treat" just because. "Living my life for the last two years for my mother (which I have; tried to get our life together working, and her life, for the last eight months, back on track), has been crippling. And I feel like I'm kind of free now and I'm getting back to me and imagining again.

"Who else's morning started out as fun"—I arched my eyebrows conversantly—"as mine did? Y'all, okay, so I kind of expected"—I paused to get something out of my eyelashes—"to not have a great day. My primary doctor, who I would normally call for a refill on my meds, has changed specialties. So I don't have a primary doctor anymore. First time that I've had one that's gotten to know me, and she changed specialties. So I'm gonna hunt her down and be like a stalker patient because...what?"

I laughed, confused and sad. "So anyway, try getting my mom to turn the phone back on, still two days away from the bill being due. Wouldn't do it. So I said, 'Look, if you're not gonna do it, I'm gonna turn the internet back off, because that's the only way I can guarantee my phone works, because our deal was $45 and turning my phone back on, and you didn't honor that part. Bye, Internet.'"

Mom came out of her room when I did that. She started recording me with her phone too.

"The family needs to understand that you're walking away from this knowingly, that I pay $200 a month every month to it."

She interrupted. "That's all I'm asking for. Pay it. Pay it!"

"Mother. I can't pay for something that you've turned off. I refuse to pay for something that I'm not using."

She scoffed. "Then give me the money, and I'll pay it. K?"

I repeated my disgusting insult from earlier. "Kiss. My lily-white ass. And you guys heard me. I'm so fucking done. I'm so done. So I'm gonna take my phones and go turn them on at AT&T or somewhere else. I'll try T-Mobile first 'cause God knows they know the story. Um, so basically, they're just paperweights right now while I'm off of Wi-Fi, which is fine with me, because I have Wi-Fi everywhere. And thankfully, I remain in control of that. So, uh, that's where we stand now guys. She's probably gonna lose phone service in a couple of days. Um, I don't know if that will be enough to clue her in to how sick she is? So that's gonna be less than a minute, which will be TikTok-length, which means I'm posting it now."

I said that to piss her off. She hated social media and simply sneered when I said that.

In bed that night, high as a kite, I made a TikTok with T Swift singing over me. "Another day in the books. I'm very very tired. Very tired. Um, I'm taking a personal day from work tomorrow, which doesn't happen very often. But I am not thinking very clearly, and I think I'm gonna spend tomorrow singing and trying to get back to myself a little bit, because this has been a hard few weeks, and I'm ready...I'm ready for a change."

I furrowed my eyebrows.

"God bless. I can't believe I'm back here again."

January 25, 2023

2:24 AM: Pissed, I said, "It's almost to the point of being a joke. Almost three months in this apartment, and I think I've slept through the night twice. Only once that I know for sure, so I'm saying twice to be generous."

I stared at myself for a few seconds.

"My hair looks good."

I stared for a few more seconds and scoffed.

"What a life, man."

At ten, after I had been crying, I said, "You know the worst part about all of this is these dogs. They just don't understand. So Ruby's sitting here, and here comes Cookie, just confused. When we went to go take a nap, I brought her with me, and my mom decided to leave and take her with her. She is now on the phone with somebody, telling them that I essentially kidnapped her dog. Um, I pay for the dog food. If I had to, I'd pay for dog bills. I mean, vet bills. This is my dog too. I don't...my life is a fucking joke right now, y'all. A fucking joke. I'm twenty-two years old again. This is what's happening. In my life. And I made these decisions. For myself. To try to help her. And I'm getting fucked for it."

A few moments later, I asked her when she was moving out. Whatever she did to the dogs made me so angry, I called it the final straw and asked for the divorce. I then spent the day watching three Harry Potter movies and sleeping, which made me feel better, but I took another personal day the next day.

January 27, 2023

So my aunt found out something else my mother was doing to me and asked what her motive was, "I wonder what her motive is?" and I said to look out for number one as it always has been. And for some reason, I hadn't really thought about it that way yet (my mom is very selfish. Love her dearly; she's taken care of me in some bad times). It's a bad time for her, and she's not letting anybody help. Um, or herself help. So after a few months of dealing with this, I'm at the point where I don't want to care about anybody. If this one person can't care about me, this one person who I was supposed to trust implicitly in my life... this is why I'm gonna need therapy this round.

January 30, 2023

I held up my hand, which was covered in shards of glass and opal.

"This is the inside of the opal necklace that my mother bought me for my birthday. I think it was my fortieth birthday, so it's been a little over a year, and she bought me this necklace"—I reached into my shirt for the broken bulb on a chain—"because I tend to break opals. And are you fucking kidding me? It broke in. My. Shirt. Today. In my shirt. Did I knock something into it? Thankfully, I haven't found any cuts yet but still finding little pieces of gem"—I gestured toward my boobs—"opal. In some kind of liquid. And glass. That's how my day is going."

January 31, 2023

I got woken up today by a social worker checking in on my mom, who was apparently at work, which is good for her, I guess. So I answered a few questions about that, and he left. And then about an hour later, she called with T-Mobile on the line.

I rubbed my eyes with the backs of my hands like a child, completely exhausted.

"And finally released my phone. So I have control over that again. But other than that, nothing, no resolutions. I don't like this life I'm living. Time to change some things."

February 1, 2023

Bad stomach pains started again, and while it wasn't new, it was unpleasant, and I didn't need it. I vowed to take better care of myself.

February 2, 2023

I'm so sad. Again. Why is it that I feel so good at work and I can't keep that going at home? One of the things that happens when my mom gets sick is, she gets "messages" from the tv and music. (Happens when she's healthy too, but she doesn't listen when she's healthy!) Tonight, she stayed up two hours past her regular "bedtime" to watch Enough with JLo. I am more than a little scared. I understand she's sick, but I don't understand how she doesn't understand that by now. She's been through this enough. Why is she doing it again?!

February 6, 2023

I cried and said, "So this is what stimming looks like. It was a bad day."

February 7, 2023

I worked and sang a lot of Valentine's Songs.

"Today was a good day...but there were no interactions with the madre. Seemingly went to bed at about 7:30, left the house at seven thirty this morning."

I shook my head slowly, thinking.

"It was a nice, peaceful day by myself at the center. And now I'm sparkling and shooting everybody 'Rainbow' love."

I opened and closed my fingers a few times in a sprinkling gesture, then flashed the "I love you" sign.

February 12, 2023

Tried to host a Super Bowl party on TikTok and got banned from live (again). Instead, I had to battle my very manic mother watching the game and commercials with me, laughing and talking to the TV. I heard a ref say something about rising above and staying calm despite your situation (#clairaudient).

Mom sang "and the caissons go rolling along," to a USAA commercial, then said, "I'm an army of one and I have to harden my heart to that," and I knew she was trying to bait me, because of course, she's not. I mean, hello, she's living in my house. But I know that's how she feels right now, and it's sad and it's scary…

February 15, 2023

I'd known for a couple of days that mom had been on the verge of combusting. She was in a mood to fight that night, and I just wasn't. I couldn't anymore. She busted through the lock on my door. (I had rigged two command hooks and a scarf to my sliding farm doors. Of course it was okay for her to have the lock because she was the mom.)

"And now she's in there," I whispered, "yelling at her music, and I can't drown it out. I've got my TV on. I don't think she knows I'm home right now. Thankfully." I rolled my eyes. "I was able to sneak back in the house without her knowing. But I don't want to live my life…tiptoeing around my house. She's like dynamite. I'm scared. I don't wanna be here."

Texting with my aunt later, I detailed my mother's fun with music. She started off doing the "YMCA." Then she switched to some kind of movie score-compilation (went to Psycho after Star Wars and she laughed really hard) and said, "Of course. Oh man I love that movie. I could watch that a 1000 times."

February 17, 2023

Mom asked me to watch TV with her and I said yes, knowing I could retreat to my room if she drove me crazy. Feeling kind, she said it was my choice, so I picked The Greatest Showman because I'd just been talking about it with a friend. She got super excited, pumped the air with her fist, and said "Whoo I am on." She then said "gorgeous, gorgeous man" to a YouTube ad. By "From Now On," she was rocking fully, keeping up a dialogue, "Hot August Night. I'm gonna start from the beginning, folks. Prologue, Crunchy Granola Suite. Dialogue, Stones. Stones, Stones, Stones, Stones, I can't say it anymore."

February 18, 2023

Late afternoon, Mom was out of the house and I got scared shitless by someone knocking really hard on our door, thinking it was going to be cops telling me they'd picked her up. There was a fire in the wall behind my bedroom. She stayed out till past 10 that night, which was super unusual.

Febraury 19, 2023

Mom didn't come home the night before. Cookie, Ruby and I were scared and lonely.

February 22, 2023

She missed her birthday!

February 27, 2023

She went on the hunt for Neil Sparkle at his "Brooklyn Roads." She was in a hospital in Syracuse for a week, then that night showed up on our doorstep like nothing had happened. It was almost nine, and I was going to bed soon, and the heat was being turned off. Mom was mad because she hadn't taken a shower yet, so I told her to take one before I finished the show.

"It's too cold. I'm gonna be up playing my music or my skits, whatever it is. Let me do that."

"I don't mind you doing that," I said, though I was thinking, Shouldn't you be sleeping? "If that's what you want to do all night long, that's fine..."

"That's what I'm going to be doing, but I'm not—"

"But the heater's going off when I go to bed."

"Bitch," she spat.

"I'm sorry," I said automatically, 'cause I was.

She came close, her face nearing the camera, her hands on the couch where I was sitting.

"Why are you so controlling, honey? Why don't you let me just have this night of heat? Why don't you let me?"

"Because I can't sleep with the heater on," I said as if it should have been obvious.

"Then throw off a few blankets."

"And my mental health is just as important as yours is. So I'm gonna take care of me this time."

She stalked into her bedroom, waving dismissively, and said, "Whatever. Good night."

"Good night, Mom."

She then turned back around, shaking her head in disbelief.

"Yes?" I asked.

"You will never learn," she said.

"Neither will you," I replied, my voice pitched high, struggling against tears.

"Not until someone clobbers you over the head."

"You have."

"You will never learn."

"I already have."

She turned to go back to her room.

"No, you haven't. I guarantee you. I guarantee you that. One-hundred-percent-authentic guarantee."

"Sounds like a threat," I said to the camera.

"It is a threat," she said back, from her doorway. "Sort of. But it's also a promise. Both."

NOT THE F——ING GILMORE GIRLS

February 28, 2023

I got up to take off the dangling command hook "lock." Mom was already up (still up?), and she danced around the kitchen as I made the dogs breakfast, the sash from the winter coat she was wearing inside (dramatic much?) tied around her head. Cookie's new habit of chattering was on high power, and I spent the day on the couch with her while Mom puttered around the house. By 6:30, she'd somehow managed to withhold Cookie from me, but to make matters worse, Ruby wouldn't go in my room with me.

March 1, 2023

In the evening, she asked if I was staying around the Manchester area for work, and I said, "Well, yeah."

I was unwilling to let her know I was staying in the same complex. "Where are you going?"

"I don't know yet," she said dismissively. "I'll figure it out."

"So you're just gonna throw your stuff in storage and—"

"Hit the road, Jack?"

"Hit the road, Jack?" I repeated.

"I have no other course of action," she said, loading the dishwasher.

"Okay," I said scornfully. "Sounds like fun."

"Well, it can be. It can be a lot of fun. It's what I've been doing for the past couple of months."

At 9:45, she came and got Cookie out of my lap.

"I said I was interested. I said you could make the decision," I said, sounding panicked as she took my therapy dog.

"No, no, actually, you didn't."

"You're such a liar," I deadpanned.

"Oh, Courtney, you're so mixed up, honey."

March 2, 2023

At 5:34 PM, standing in my bedroom door, I started the phone, amusement in my voice.

"I'm gonna beg your forgiveness for what?"

"All your sins," she sighed smugly.

"I've already asked my God," I said, sounding just as smug. "I don't need to ask you."

She stared at me.

"My God's got me," I added.

"I know He does," she said, surprising me.

"I hope He's got you too, 'cause I'm afraid of you on the road."

"Honey, I know He has me."

"Oh yeah?" I interjected hotly.

"I've always known that."

"Okay."

March 6, 2023

At 9:09 AM, getting ready to leave (for work?), she wanted me to do the dishes for her while I was off.

"We are going to sit on this couch till the day we die."

"No, we aren't," I countered, certain that I was about to start getting my life back.

"Yes, we are, obviously, since you won't do the dishes for me. If you can't even do the dishes for me, then I certainly can't pack up, can I?"

I ignored her, knowing I'd do the dishes at my own pace on my day off. But then I said apologetically, "Then you're gonna be evicted."

"I'll live with that."

Clearly, she didn't believe me.

"I'll come back and sit on the couch until I die."

"Okay. Bye, Mama."

She left, leaving the front door wide open to the snow.

That night, I tried to ask her again how Friday (moving day) was going to go. She very calmly explained that she had a storage shed that the movers would be taking all her stuff to.

"Okay. I need the address for the shed to give the movers so we can know what's happening."

"Look up storage sheds—"

"No, YOU!" I said, cutting her off. "You. You pick your storage shed."

She thinned her mouth and leaned back into the couch, ignoring me.

"Mother, I'm not doing this for you. You do understand this is your choice. I did this for you in November. You do understand that, right?"

She continued to ignore me like a child.

"Okay, so this is how this is gonna go on Friday, right?"

"Twenty-First Century Fox," she read.

"Right, you're gonna ignore me?"

"Yep."

"Okay. Well, then..."

March 7, 2023

Mom left the house without the dogs.

March 8, 2023

Mom stood outside my bedroom door and used something to knock down my newly rerigged command hooks lock. She then stood outside and played a song that sang "Pleeeeease release me" while the dogs barked in confusion from the end of my bed. Half an hour later, I ventured out to brave a conversation.

"Ocular dexter that are falling out by the moment," she was saying.

"I don't know what that means."

"That means, in my right eye"—she tapped her left eye—"my eyelashes are falling in..."

"So when the movers get here Friday, you want all this stuff trashed?"

"I'm growing aggressively older, and the grass won't pay no mind."

"Right. That's what I'm hearing?" I asked, trying to bring her back to the present.

"What?" she said innocently.

"So you want all your stuff trashed?"

"No..." She looked around the living room.

"Because I'm not gonna take it."

"I believe I told you that the family was gonna help move stuff."

"But they're not."

"Or that you have a mover."

"I do have a mover. I would like to be able to tell the movers what to do with your stuff. But if you don't have a plan, then I'm going to tell them to trash it."

"That's good."

"So if you don't have a plan for it and you don't have your..."

I gestured, lost for words, and she nodded and said, "Right."

"It's gonna go in the trash."

"That's okay."

"Okay," I said, sounding sad. "So do you remember this is what you did to mine and Jimmy's baby stuff when you moved from Texas to Connecticut?"

"Well, I saved the important cups. The important sterling ones."

"Okay, but you realize you're trying to do this to everything you own? That's what you're trying to do?"

"Yes. Yes." She sounded exhausted. "And sort of live like Jesus."

"Okay. Okay. Good luck. I wish you the best."

March 9, 2023

She went Godzilla on the apartment, dumping over everything I'd managed to pack and breaking every glass item in our kitchen as she chucked them at my head (the first one was a Pyrex glass measuring cup. I ducked.).

March 10, 2023

  I was safely in the new apartment with both dogs. I moved everything she hadn't wrecked as quickly (and expensively) as I could into a studio apartment. I knew when she got out of the hospital (the cops came real fast when I called as she was exploding our kitchen.), she'd need all her stuff, but I was prepared to "store" it until then.

March 11, 2023

  I hadn't watched "Modern Family" since my mom started getting sick because it just relates too much and I somewhat hoped that we'd finish it together when she got better. So I turned it on tonight telling myself that if it was a relatable episode I would keep watching it, and it's freaking spot-on relatable. This is my brother, my sister, and me in this next clip (as adults. Unfortunately we didn't figure this out until later in life.):

HALEY: You know Mom's just gonna want us to apologize.

LUKE: Well, we did kind of ruin her Mother's Day.

HALEY: No. She ruined her Mother's Day. She took us to a place she knew we wouldn't like, and then we complained for like a second, and we're the bad guys?

ALEX: That's a good point. You ever get the feeling she does this intentionally?

LUKE: Why would she do that?

HALEY: So she can make us feel guilty.

ALEX: Exactly. And the next time we're choosing what to do, she gets her way again. And the next time, and the next time, and eventually it's Mother's Day every day.

LUKE: Wow. Mom's really smart.

HALEY: Well, not smarter than me.

ALEX: Well...

HALEY: I say we don't apologize this time. Let her know we're onto her little game.

ALEX: *We could change the way this whole family operates.*
HALEY: *So no one says they're sorry, got it? Keep your mouth shut when she comes back.*
LUKE: *If she comes back...*

March 16, 2023

Wearing a "Lucky Charm" shirt, I sang "Lucky" by Chapin, and then spent a lot of time doing St. Patrick's Day filters, decked out in rainbow sleeves and another Lucky Charms shirt.

March 19, 2023

ME: *Hi, Mom. I don't want to have any more conversations until I heal some. Please respect that. Take care and I hope I'll see you again. I love you more than you can possibly know. And I believe that's true.*
MOM: *I need my Mac and ring. You do not have to talk to me for another decade; I will respect that. But I must have my Mac and ring. Absolute must, no matter how you "feel" about that.*
ME: *I'll contact Rachel to see how to go about getting them to you.*
(*Rachel was a mediator who worked for the state.*)
MOM: *I've already told you, but in any event, please do not make me take you to small claims court.*
ME: *If you feel that's best, go ahead.*
MOM: *Obviously I don't. Can't you just do what I am begging you for a simple twist of change.*
ME: *Absolutely not. I spent two years doing that and still got gutted. So no. If you'd like to take me to small claims court to have a judge tell you that you'd be a hero for paying your family back the $17,000 I bled through in three months. Otherwise, I'd surrender the computer and ring for now and call it a day.*

Have a good night, stay warm and please stay safe.

Mom: *Okay. Talk to you in 2033. Maybe. Don't ask before then.*

Me: *I won't be. But I hope you will. Heal well.*

(A few days later.)

Me: *Hi, Mom. We have a few more things to exchange before you take off on your journey. Are you still at Manchester Inn and Suites; can I make a drop off tomorrow?*

Mom: *Nope I am staying at the Red Roof Inn in New Britain until Thursday waiting for my doctor's appointment. What do I have of yours to "exchange?"*

Me: *Well, nothing I guess. True. Katherine just took some of your clothes home to launder, so I'll get a bin packed and leave it at the front desk of the Red Roof Inn.*

Mom: *Please include all my jewelry but most especially my dolphin wedding ring and my Mac.*

Me: *I still don't know what wedding ring you mean. I will not be including the giant black thing of jewelry. It will not fit in your car. You can utilize my apartment as storage until you're ready to pay movers to get into a storage shed or your own place.*

Mom: *Didn't ask for the black thing, just the jewelry. And I mean the 18-karat gold wedding ring with 3 dolphins on it that I pointed out to you last time I saw you as it was on the kitchen counter. It is priceless to me.*

Me: *Next time something priceless is in the kitchen, don't demolish the kitchen.*

Mom, the next day: *Any idea what time you're "exchanging" my bin of stuff today? I'll work on movers to move all my stuff taking up room in your apartment on my end. Oh, and I'm taking Cookie with me.*

When I didn't reply, she yelled: *Hello. Again any ETA? Courtney, answer my bloody texts. I need* your address and day you can let me and the movers in immediately!

ME: Hello. I'm sorry, I'm at work. Your stuff is in the lobby. I was not able to bring it; enlisted help. Please go retrieve it ASAP so it's not sitting there asking to be stolen.

MOM: Done. But give me your address and date I can move my stuff to storage ASAP. Plus your phone isn't set up for voicemail retrieval.

ME: I can give you the phone number for the moving men you'll need to use, but I will not give you my new address. Marcus and the guys are prepared to move you into whatever storage whenever you're able to pay them. They take Venmo or card over the phone if you want to go ahead and schedule them, Marcus can get in touch with me to schedule my part.

MOM: Okay, give me Marcus's number. Will I need to bring police as well to make sure I can take all my stuff? Left a message for Marcus. No brandishing of knives allowed as I take the large TV, the Boos table, the cedar chest, just as examples. I will leave you your bed. That and a few bookcases.
And Cookie.

ME: I'd prefer a police officer be there. But you're not welcome, so you can give Marcus a list of what he needs to take.

MOM: Nope, I will be there with Marcus. And where is my jewelry? I'll use the hideous necklace you meant for Mom in the meantime.

ME: You're a dick for opening that. A lot of thought went into that.

MOM: Same as all the thought that went into returning my jewelry.

ME: Well, none went into that. When you trash the kitchen and something priceless is there, that priceless object might get lost. It also might be in the black thing with the rest of whatever I could salvage. As I've said, you're more than welcome to leave anything there that's already there. It isn't taking up space and I've managed to make my new place pretty nice.

Mom: You are making this exchange virtually impossible for me. I will be there with Marcus and if you need to call the police, do so. But Courtney, how can I get my stuff if you won't let me?

Me: I am letting you. Not sure what the problem is. Make your list. Marcus will do the work. All he needs is an address to deliver the stuff to. I'd suggest emailing Rachel. I've emailed her as well.

Mom: Okay, any word from Marcus? I've left two messages to no avail. If you would simply hand over my jewelry and Cookie, I will leave you with everything else. If you want me to move it, you will simply need to provide me with your address and I will move it. Otherwise, meet me somewhere with my jewelry (not the black box) and my dog and I will get out of your hair completely for the next decade. Not a promise or a threat. Both I guess. Even Kath agrees I might have to stalk you from work at this point of no return.

Me: Hi, Mom. I have had no word from Marcus, but I'm not the one who's trying to move again. I can "hand over" what jewelry there is to save. I didn't bother making sure there were matches. Cookie is staying with me. You will see me in a custody battle for that.

Mom: Okay. I'll go to court tomorrow while I'm at the doctor appointment and file a claim against you.

Me: Sounds good.

Mom: Coolio. But how do you get me my jewelry?

Me: I won't be getting you anything else. I've done everything I can. A thanks to Katherine for doing your smelly laundry would be nice. I'll mail the jewelry to your next semi-permanent location.

MOM: *Fuck you. I'll include it and all my furniture in my claim tomorrow.*

ME: *Sounds good.*

MOM: *See ya soon, you bloody piece of human waste.*

ME: *Why yes. I'm a piece of yoj.*

MOM: *Yoj? Who is Yoj?*

ME: *You are Yoj. Like what it would be like if you called Jimmy a "son of a bitch." Yep. True too.*

MOM: *Fuck off, you absolutely insane woman. When I get married, you are not invited.*

ME: *Cool. Same.*

MOM: *You will never get married. Hate to say it but you are way too controlling and way too much a bitch for any man to commit to you so that won't be a problem for me.*

ME: *You don't hate to say it. I think you enjoy saying it. I think you're wrong. So do the people I'm in a relationship with. So goodnight, mother. I wish you a safe journey. Good luck at the doc tomorrow.*

MOM: *More to the point, good luck on my filing a quick claim for Cookie, you fucking dog waste. Not even human waste. More like gorilla waste in your fat ass case.*

I am so done with you. Fini. Finished. Never ever ever again. Not 2033 not 2044 not 2055. You just die and I'd be thrilled. Like kill yourself tonight and I will laugh till I die.

I suggest lots of Tylenol PM, plenty of your vape so you fall asleep and slit your wrists. And hang yourself, and I will laugh till the bloody world kerls off its axis!

Keels, not kerls.

I do not know other words to tell you how completely I am done with you, you absolutely clueless bitch. I am getting married very soon and you cannot come to my wedding.

Okay, I hired a lawyer for obtaining all my stuff as well as Cookie. You will be served with a court order as fast as possible at your work.

ME: *Okay, sounds good.*

MOM: *Kath just told me they'll move out everything I list as mine (all the stuff in your apartment) into a storage shed and give me the key. She said they will make sure I get Cookie.*

ME: *Okay, sounds good.*

Hello. Movers are scheduled to be at my house on Sunday. They're using your email so you can go ahead and set up payment with them. If they don't have payment, they will not be there. Again, I wish you safe journeys. And eventually, a calm mind.

April 2, 2023

I spent weeks playing with dogs and filters, healing as best I could. But the hits kept coming.

One filter: "Why are you still single?" It landed on "You're not, you're in a relationship with yourself."

The depression got the better of me today. I spent a lot of time sleeping and a lot of time watching "America's Next Top Model," which was just "pure joy." I planned to do it again on my next day off. I just was not ready to face the real world yet, and it was disheartening. But I'd get there, and I knew it.

April 9, 2023

Another filter flipped by; the game at the top said, "The cause of all my problems is..." The sound playing said, "The cause of all my problems? I am pretty sure that the cause of all my problems is me. Oh well..." The spinner landed on "My parents," which made me laugh.

Then I saved a meme that said, "Someone once said, 'You know you have a big heart when you feel bad for doing what is best for you.' And I felt that."

But I got to go over to Katherine and Fritz's for Easter dinner, and they made me an Easter basket, and we had delicious food, and I felt so overwhelmed with love, I almost felt guilty.

The final piece in my healing journey is learning to let people love me without feeling like I have to repay them. It's really hard.

April 11, 2023

    The dogs and I went over to Melissa's to help her paint. The next day, I got a package from across the pond when my cousin Rosie sent me snacks.

April 16, 2023

    Went to go see Tina with Katherine. If fell flat to us, which was disappointing, but it could have been the size of the theater.

April 29, 2023

    It was a really joyful day despite being filled with uncertainty, and now I'm home with my dogs and... still smiling. I have such a good feeling, so we're just going to go with that. Positive thoughts, prayers, hope, all the good thoughts you can manifest...we'd love it.

May 2, 2023

    I started making a schedule for TikTok and business plans for my coaching business.

May 3, 2023

    We learned that despite our best efforts, including training for an entirely new "Jenny" and being promised we'd all have opportunities, Jenny Craig went massively out of business. They told us with an email. At midnight. I took it very personally, after five years, and I can't imagine how my coach felt, who'd worked there for 22 years.

    "Lights are all off, offices are all empty. We are sad. We are very very sad. We are very sad. Don't give up. You've still got this. There are people out there who can help you. Don't be afraid to ask for help. May come from an unlikely source, but it's there. Love you all."

May 4, 2023

    I made a TikTok of Skipper pictures. "Looking at these pictures and video (look at that smile) just makes my heart so happy when I'm so sad right now. These babies were like my kids, and I'm so thankful to their parents who shared them with me for so long. I may never have any kids of my own, but...just look... look at that. Precious."

May 6, 2023

A third blow on the dandelion filter, this one revealed, "Good news is coming," and I nodded sagely.

May 10, 2023

Spinning filter said, "What is the universe trying to tell you?"
"The universe has my back!"

May 13, 2023

I made my mom a Mother's Day TikTok that she will never see.

May 17, 2023

I made a healthy ham and cheese casserole because of 8OHD on TikTok. (If you don't know him, look him up. He's amazing too.) He's a grow host on TikTok and a mental health technician and nurse. His energy is balm to my soul because he understands how hard it is to deal with mental illnesses. He's like a giant bear hug through the screen.

May 20, 2023, 4:44 PM

Filter for "daily affirmations, do I slay today?"
Answer, "I am the sunshine even when it's raining."
I beamed.

May 25, 2023

Found and fell in love with QueenHayleyBelle on TikTok.

May 27, 2023

Had a panic attack and said I felt like I had nobody, which I knew was untrue. But I woke up in the same anxious mood the next day, and cried for the first two hours.

May 28, 2023

8:39 AM: "Rocking with this girl"—I showed QueenHayleyBelle—"and trying to find some joy because today is Sunday, and tomorrow is a holiday, and I can't do anything till Tuesday anyway! I am dangerously close to having a mental breakdown myself, if I haven't already. But..."

I paused to catch my breath.

"I'm sad. I'm so sad. I'm so sad. And I'm tired. And overwhelmed. And stressed out." My voice broke. "And I have friends on here that keep reaching out to me, and I just want to hug you all. And I can't. So I love you, guys, and thank you for the support, honestly."

I went to get some "stuff" for my nerves, then spent the rest of the day watching musicals.

May 29, 2023

Memorial Day concert and I got to battle DadBod on TikTok, and he kept calling ME a legend!!

June 1, 2023

Pride concert, the comments made me feel like I was starting to get big... I had real trolls!!

BRIXTON: *Your life is sad*

GIDEON: *Okay, I appreciate you too. You make my heart calm down.*

ISIS: *Green lipstick, noooo. Not working out for you!*

(I remember my response to that one: "Did it get you in here? Then I guess it's working fine.")

GIDEON AGAIN: *You are so cute and amazing with a sweet voice. You can send her gifts for this sweet voice. Let's help this live to improve* together. You are wonderful. I fall in love with your music and you are singing. God this woman has a pure voice.

June 2, 2023

I had to stop my live to go throw up. Twice. Then I had tater tots for dinner.

June 3, 2023

Amazing Saturday "concert," my first big gifts, from Paige and Katie.
MEL: That's sooooo awesome
KATIE: Clearly you are loved!! Paige, you picked a lady that deserves good things.
PAIGE: I knew as soon as I swiped on and I waited till the end, she really does deserve them.
KATIE: I agree... something about her.
PAIGE: I think I've been smiling this whole time. I have a few more, but please don't cry love
MELISSA: I love this song.
Paige sends another galaxy (gift on TikTok).
I was on such a high from that show of love, I stayed up late to party with Raynie and Daniel, TeamSouthernLove, for their 100,000th follower. I even got coffee and popcorn, preparing to stay up and have fun with my friends.

June 5, 2023

2:24 PM [I posted a twenty-eight-second video, likely taken right at 2:22.] We had another fantastic live today; I am just so thankful for each and every one of you. And out of 10,000 people, 10,000 friends, I hope I get to know each of you individially. I'm so thankful.
At 5:55 PM, I posted a rainbow meme that said, "I speak my mind because it hurts to bite my tongue."

June 7, 2023

> I'd been spilling my heart in my live to the six or so people in there, and I got banned for hateful speech and bullying again. Starting to panic, I took to a video.
>
> "I don't know if I was bullying myself? If I was, then I'm sorry?"
>
> My voice cracked. "Um, I hope the appeal goes through. I don't want another week of not being able to go live. I don't think I can take it!"

June 8, 2023

> Please do not worry, yesterday's meltdown video was out of pure frustration. I am okay. Suspension sticking though.

June 9, 2023

4:44 PM! I got a little lightheaded for that one. The magic is here.

> You guys, I am on my way to New Haven to see Jeremy Jordan in a concert, and I freaking cannot wait. I think I might be leaving like an hour earlier than I need to be, but I'm almost praying for a little bit of traffic, just so there's a reason for me to leave this early. Ahh, so excited!!
>
> Down in New Haven, I got a shake sprinkled with rainbow for Pride, decked out in my rainbow t-shirt and hoodie. Still early for the show, we walked around Yale campus, admiring the trees.
>
> I took a taboo recording of JJ singing "Bring Him Home" for my mother. Unfortunately, I couldn't show him, but you could hear him okay. My TikTok that night used "Broadway, Here I Come!" (If you haven't seen Smash, I highly recommend changing that! But if you can't find it—it's hard to come by—watch Joyful Noise. Just pure magic.)

June 13, 2023

    We had a crafting-and-movies-in-bed day. Not sure why the depression was getting stronger, but we were tying to overcome.

June 14, 2023

    "We're back. I, like, almost don't know what to do. It's been a really weird week."
    I sing for a few seconds to the song playing on my computer.
    "So we're gonna sing and paint the dresser, and y'all come hang out. I'm almost like nervous. What is wrong with me? Can't wait to see y'all!"

June 16, 2023

    Last Friday, we went wildin' Broadway-style. This Friday, we wildin' from bed with popcorn, coffee, and our shows. If either sounds good to you, won't you be my neighbor? #newenglandvibes

June 17, 2023

    [After giving a Pride concert on TikTok, I was full of confidence.] So y'all wanna know how I know I think I'm ready for…my future person? My forever person? (Or people. Forever people. #allaboutthatpolylife.) I am 100% okay being alone, and I just make myself laugh. And enjoy my own company. I'm really pretty awesome. And after days like today and yesterday, it's nice to feel that again. So thank you to everyone who has participated in helping these last few days.

June 18, 2023

    Father's Day concert on TikTok. Naturally I cried a lot. Then I got banned again, and this time I thought it was the word "hate" itself. This time I was just angry, so sick of being called hateful.

June 19, 2023

  I spent the day sick in bed then went to the first Haven's Harvest Summer Series dinner. I fell completely in love with their mission; it went perfectly with what I wanted to achieve here.

June 21, 2023

  [I posted photos of a beautiful man wearing a Stitch T-shirt and rocking the floral garland gift on TikTok.] Love when handsome, masculine men can be comfortable in their skin. You go, Andre (80HD). Love you big.

June 22, 2023

  "Okay, so I went to the grocery store this morning and..."
  I paused, smiling to myself. "I'm just so hopeful and so excited for what Connecticut is going to bring me now that I'm"—I sighed—"single again. Let's just think of it that way. So we are gonna make color-changing s'mores with white chocolate popping candy. How much more Coco can these get?"

June 26, 2023

  I had the best little surprise in this morning's live; we were talking about manifesting what you wanted, which naturally I believed in all my life, and my Pinterest board is my manifestation. That is my...this is my dreams right here, literally. And so I just jumped in and went to go pin a "New Hampshire's ice cream trail," the name of the pin promoted by "visit New Hampshire." And so I went to go pin it thinking, "Oh my goodness that would be such a fun TikTok trip," like let's take a trip with my people, and went to go pin and my New England board is called New England dreams instead of New England living, which is what I thought it was called, and I'm just so here for it. I've been here for 2 1/2 years, we're going to make this real.

NOT THE F——ING GILMORE GIRLS

June 28, 2023

I used a sound on TikTok: "What you're looking at, baby, is a motherfucking legend in the making!" The CocoPhoenix has risen for the final time.

June 29, 2023

News broke officially that Jenny Craig would be coming back to business. Later that night, I magically bounced in on one of my favorite glow hosts on TikTok (MrTurksDelight), and it happened to be his birthday. I was a big lover of birthdays, so I told him to put up what he wished for, and if I could grant it, I would. He asked, and he received. It was pretty amazing. I was crying; he was crying.

June 30, 2023

Another of my favorite hosts, TheNarrowRoadFamily, became a regular and important part of my day. In one video, I'm whisper-singing along to the music in his room, and I asked, "Why do I whisper-sing when I'm singing along?" Six months later, I can answer that question: I was trying to live small. Always. No matter who it's been for—neighbors, my mother, roommates, or friends—I always tried to be quiet. Sad and stopping today.

At 3:33 PM, I took a screenshot of my answer to a healing song on the Awkward Yeti's Facebook: "Southern Cross" by Crosby, Stills, Nash & Young. I haven't figured out the magic in that song yet, but the time stamp just gave me more faith that it's there.

After listening to this song three times on February 15, 2024, I finally saw my version of the song is four minutes, forty-four seconds. The magic is here!

July 1, 2023

Got banned again, giving a 4th of July concert on TikTok live.

July 2, 2023

My throat hurt, and I wanted someone to live with me again. Be my support. Look at my throat.

July 4, 2023

TikTok, which was sung to the tune of "We Will Rock You," and I lip-synced to, "People like to say I got an attitude, but the vibe I give off really depends on you. What you give you get back, and that is a fact, so if I was a bitch, then you deserve that."

I suppose this was where TikTok began to simultaneously take off and take on a darker side for me. Samantha used the same sound, which was such a thrill for me because I loved her so much. Later, she was a huge bitch to me, and I didn't know what I did to deserve it. I spent months crying about it, wondering what I did wrong. (She wasn't the only friend to abandon me, but I took hers the hardest.) I mourned her with the help of other friends and... my dogs. But again, the hits just kept on coming.

July 7, 2023

I went to New Haven to help package coffee with Haven's Harvest. There were posters in a room that depicted New Reach, a program trying to "end homelessness in Connecticut by making it rare, brief, and one-time."

Later, I saved a meme that said, "Laugh when you can. Apologize when you should. Let go of what you can't change. Kiss slowly. Forgive quickly. Play hard. Take chances. Love with all your heart and have no regrets. Life is too short to be anything but happy."

And another one, "People are often unreasonable, irrational, and self-centered. Forgive them anyway. If you are kind, people may accuse you of selfish, ulterior motives. Be kind anyway. If you are successful, you will win some unfaithful friends and some genuine enemies. Succeed anyway. If you are honest and sincere, people may deceive you. Be honest and sincere anyway. What you spend years creating, others could destroy overnight. Create anyway. If you find serenity and happiness, some may be jealous. Be happy anyway. The good you do today, will often be forgotten. Do good anyway. Give the best you have, and it will never be enough. Give your best anyway. In the final analysis, it is between you and God. It was never between you and them anyway."

July 9, 2023

"Hope this is more noticeable since it's in red. I'm having a little bit of a crisis of faith, which doesn't happen to me very often. I'm..."

My voice broke. "I...I skipped applying for jobs this week, so I don't get $460 from the government because I skipped. I missed it because anxiety. Whatever. I forgot...plain dang forgot. And it's $460 worth of forgetting that I can't afford. It's been suggested that I hold a fundraiser, and while the idea is beautiful, it makes me feel unbelievably guilty because who am I? Who am I to ask for a fundraiser? And then I said, 'You know what? I have things I can sell, myself being the first one, my website, my fingernails, my Color Street, my handwriting, my wreath-making. There's all kinds of things.

"So I'm wondering, if I put this out to my friends and my family who I know have my back on here, can we do some kind of fundraiser? It's trying to get money for me. I'm not gonna sugarcoat it. I'm...well, especially without this $460 check, probably $1,000 short of rent easily that's due tomorrow, or I'm starting to be late. And when I say I have a crisis of faith, God has never failed me ever, and I've never known where it's gonna come from, and that's where the panic comes because this is not...

"I've told everybody this is not gonna be where my money comes from. I'm not trying to make this my job. I'm not...I'm trying to make weight loss coaching my job. I am a weight loss coach. I'm a cheerleader. And I...I can I can sell that. You just gotta sign up for the website. So anybody that you know that's trying to lose weight, anybody that you know that's into fingernails, I'll do my manicure online! All ideas welcome."

July 11, 2023

I cried over Chicago Fire and asked my followers if they got addicted to characters like that. I felt like I was watching my friends' lives unfold. Was that normal?

July 12, 2023

Second Haven's Harvest Summer Supper. On the drive home, "I'm sitting here jamming out to my favorites playlist, which I always kind of think of as being in God's hands because, well, I feel like my whole life is, so I'm listening now."

My voice broke. "And the songs are just so fucking amazing right now, you guys! And I'm sitting here happy-crying because I'm so thankful and so blessed and overwhelmed and tired, and it's been a long, beautiful day again. And it's just stunning, and I just want to say thank you again. And I'm gonna post this before I get in bed, and then I'm going to bed, and then I'm going to be bright-eyed and bushy-tailed for box battles in the morning. So let's freaking go, and thank you all for everything you ever do for me."

July 13, 2023

One of the best lives we'd had. Listen to what this sweet woman Stephanie Lee said about me and my room: 'Great love in this live, and I love it, and your vibes and energy is out of this world. I've never seen you the past three days have any type of negativity, cockiness, bad vibes, nothing. Like, you are honestly an angel, and thank you for allowing everyone to hang out with you. Thank you for allowing everyone to make the coins that they make, whether it's to give back, whether it's to keep for themselves to buy themselves a coffee or a meal or whatever it is.

'Me being home and literally being on bed rest from having knee surgery three days ago (I've been out of work since March, dealing with a torn meniscus, and that's why I had surgery). But honestly, forget about that. I just want to say thank you, and you're absolutely amazing. Don't ever change for anybody because your vibes and energy is honestly just there, dude, like, there. And you are loved. And if you need anything, inbox me. If I can help you with anything, I will.'

The comments scrolling by were magical as well, including those of my beautiful partner-in-crime Amber. People were praising both of us for our hearts, and I'm surprised I wasn't weeping.

July 14, 2023

"At the beginning of this miraculous week—miraculous!—I promised myself that I would listen to myself and listen to my God and listen to my dogs and listen to my body."

I yawned.

"And not overdo it! And so while it's amazing and fun and crazy, I am exhausted! So I went and tried to go into Brandon's room, and when he didn't come live, I passed out. So now I'm gonna go support everyone who was supporting me this morning, and we'll see everyone at 8:00 AM tomorrow morning. Let's go!"

That night, I received a message from someone I wasn't even friends with yet: "Yesterday was my first time in your life, and you said, 'One day at a time, do something fun. It's your choice.' It legit stuck with me. I switched to stay-at-home mom with three kids, and I've never been without work. So I think it was taking a toll on me that I'm just at home all the time, but your words are just so powerful. We did face painting and played soccer yesterday, and we enjoyed ourselves bc of your words."

July 17, 2023

    I had my first "scheduled" battle with the agency on TikTok. I won it, thrillingly.

July 18, 2023

    "So I think I told you, I'm a pretty big numbers person. So 444 is where it started, and Amber said, 'Ooh, I love Coco's angel numbers.' So I looked up what it meant, and it said, 'A sign I'm heading on the right path with the right partner (or partners).' Completely moved, I threw her some roses since she'd become one of my partners. Then while I was marveling over the 444, someone gifted me again and got me to 555, which naturally I had to look up too: 'Changes are underway, so have faith in the adjustments you're making.'
    And then Amber added 'Coco at another angel number' and just thrilled me further. God bless her." (#cocosangels was one of my favorite hashtags. These women [and some amazing men!] became so important to me in a matter of days.)

July 21, 2023

    We hit Rising Stars Number 13 (in the country) for the first time. I was in contact with my leasing office that I'd have the money soon (I still hadn't paid July rent).
    The only reason I'm adding this one was because of the time stamps. Scam-city, but I appreciate my response even now: His name was @anointed_money29 and he started by asking if we could be friends. I replied with "I don't know, can we?" He said "yea I really wanna be your friend. Please don't say no please." So at 4:44 PM (therein lies the magic of course), I replied: "I don't know. I don't know you at all do I. Because of your screen name, I want to say no because honestly I think you're a scammer, but I also am quick to decide and TikTok is a different game, so you'll need to answer that question yourself. I'm a friend to everyone. If I'm mean to you, you deserve it."

In the evening, I took a TikTok with my chewed thumbnail and wrote, "Anxiety. If I don't hold something, I do something to hurt myself. Accidentally. But I know. Get something in your hands." In the next frame, I showed my Smokey and my baby blanket, which always stayed cool, balled up in my left hand.

July 22, 2023

I posted a meme: "One morning she woke up different. Done with trying to figure out who was with her, against her, or walking down the middle because they didn't have the guts to pick a side. She was done with anything that didn't bring her peace. She realized that opinions were a dime a dozen, validation was for parking, and loyalty wasn't a word but a lifestyle. It was the day after that her life changed. And not because of a man or a job but because she realized that life is way too short to leave the key to your happiness in someone else's pocket."

July 23, 2023

I got an emergency text at 2:43 AM, from Chantal, who I barely knew yet, but I trusted and loved already... "SOS!!! I need Amber Lee's number. Smitty took pills and we need to make sure he is ok. Does she have his number? I'm on the phone with Chelle."

I wrote back that I'd texted Amber, then I spent some time searching rooms of people who were live on TikTok to see if I could get anymore information. I didn't know Smitty yet either, but I had been watching Chelle because she had some crazy tendencies and had been known to lie.

It turned out to be true, and the scare brought me and my "sisters," or "Angels," closer together. We got to know Smitty and he became super important to me too. But all that glitters is not gold.

That evening, I saved this meme: "She is the Phoenix who has risen from the ashes to which she has been reduced...this time wiser, stronger, and more powerful in her own right. She is the fire, looking for someone to warm...to enlighten...but never to burn... she is a bird in flight, that one can only see if they believe in her... she cries tears that can heal wounded hearts, sounds, and bodies... in her rising she is cautious and aware of her own vulnerability...yet still just as inquisitive and observant as she ever was... she is a little dark and very mysterious...and overlooks nothing...contrary to the shallow minds of the world... she is alive... she does exist... she is the Phoenix... and she has risen again..."

July 26, 2023

    I made a short TikTok chanting, "Let's go, Rangers, let's go."

July 28, 2023

    I stared blankly for a second, smiling vacantly.
    "We were up late. Toxic bock battlesss...yep. Need to help...yep. I'm sleepy."
    "My words do not exist yet" were typed across the screen.
    After my own live, I sent GoGang (MrTurksDelight) a Leon the Kitten, and I wish you could hear this in his accent. (Actually, you can if you go follow me on TikTok! Have I even said that yet? CocoPhoenix1313.)
    "Oh my gosh! Coco! Oh my God, what is going on today, people?"
    His hand covered his eyes, overwhelmed and excited.
    "No! No! You guys are gonna make me cry again. Man, I don't like crying, bruh. Don't make me cry. I can't believe it! I can't believe what's going on today."
    He raised his hands, utterly perplexed.
    "Please, someone say you screen-recorded that. My heart's beating bro. Oh my God. Oh my God, Coco."

I laughed, totally peaceful.

"CoCOOOOOO!"

He makes a Leo the Lion growl face, and I laughed harder.

July 29, 2023

I danced to Amber Lee's music while she ran her live. Then I had a blast in Brandon's live, dancing to Meghan Trainor. Next, I made a video that said, "I'll hear it. Also, remember, actions speak louder than words." And I used Gwen Stefani's "I heard that you were talking shit, and you didn't think that I would hear it."

This was where I really started getting cocky. We were making money. People were hearing about us. I had real supporters. All was glittering. Still...

August 3, 2023

My grandma died, which was neither a surprise nor terribly sad for me. The sad part came in not being there for my mom, who called me for the first time in months and hung up before I could answer. I believed that was her way of telling me Grandma died.

My aunt Katherine wrote a eulogy on Facebook.

"After a tough 10 days post-fall / broken hip, my mother passed away early this morning in California at the age of 95. My siblings and I had been by her side 24/7 and my sister Beth was with her the moment she struck out for the territory ahead. She was a complicated woman, a lifelong republican, full of piss and vinegar, humor and sarcasm, love of country and family. She was a force, teaching her children tolerance, open-mindedness, and table manners. She will be missed for her spicy attitude toward life and her trenchant observations about the world. RIP Marie-Ruth."

August 4, 2023

On my live that morning, I got super dizzy and felt sick. One of the people in my live, Jiggy, who had become a really good friend, was a traveling nurse, and he came up into a box to talk to me about my symptoms. They made me go to urgent care, who in turn sent me to the ER so I could avoid the eighty-dollar charge.

I started to panic almost instantly despite the emptiness of the waiting room, and I had to breathe myself through it. The nurses there were very kind (Manchester Memorial Hospital), and everything went wildly smoothly despite the ER Internet being down, like we were in an episode of Grey's.

One of my nurses was named Samantha, and Samantha Eve, whom I considered my head angel, was the only person I stayed in constant contact with while I was in the ER. It felt good to know people cared about me and were concerned.

August 8, 2023

A TikTok filter asked what I was made for and answered, "Encouraging dreams. Embracing life's beauty. Bringing warmth. And encouraging dreams endlessly."

Ugh, this was where it started to get ugly. A girl I had been watching, someone being accused of being fake and a scammer, came into my live and tried to start some stuff. I messaged her on Facebook.

"Hey, chica. You doing okay? Some people mentioned you might have been having a rough morning. Hope you're okay, and you know you're always welcome in there."

She answered, "I am actually not okay. I came in and was commenting and didn't know if anyone saw me because nobody said anything, so I felt unwelcome. It hurt my feelings a little. But what hurt me even more is the fact how you talked about me when I left."

My head spun from that one, and I thought back over the morning. Never one to talk about people behind their backs, I knew she had either lurked outside the room and made up her own conclusions, or someone inside the room took what I said and twisted my words.

So I said, "Aw, I'm sorry you felt unwelcome. Sometimes, we miss chat. It doesn't mean you're unwelcome. I don't know what you heard was said, but I wouldn't say anything behind your back that I wouldn't say to your face."

It blossomed until I was being called a bully and rude, and I made an angry video.

"Most of the times when I make a video like this, I'd tag my family. I'm not gonna do that this time. This one hurt me. And I'm gonna sing about it. The next time anyone wants to come for me or my family? Do it to our face."

I shrugged, my anger apparent.

"I have always said I would never say anything behind your back that I wouldn't say to your face. If you're feeling unwelcome in my room, there's a reason. So hold that mirror up. Question what you might be doing, because all we are"—I drummed on my chest—"in my room is a reflection of the energy that you give off. That's it. We. Are a. Reflection of you. Got it?"

I winked angrily and started the music, "Rumor Has It" by Adele.

Later that evening, I posted, "Jesus answered, 'Most certainly I tell you, unless one is born of water and spirit, he can't enter into God's kingdom!'" I added, "It's not often I feel led to post 'God' things. It's just never been the way I choose to lead, because it almost feels cocky. 'I have God, ha!' But y'all. This. Weekend. Through today. Has been. A battle. So. Warrior up. Always."

Comments appeared on the video that said things like, "Done what to myself?? This is childish."

I recorded my reply: "Do you really want me to continue to address this, my dear? 'Cause I will. But like I said, I prefer you do it face to face. This"—I circled my hand to indicate social media battling—"is childish. This"—I circled my hand again—"is silly. I will be live tomorrow morning at 7:30 eastern if you care to have a conversation with us. We will see you there. Or we won't. Good night."

One guess if she ever came to talk to me like an adult.

August 9, 2023

The haters kept on coming. We kept getting hits from unexpected places.

August 10, 2023

I took the day off to listen to music and sing, and in the afternoon, I posted a happy video that said, "It's a wonder what a day by myself with my music and my God will do for me. New adventures await. If you want to see me, drop your state in the comments!"

This was where I started seriously thinking about driving to California for Grandma's funeral. I had received my eviction notice, and I dreamed of putting all my stuff in storage and getting on the road for a few weeks. Driving across the country had already been a bucket list item of mine, but I really wanted to have an RV. But nothing sounded better to me at the time than me, my dogs, and the open road.

August 14, 2023

TikTok put me on a shadow ban for "bullying." Apparently I received multiple complaints against me. My agent advised me to wait it out, quit talking about the drama on my live, and try to get back to normal. I tried.

Somewhere around here was when I lost most of my "family." People I'd considered sisters and brothers, exchanged I love yous, songs, tears, and laughs with, completely abandoned me. Jamie made it seem like they thought I was having a breakdown, and I kept asking for them to prove it, show me what I'm doing. And no one could. Not a single person had a screen shot or a recording, any other form of proof. My ride-or-dies suddenly blocked me and wouldn't speak to me in other lives, and I felt hopeless and sadder than I'd been in months.

But it was when I started fielding questions from other hurt people that I got angry. The exact thing we'd been trying to avoid, these people who preached mental health and love for everyone were suddenly at the center of it, and I hated them for it. Their "love yous" and "this family is so awesomes" suddenly sounded hollow and fake. They were nothing but the high school mean girls (men included) and they sucked.

August 25, 2023

One of the people I'd considered family who had been helping spread the rumors, which by then I had learned was that I was reporting people's profiles and getting them banned, came in the live to say that he was sorry and that he loved my face.

Later, I used TikTok magic to contact a guy I'd dated when I'd first moved to Connecticut and always had a sense of unease about the end of our friendship. While we were dating, I had huge dreams of what my TikTok channel could be with him, but he was sorely lacking in other ways. So to protect my heart, I completely wrote him off. But not a day went by where I didn't think of him, so I began laying the bricks to build my dream house.

Luci, a TikTok chum who lived in Connecticut, got in contact with him as a client. He contacted me, and I tried to get him interested in building his business on TikTok. Knowing Sean the way I did, my anxiety stayed high despite his enthusiasm in the beginning.

Late that night, I saved a meme that said, "You should be flattered. There was a group effort to take you down, and you are still standing."

August 26, 2023

    I posted a meme: "This is your life. You are the only one who decides how it goes. You are the only one who can give yourself the joy, the love, the hope, the money, the experience, and the existence you crave. You are not stuck, you only think you are stuck. You are not broken, you only think you are broken. Everything you judge, everything you see, everything you interpret, everything you fear is all a projection. This is your life, and if you want to change it, the first step is realizing that you had the power all along. The first step is saying: I am willing to see this change." By Brianna Wiest.

August 27, 2023

    I posted another meme: "Please understand this: Bad chapters can still create great stories. Wrong paths can still lead to right places. Failed dreams can still create successful people. Sometimes it takes losing yourself to find yourself."

August 29, 2023

    "Our generation thinks it's cool not to care. It's not. Effort is cool. Caring is cool. Staying loyal is cool. Try it out." —Post Malone

    That evening, I was hanging out in JR the Truth's room. Then I went over to Shady's. A phone number I didn't know called, and I ignored it. JR texted me and said, "Call me. You're being challenged." Penelope, someone I'd once considered a friend, was throwing down the gauntlet, and I didn't have the stomach for it. So I wrote back, "LOL. How did you get my number? That challenge wasn't friendly, and I'm a little bothered that you didn't see that. Love you, and I'll be supporting you, but I'm not ready for a battle against someone I called family."

    He answered, "I'm a nobody with nice hair. I have my ways of getting VIP contacts. And np. It was an exhibition match."

From that point forward, I no longer felt comfortable in JR's room either. And in a few weeks, he would block me too, along with a whole new slew of people.

August 30, 2023

I posted a meme: "And suddenly, you know... It's time to start something new and trust the magic of beginnings."

I posted on Facebook: So much this. People need connection. And they don't care about your clutter or mess, you live there, like really live. Queso is Always a meal. "Could we please bring back the lost art of the simple get-together? Fancy dinners are great. Themed nights are so fun, but it is hard to plan that stuff. As a whole, we're really not craving over-the-top celebrations. We're craving connections, but we've gotta make it easier and lower the expectations. Lower. Nope. Even lower.

"So invite some neighbors to hang out in lawn chairs. Get out a pack of cards. Throw down your leftover Christmas paper plates, shove the clothes and toys scattered around in a coat closet, light a candle, and call it good. It doesn't need to be Instagram-worthy to be worthy. Being together is enough. Love, Amy. Also queso is a whole meal. I said what I said."

Later, I posted a meme: "The body can literally reject someone's energy. Your anxiety will start acting up anytime bad energy disturbs your spirit. Listen to your body."

And this one: "How empaths can trigger people: Empaths can truly be hated simply because, without intending to, they can energetically mirror back the entire inner angst and lack of personal integrity of another, exposing an unwillingness to face their own dishonesty, greed, hatred, and desire to hide from the truth as well as from themselves. This can happen completely outside the empath's conscious awareness as they tend to keep sending out light which can irritate another's demons while being perplexed at the reactions. It can literally drive those who thrive on inauthenticity out of their minds."

August 31, 2023

The day I realized I still had some real friends, I ventured into Whiskey Dadbod's live just to say good morning, knowing there would be people in there who disliked me now. Amber Lee was up in his boxes, and I scampered out almost as quickly as I had gone in, unable to bear her sweet voice when she wasn't speaking to me. About half an hour later, I was running my own live, and Whiskey showed up and sent me a message that said, "I really, really hope that what happened this morning wasn't true. I've stayed very neutral during all this, and to use my live to do that makes me really upset. I don't care whatever is going on between all of you guys, but please never, never use my platform to do something like that."

Moritified and obviously having no idea what he was talking about, I panicked.

"Whiskey, what do you mean? What happened?" I asked in my live.

He wrote in the chat. "Amber Lee got banned right after you'd been there."

I assured him it wasn't me, and for my own peace of mind, I texted my agent, who was also Amber's agent, and she told me she hadn't gotten banned. So there were two lies being told.

To add insult to injury, someone came in and said, "Someone said you were talking rude about Brandon."

I made the literally hardest eye roll ever. That one I simply blocked and ignored, grinning the whole time. I was done letting the haters get to me. I had lost friends and family and survived it; let the trolls come.

I shared something written by Cody Bret on Facebook: "If you can take the person I'm in a relationship with, please take them. If you can ruin my friendships with a rumor, do me a favor and please ruin them. If you can shake anything against me in my life, please do it. I don't have the time and energy to fight for things that are easily persuaded. If it doesn't bring me peace, fulfillment and love, I didn't have any room for it in my life to begin with."

I posted another meme: "Life might be unfolding much differently than you had thought, but don't let that ruin your mood. Your new path has the potential to be more amazing than anything you could imagine."

To cap off another yucky family drama day, Cristina, a sweet young woman taking care of her ill mother, messaged me.

"I just feel like Samantha and them are mad at me or something. Not that it matters, but they haven't been spreading love to me, so I stopped giving to them. It's whatever. I'm not guna pick sides between them and you. I have nothing against you, and u haven't done anything to hurt me."

I wrote back, "I did nothing to hurt them either, my love. I'm very sorry to hear they're doing that to you. They've gotten very cliquish and it's gross. But please protect your heart. If it's any consolation to you, we miss you a lot in my room. I lost a lot of 'family' over the rumors going around, none of which are true. I managed to get one squashed before it started this morning, so that's fun. Social media sucks. Don't be afraid to take a breather."

September 1, 2023

Meme: "I make like a friendship farmer and fertilize all my easy, joyful friendships. The other ones? Well...nature can decide what to do with those."

I posted a meme: "Have you ever gotten in a fight with someone because you told them what was bothering you and instead of them apologizing, they find a way to make you feel bad about it? So you are left regretting even saying anything."

I posted another meme: "You get to a point in life where you don't care who's mad, why they're mad, and who all they are recruiting to be mad with them. It's peaceful over here."

I posted a meme of a hippie in flowers cartoon: "I'm mostly peace, love, and light...and a little go f*&$ yourself."

"A bottle of water can be .50 cents at a supermarket. $2 at the gym. $3 at the movies and $6 on a plane. Same water. Only thing that changed its value was the place. So the next time you feel your worth is nothing, maybe you're at the wrong place." —Kobi Simmons

September 3, 2023

Queen Hayley Belle was hosting boxes, and I popped in to say hi and she invited me up. I don't know if the prayer that she'd ask me to sing "Power of Love" came before or after she asked me into the boxes, but either way, it was answered. Performing in front of 56+ people in a room that was not my own was insanely exciting.

September 4, 2023

Whiskey called to tell me about the Labor Day "meet-up" in South Carolina that I was supposed to have been at, but 90% of the people hated me now. I don't remember how we got upon the subject, but he said there was someone he'd talked to who wanted to make amends with me. I knew without a doubt it was Amber Lee, and I learned she hadn't even gone up to SC, but she had told Whiskey how much she missed me and our talks. I felt so happy, and later that night, she unblocked me on TikTok and messaged me a sweet, short message. I responded in kind, and that's all it took to know she was my friend again.

September 6, 2023

    I was supposed to get on the road to Cali today, but something made me wait one more day. Instead, I did errands and received horribly sad news.

    I was driving home when MamaMoose, one of the "sisters" who'd completely shunned me, called. I panicked, thinking I was about to be put on the air on a TikTok live joke, and I braced for the worst when I answered, "Hello."

"Coco, I have some bad news."

"What," I said, filled with dread.

"Amber Lee was in a car wreck. She didn't make it."

    Nothing could have prepared me for that, and I stuck with the "TikTok live joke" theory. I was silent, my head spinning, wondering if I could have really finally gotten into the darkest side of social media. Who lied about shit like this?? "Sydney, are you kidding?"

"No," she answered, and I heard the truth and burst into tears. She soothed me for a couple moments, and by the end of the call I had hope that as sad as it was, Amber's death would be the glue that brought us back together.

    At 4:43, she texted from a number that had blocked me: "Make sure not to say anything on TikTok yet. Tay doesnt want it on TikTok yet."

    And at 4:44, my Angel girl, I wrote that the rumor mill had already started. I cannot believe what this family went through on TikTok... can you imagine what Kobe Bryant's family went through? Or Matthew Perry's?

September 7, 2023

    I woke up like normal, shockingly. My eyes were swollen into red folds, and I made a video, hoping the crew would come mourn with me as I drove to California (when I'd first started planning this trip, Amber was going to be my eyes as I drove. She was my number one mod, I trusted her implicitly, which is why it hurt so much when she'd given over to the rumor mill. But all that mattered to me anymore was that she and I had spoken the day before, and we were good. I thought of her as being my eyes from Heaven, my true guardian Angel, and I cried a lot in those first few hours.). But they didn't.

I had a few "faithful" friends (put in quotes cause they've since jumped ship too) that rode with me, listening to me sing and trying to drive the room. It didn't work very well, but I made enough to stay in a Hilton that night, and when we got to Pittsburgh, there was the most perfect double rainbow you could ever imagine over the hotel. I freaked out live on camera, constantly shocked by God's promises.

September 8, 2023

I started the day by singing "Power of Love" in the hotel parking lot, and we got on the road early:

"It's only 7:35, which is only a couple minutes later than I normally would have gone live, so... our normal life is progressing...which is a little bit shocking. We have about eight hours, nine hours, in the car again, so come in and enjoy some boxes and music and friends and support."

I did more "Power of Love" at a rest stop and then got to Paris, Ohio, before five. As I chilled with the dogs, I saved my Bible verse from the day: "I tell you, keep asking, and it will be given you. Keep seeking, and you will find. Keep knocking, and it will be opened to you."

Bank balance included "777." One of the suggestions if you kept seeing that number was to slow down and enjoy your journey.

September 9, 2023

I did another "Power of Love" performance for the morning crowd: Today is a ten and a half hour drive, y'all.

NOT THE F——ING GILMORE GIRLS

My angel in my head, I decided to pull off for my first solo sightseeing. My live had ended (I don't remember if it was on purpose or if it was signal-related), but the allure of the World's Largest Gift Shop and Candy Factory was too good.

"First of all, y'all would never believe how it smells in here," I started, showing bins of taffy in any dreamable flavor: vanilla, carrot cake, apple pie, popcorn, pickle...

"This is gorgeous. Berries and cream, caramel apple—this is amazing. I feel like I'm going too fast to see it in the video, but... Eggnog. Are you kidding? Blueberry muffin. Oh my God."

I continued around the tables, in awe. There was peanut brittle and fudge and more, oh my! Cotton candy in a thousand flavors. A wall of regular candy. Bins of retired candy. An entire cooler devoted to food-flavored sodas. And an insanely gorgeous bathroom, which I was not the only person photographing.

Even with that stop, I made it to Oklahoma while it was still light outside. My air-conditioner had given out somewhere in Missouri, and my poor car, dogs, and I had battled nearly one-hundred-degree heat for a few hours. We got Whataburger for dinner, which we all but inhaled, and marveled that there was a weed store next door.

In the evening, I checked in with Brandon, who'd loved Amber. He said he was doing okay, that a lot of stuff outside of Amber had been going on. Since we were still in the same agency, I asked if he'd keep me updated if he heard anything, that he and a few of his mods were the only people I still trusted.

He replied, "At this point, Coco, don't trust anyone but yourself," which alarmed me, but I still listened to my gut. I never had a reason to distrust him. But I'd keep my eyes open.

September 10, 2023

Per usual, I started off with the song in the parking lot, then jumped in to Queen Hayley's live to say good morning to her before getting on the road. She was doing my song and I knew it meant our journey was safe.

Also, Venmo balance was $44.44.

I put up a background with Amber's face in the corner, and said everything that I made on top of what it took to get me home would be going to her husband for the funeral. I caused an uproar, and when I got to my destination, I had 75 texts.

My left arm and neck got mega-sunburned, despite me trying to keep my arm covered.

September 11, 2023

On the road again, I tried using the same picture and caused an even worse uproar. I thought I'd gotten "okay" with Amber's husband, and he knew my heart and my intention, but it didn't matter. I was the bad guy for "using" Amber's image for my gain.

I also had a pretty huge misunderstanding with my aunt, which resulted in me deciding to camp rather than stay in a hotel. Having made great time, we were now in Arizona with quite a bit of time to kill. Flagstaff was gorgeous, and a quick storm broke the heat by ten degrees, and we spent three glorious days doing nothing but reading and trying to heal.

September 13, 2023

I posted a meme: "Imagine being bitten by a snake and instead of trying to help yourself heal and recover from the poison, you're trying to catch the snake to find out the reason it bit you and to prove that you didn't deserve that."

September 14, 2023

> We made it to Cali thanks to my brother, who had to come to my rescue because gas prices nearly doubled when I hit California. I felt even more sick after that. Always the one needing to be rescued, why couldn't I have just made enough to cross the country all the way?
>
> The beach was beautiful and the smile was real, even if the heart was bruised.

September 15, 2023

> I posted a video saying I was going to go live, but I never did on the west coast. I took a much-needed mental health break and stayed almost completely off the app for two weeks.

September 16, 2023

> I posted the verse from my Bible app: "For I consider that the sufferings of this present time are not worthy to be compared with the glory which will be revealed toward us."
>
> I posted a meme: "I am too busy smoking my own grass to notice if yours is any greener."
>
> Grandma's funeral was in the morning, and we went over to Uncle Jimmy and Aunt Helen's for the reception. Their backyard was amazing, and at 12:22, I was taking footage of it.
>
> A bunch of us gave speeches about Grandma, some of which were funny, some poignant. Susan started them off as the oldest daughter of the departed.
>
> "When she was twenty-three years old, she was in Austria. She couldn't speak basically a word of German. She could say 'Danke,' and that's about it. She was married to a man who, you know, belonged to the US Army. He was never home. He was certainly not home when she had me. Um, tended by a couple of amateur doctors. I mean, they weren't fully qualified."
>
> Someone asked if they were German.

"No, they were military doctors, and does the military really need ob-gyns?"

We laughed as she continued fondly.

Katherine went next.

"She went by a lot of names, and she was a different person to each one of us, and we each have our own memories. You know, the grandchildren did not have a traditional grandmother..."

Next were Ben and Asher, some of Grandma's great-grandkids. They made us all laugh.

At 3:33 pm, it was Ryan's turn, and he had the traditional Grandma stories. He also had some adventure stories about Grandma snorkeling in Hawaii.

"Grandma was always down to do it. She was always ready to go. On the cruise, I saw Grandma in her underwear. Grandma in a white T-shirt. That's not something a grandchild should ever see. Grandma always said we are all here because of her. To Grandma, we are all here because of you."

Jimmy went next.

"I am the oldest grandson. I didn't live the closest to her, and I didn't know her the longest, but she probably cared about me the most, so..."

We all laughed again as he continued, talking about our family taco recipe, which had evolved since Grandma started it, and his most prized possession, a dagger our grandpa Jim had owned.

Auntie Elizabeth was up, third in line of daughters.

"Mom was one of my best friends. It took a while to get there, but it was worth the wait. We talked about politics and the state of the world. I got to hear about her first orgasm with Jim. It made me squirm. But I suffered through it."

Kevin, the second-oldest grandson and dad to Asher and Ben, went next.

"My first memory of Grandma, I was staying at her house all alone. I have no idea why. Probably six, seven, eight years old. Um, that house was pretty scary. It had Jim's haunted room in the back..."

Jimmy, Grandma's only son and the youngest child, said emotionally to Beth,

"You say that she was your best friend. She saved me."

He shrugged, picking at his hand. He continued, also making us all laugh through the tears.

"I'll tell ya, I wouldn't have what I have today if it weren't for her."

"Why?" Katherine interjected.

"'Cause she was strong, she was smart, she had a wicked sense of humor, she was engaging, she was charming when she wanted to be, but she was as tough as anybody you've ever met."

And finally, Alie, as one of the youngest grandkids, wrapped up the show.

"I just think we should all take a step back and look at how amazing our family is. We haven't done this gathering in years, and Thanksgiving is her favorite time for us all to get together. She's made some and raised some really amazing women and my dad, and we're all so strong together. And cousins-wise, like, we are all very strong individuals. So I just wanted to toast to that."

I spent as much time as I could hogging my baby cousin Dani. We all picked paperweights, and the sisters exchanged jewelry, some of which the grandchildren absconded off with. It was a pretty good day, a true celebration of life in the only way she would have wanted it, with her family, except my mother, whose absence I felt like a splinter in my heart.

On the drive home to the Airbnb, my car began choking. I ignored it, praying it was just tired, praying it would at least get me back to the beach house. It did, and then it completely gave up the goat when Katherine and Fritz tried to take it for dinner the next day. Naturally, I was relieved it happened then and not on the road somewhere but again mortified that I had to be rescued. My uncle Frank came to check it out, couldn't get it started, and had it towed to a shop he liked.

They fixed it, and I got back on the road and almost died on a hill in Thousand Oaks. Of course I was in the left lane, and of course it was rush hour. When my car wouldn't go above forty, I flashed my hazards to warn people, switched on my blinker, stuck my arm out, and prayed real hard as I crossed five lines of California traffic and basically let the truckers push me into a weigh station, where I stopped my car and burst into frustrated tears. When I called Frank, he knew exactly where I was and came to my rescue a second time.

Finally, finally, I was back on the road, with a thankful heart—my aunt Margaret had yelled at me about some of my recent life choices, and while it was shocking to know someone still cared, it felt really good—and a healthy car.

September 21, 2023

On Copper Mountain near Vail, I hit traffic for the first time in 4,233 miles, literally. I was nervous because of my angle and anxious to get to my dad's, whom I hadn't seen in a really long time and had barely spoken to that past couple of years. But that still small voice had told me to visit him, that he was getting older, and who knew what could happen? My brother had told him not to discuss politics, and we would be fine, and it was true. We had a great time. We even met Lisa, Matt, and Allie for dinner at Chuy's, a little taste of Texas.

September 22, 2023

I posted a quote from my motivation app: "You've never needed someone to complete you. You just needed someone to remind you how amazingly complete you already are."

"A healthy relationship is one where two independent people just make a deal that they will help make the other person be the best version of themselves."—Lewis Howes

I posted the verse from my Bible app: "The Lord is my strength and my shield. My heart has trusted in him, and I am helped. Therefore my heart greatly rejoices. With my song I will thank him."

September 23, 2023

I was on the road again. I just told my dad about birds' uncanny ability to poop right in the center of my vision on my windshield. No sooner had I gotten back on the road after my first gas stop than those abilities were proven.

At 5:55 pm, I received a text saying "You can do it" in response to me saying, "It's gonna be a twelve-hour shift tomorrow. But it'll make my drive home eight hours, and that sounds amazing. I can do it."

I stayed at a Kansas City KOA that night, newly addicted to car camping. There was a storm just as we stopped. Then it was gorgeous.

September 26, 2023

I shared a tweet from @Theminis: "I don't think young ppl realize just how hard it is for millennials of a certain age to refrain from posting song lyrics as cryptic emotional status updates."

September 29, 2023

Karaoke to "Crowded Table" by the Highwomen.
5:55 PM: I saved a bunch of "autumn" pictures, still high from the road trip camping weather

October 1, 2023

Karaoked "Handle with Care," my new theme song, for my "series" "Dear Future Person" on TikTok.

I saved a meme that resonated with my constantly grounded teenage heart: "A therapist said if you self isolate when overwhelmed you probably had to solve a lot of your problems alone as a child."

October 2, 2023

> "May all that has been reduced to noise in you, become music again."

Writing my life story has me in all the emotions.

October 4, 2023

I shared a quote from Pinterest: "I wonder how many people believe that I'm a horrible person, because a horrible person said so."

October 5, 2023

"One year from now, I want to be able to look back at my life and say, 'Girl, you really did believe in yourself & it worked.'"

I shared a cartoon of a bunny and a unicorn sitting on a log, the bunny holding his paws out with sparkles in them: "Here, you can borrow my belief in you, until you can find yours again."

October 9, 2023

And along came the magic we will call Papa Bear. Upon returning from my road trip, I was so sure I knew what I wanted, so sure that God was in charge completely, that I gave my number to him easily. After he texted me, we got into "life goals" quickly, as you do with online dating, and I told him my "ultimate dream": Throw every extra cent to a down payment (or whole amount?!) for the RV. Use the RV to move around the country, camp, and visit people for about six months. Then be back in CT with hopefully another down payment for my house, where I'd love to spend autumn of next year and every year after. We will see when it happens.

PAPA BEAR: I love that dream!! It all starts with a positive attitude and a degree to achieve your goal. I'm guessing full-time employment will help you achieve your dream faster. I wish you all the love and luck in the world!

"Lol well thank you! My TikTok platform is all about manifesting so... What about you?"

"I enjoy watching TikTok vids. What do you like to do for for fun? And more importantly, what are your plans this evening?"

I admired his language so much. We continued texting flirtatiously...

October 10, 2023

I asked, "For argument's sake, let's say I'm talking to someone else who I think might be a much better fit for the future. But I want to hear about your life anyway. Are you in the market for friends for life?"

"Yes, sweetie," he assured me, immediately putting me at peace even through text. "Being friends is serious and real for me. I don't take it lightly. So many fakes, flakes, and backstabbers and selfish people who only care about themselves. I like to consider myself true friend material. Just has to be fifty-fifty."

Later, he asked me to meet him for drinks and trivia the next night. We started throwing out ideas for team names, and something he suggested rubbed me the wrong way, and I let him know. After a few more minutes of banter, I was honest with him.

"Look, I'm kind of having a bit of a panic attack. I expected the sense of humor reply when I said no. But now I'm worried that something I do tomorrow is going to bug you, and I'm going to spin out, and I might not be altogether ready to meet in person yet. LOL."

"Okay, quick observation," he said, "you're a severe overthinker. It's okay not to know what to say. Be yourself."

October 11, 2023

We had a great time on our first date at a bar to watch a Latin jazz band, even with my panic attack when the money I moved to my bank account immediately evaporated into waiting bills, leaving me broke for the night. He was so sweet when I told him; he put his hand on my knee and told me not to worry about anything for the night.

October 12, 2023

    Karaoked "Maybe This Time" for my TikTok Series.

October 13, 2023

    Papa Bear replied to my "Depression sucks."
    "I'd like you to seriously start declutterring your place. By having a clean and organized space that is decluttered, it will do wonders for your mental health and allow you to be more organized for your social media efforts and also increase your pride in yourself. Think about it. You need to make some decisions about things you need and things you don't need."
    What he didn't know, because I still had stuffed animals from my childhood, was this was the essentials. I had streamlined again and again in an effort to live as small as I could. Those stuffies, as he called them, had been in my car for three years; they were only inside now because I had just returned from a road trip.
    "No," I said, for the first time feeling like that would be the end, and I would push him away by standing up for myself. "You are not going to come in here and tell me to get rid of the one thing of my childhood I think well of. Sorry."
    "Okay. I get it. Can you keep two or three of them perhaps? The most special ones. And keep those two or three in your bed so you interact with them daily, a healthy reminder of the past," he suggested.
    "No. Sorry, but this is not the conversation for you to have with me. We can revisit if you're still a part of my life when I find my permanent place of residence," I said firmly.
    "Okay, sweetie. Didn't mean to trigger you or give you shame. Just trying to give you helpful ideas from an outsider perspective."

NOT THE F——ING GILMORE GIRLS

October 14, 2023

I went over early in the morning that Saturday to help him take some loads to his new place. His mood was dark, and the energy in the apartment was black (he was leaving a relationship), but I muscled through, Bonnie's and Laurin's voices in my head from the first year I met them: "That's what friends do."

We did a good amount, and when we left the apartment, his energy changed immediately. My heart lightened, and unloading at his new house was really fun. We ran a few more errands before I went home, and I kept praying he didn't offer me money for helping him despite his knowledge of my finances. But that was exactly what he did, and his explanation when I had a panic attack (as silently as I could manage) was so perfect: "Friends help each other out, right? You helped me move. Can I not help you by paying for your gas and dog food?" He was so right, of course.

That night, after I was home, I sent him a long text.

"I'm afraid I'm gonna ruin this before it even starts. That's why I keep having panic attacks. I'm 100 percent convinced I'm gonna do something that's gonna irritate you enough you're not gonna talk to me anymore. I need you to know it's been pretty awesome to be able to hang out with you without having to talk constantly. I feel safe with you, and this is all me. So please, please…just be patient."

He replied kindly, saying, "You're fine! I do have patience. Try not to get worked up or overthink anything. I'm a laid-back, easygoing guy. If you can be just as chill and laid-back and cool, we'll get along fine."

October 15, 2023

Karaoked "Bad Reputation" for Episode Three.
I posted a meme: "It's not unusual for an abuse survivor to be enormously sensitive to things like

someone's tone of voice, a look in their eyes, or tiny quirks of body language. They've learned avoiding tornadoes is about detecting the smallest shift in the wind as early as possible."

"Sometimes even the thought of being rejected is so upsetting to trauma survivors that we quit asking for things or expressing what we need or want. It's not even that we think we'll actually be rejected—it's that the thought is so upsetting we slam into freeze/flee mode." —Dr. Glenn Patrick Doyle, @DrDoyleSays

October 16, 2023

I posted a meme: "I like clingy people. I would rather have someone who blows up my phone and shows that they care than someone who texts back 10 hours later."

October 17, 2023

I posted the verse from my Bible app: "A man's heart plans his course, but the Lord directs his steps." Karaoked "You'll Accomp'ny Me" for Episode Four.

October 19, 2023

@DrDoyleSays: "'I have to keep you entertained (or turned on) so you don't turn on me or abandon me' is a mindset so familiar to so many complex trauma survivors that a lot of us don't even realize it in so many of our relationships."

"Feeling dismissed by someone important to us can be a serious trigger for complex trauma survivors. It's more than feeling 'invisible.' It's feeling we are seen—we're just not important enough to be taken seriously. Yeah. That'll bring us back to some not great places."

October 20, 2023

4:44 AM: I woke up and screenshotted my watch.
3:33 PM: Aunt Katherine and I were at the Taylor Swift movie, and I was seated in #13, mine and Tay's lucky number.

NOT THE F——ING GILMORE GIRLS

October 22, 2023

Venmo balance ended in 333 again.

October 23, 2023

Rangers win and proceed to the World Series, my 42nd birthday! I knew this was our year. I knew it.

Gas prices were $3.33 by my house.

October 24, 2023

The Rangers won the freaking pennant last night. (I thought for a moment, grinning.) Seven years I think, since they've been to the playoffs? Oh my Gahd. We're going to the World Series; it was the best birthday present ever (I rolled my eyes heaven-ward.) Because I needed a win. And the boys needed a win. And we are going to get the World Series (I grinned and shuddered, excited) for the first time ever for my 42nd year. Because hashtag 42, Jackie Robinson's number, it's gonna be a lucky year. We are calling this now. This is ours. We got this. Rangers fans of the world unite, let's go.

Papa Bear's tone was cold in the morning, but I happily tried to appease him throughout the day. I knew it wasn't necessarily due to me, but I still wanted him warmer. At 3:33 pm, he asked to make plans to watch game 3 of the World Series on the thirtieth.

"You asked at angel numbers," I alerted him, hope blossoming in my chest.

@DrDoyleSays: "When we're triggered, we often want to reach out—but we don't quite know what we want or need from someone else. Not advice; not exactly distraction; just...presence, without pressure. To know that what we're going through doesn't make us bad, undesirable, 'too much.'"

"Feeling like we're about to be 'in trouble' is one of the most common experiences for trauma survivors that we hate talking about, because it feels like the kinda thing a kid would be worried

about. That's because it was—and we're still carrying that kid in our head & heart."

I posted a meme: "It's showtime, babe. Time to become everything you've ever dreamed of being."

Finally, I shared another tweet by @brosandprose: "I asked my therapist why I'm so easily agitated these days, and she explained that while I'm processing all of this trauma, I'm basically navigating the world with third degree burns."

That one hurt. Literally.

October 25, 2023

> @DrDoyleSays, "Sometimes trauma survivors can get anxious AF when we actually get something we want—because we have a voice in our head saying, 'good things don't last.' No, actually—it's often more like 'good things get taken away.' Or 'you're gonna pay for that good thing happening.'"

Or worst of all, you push it away because you're just not healthy enough yet.

> 2:22 PM: @DrDoyleSays: Part of what makes complex trauma "complex" is that it's often entwined w/ our closest relationships, especially growing up. It's a real mind-f*ck for your most painful memories to involve some of the people you were most attached to or dependent upon for survival. IYKYK.

October 26, 2023

> 4:44 PM: Took a pic of a bumper sticker that said "If you're gonna ride my ass, at least pull my hair."

Sometimes, the angels have a wicked sense of humor, but that one was all meant for Papa Bear.

October 27, 2023

> Another flock of rumors came on TikTok, this one being that I was going into other people's rooms, telling them who they could and couldn't be friends

with, and another slew of friends blocked me with no explanations. Sick of it this time, I bypassed sadness and went straight for anger. The same people to whom I had sent money and gifts when I had them and offered food, not to mention endless love and support, were now calling me disgusting and deplorable.

I finally got it through my head that this was as silly as MySpace in junior high, and while it was mildly annoying, it was also wildly amusing because it meant I was getting my name out there. I just prayed that the good continued to outweigh the bad.

October 28, 2023

"Game 1 of the World Series belongs to us."

I grinned. "I fell asleep while"—I nodded, looking anxious—"the Diamondbacks were leading. Woke up just in time"—I exhaled in relief—"to see the tenth inning...fell back asleep before I found out who won it. So I panicked at 1:15 because my brother had texted me 'Shit' and that's it. And I was like, 'Oh my God, we didn't end up doing it,' but we did. We took it in ten, holy cannoli fatoli. We have three more games in order to win this, or else my nerves are going to be shot. We're doing it in four. I can't take no more!" I chanted.

I posted a screenshot at 3:33: 2 missed texts from Papa Bear, whom I'd spent the morning running errands and making TikTok footage with, generally having a good time.

Matthew Perry died during the second inning of game 2 (or I should say, we heard the news), and we lost the game. As soon as the news broke, I knew the game was lost. "We're doing it in four!" lost its excitement, but I felt like I'd gained another guardian angel in a weird way.

I freaked myself out fully and completely by being on the episode of Beverly Hills, 90210 that guest-starred Perry himself. I cried while I watched of course and posted Facebook tributes. I screenshotted a post from Chandler Bing Sarcasm that had 222K likes.

October 30, 2023

My fav cartoon, a pug sitting in a throne in the clouds, with an Angel standing in front of him, having said, "You mean..." and the pug answered "Yes. Your entire species is dyslexic."

October 30, 2023

I went over to Papa Bear's house to watch the game, excited to hang out with him, but it all started off weird. He knew what time I was heading over, but he didn't answer the door nor phone when I called.

Trying to get his attention, I stood in his driveway for a TikTok: "First game in Phoenix"—I wiggled my eyebrows, knowing that had a lot to do with the magic for me—"is tonight. Three on the road, y'all. We got this in five." I winked. "Game 3!"

When I eventually got in touch with him, I felt like he was either hiding something or lying to me, the first time I'd gotten that vibe with him at all. I left without much word after the fifth inning and several tense hours with him.

October 31, 2023

Of course, after another win, a night of sleep, and some music, I texted him, happy as a clam. Angry at the way I left, he didn't appreciate my attempt to "sweep it under the rug" when I texted "conveniently" in the morning. I was forced to explain my overthinking bullshit, where I was just as willing to move away from it. He was getting to see far too much of the real me, and I knew I was going to blow it.

"I have to imagine," I explained to him, "and prepare for what's happening. I will always take care of my own needs before leaving my house. I never want to have to rely on someone or assume just because it's dinnertime that you're gonna feed me. So I tried to prepare for all scenarios, including the one I chose, which was to feed myself and not need food from you at all."

A moment later, I added, "I understood you weren't interested in the game. But you weren't interested in my presence either. So I felt like I was invading your house."

I screenshotted my timer, which had likely been set for Papa Bear's music song choice at 1 minute, 11 seconds, at 11:11 am. His response came at 3:33, 333, with a meme of what it meant. An hour later, we both screenshotted 4:44 to each other.

I saved a poem by Stacie Martin. "There are some humans, that sparkle in the sunshine and glow in the dark. They make a trip to the moon, out of a walk in the park. When you tell them your stories, you always feel seen and heard. They make you feel safe and loved, without a single word. They role model taking care of themselves, being patient and kind. They are the color of beautiful, that you would still see if you were blind. They are the sort of wonderful, that stands out from all the rest. And if you have one in your life, be thankful and know that you are blessed."

I spent the evening doing karaoke with Snapchat Halloween filters. While I was watching The Brady Bunch, Jan and Peter fought over the TV during an important ballgame, and it made me even more hopeful for the Rangers.

Late that night, I told Papa Bear I was watching my live from that morning, trying to find the clip where I'd made the prediction that ended up coming true, that the Rangers would blow it open in the second inning (when Matthew Perry died Saturday). They did, then added five more runs in the third. We won 11-7.

November 1, 2023

I created his first video for TikTok, which he highly approved of. But then he got nervous about the music choices.

"You're never gonna have to post anything I make. But you're gonna have to trust me."

"Okay," he wrote back. "Trust is a big word. I don't trust anyone easily."

"You're telling me? You expect me to trust you. LOL."

"Do I? I only do what I do. If you ever...I will always respect that."

"Don't you?" I asked, hurt. "I'd be sad if trust wasn't part of our deal. But music cannot be a hard limit with us. It can't be. It's what I do. It's part of my magic. And if it's not resonating with you, don't post the video."

"Okay. I appreciate you saying that. Just understand, trust is earned, and everyone handles it differently."

The conversation continued, me ending up unsatisfied with how he viewed trust.

At 11:05 EST, we became World Series champs for the first time in franchise history.

November 2, 2023

At 9:30, I made a TikTok: "So. Rangers win. Kick the butt (KICK THE BUTT!), KICK THE BUTT!! That I knew they were going to. And I felt cocky."

I exhaled a laugh and nodded.

"I was like, 'oh my God, it happened, it happened, it happened!' So then I got to spend the night with two puking and pooping animals"—I grimaced and nodded again—"to bring me back down to Earth."

I was quiet for a moment, nodding still.

"There's always going to be something, guys. There's always going to be something. Smile anyway. Smile through it. Do the best you can. Love as many people as you can. It feels good."

"Don't let me ruin this, please, friend. Tell me it's okay for me to have good things happen!" I texted Papa Bear, in the throes of excitement.

"Ruin what? I'm confused?"

"Sorry. My brain is going too fast over here. I messaged you on Facebook about your songs at 3:33. I'm overwhelmed by angel numbers, which I'm so excited means good things are finally happening for me, and I'm afraid I'm gonna self-sabotage. I'm trying to not allow that to happen this time."

"You won't self-sabotage," he soothed me. "You are aware, and that's the most important part in the healing process."

November 3, 2023

I woke up to this message from a TikTok friend, Shells the Otter: "I want to thank you again for sharing your positivity and light even in the midst of life's chaos. I look forward to seeing you in the mornings now because it gives my day a kickstart and motivates me to get going." It was so deeply appreciated.

I took a silly quiz on Facebook and knew it was going to tell me "Capricorn," so I put it on screen record for proof, and sure enough: "Courtney, your soul mate is a January Capricorn." I sent it to Papa Bear, wondering if he viewed soulmates the same way I did.

10:23 PM: (Birthday time is almost as precious as Angel time!): I posted a meme with an open book: "I trust the next chapter because I know the author."

November 4, 2023

My Bible app said, "Pride goes before destruction, and an arrogant spirit before a fall," which then remained stuck in my head for over a week on repeat until it sank in.

Papa Bear screenshotted me 5:55 and "We trust each other, yes?"

I replied, "Absolutely," also at 5:55.

November 5, 2023

> I got treated to his real phone number, instead of an app, which he'd been using. I felt privileged though I didn't know he'd done that.
>
> That night, the book I was reading called Orinthia, sounded as if I'd written it as a teenager and made me laugh: "This is all so difficult to explain. I know I'll remember it when I read this, but I pity anyone else who might find this. I would just like to say, sorry I suck at writing. I tend to ramble more than I should."

It's so true. I'm about to begin the editing process on this and wonder if it even mildly resembles a story.

November 6, 2023

> Went over to Papa Bear's for a day filled with making TikTok footage, helping him organize his room, and making dinner together. It may have gone down as one of my favorite days ever, and all we did was be ourselves (he was actually working).

November 8, 2023

> I said goodbye to Amber with a video on TikTok, the first time I'd braved that.

November 9, 2023

> @DrDoyleSays "Certain 'little' things can trigger the hell out of complex trauma survivors. Someone reading a message but not responding right away can totally trip that 'I'm in trouble / I'm about to be abandoned' reflex—& once we're in that headspace, it's extremely tough to pull out of it."
>
> "The silent treatment is so traumatic for a child because it's not only a form of emotional neglect, it's a targeted message: when you upset me, you no longer exist. Done over and over, this creates a deep abandonment wound."

These two. When we were kids (and adults), my mother had a terrible habit of doing exactly this when she was angry. Being left on read is one of my biggest triggers. It scares the shit out of me every time.

> I posted a meme: "Crying releases stress hormones. Swearing increases pain tolerance. Anger motivates us to solve problems. Silence and smiles aren't the only way to respond to pain. Sometimes it is good to howl."
>
> And finally, a tweet by @butchanarchy: "Being estranged from abusive parents is weird because you still get the 'I miss my mom' feeling when you're having a hard time except instead you just miss the idea of a mom you didn't actually ever have."

November 10, 2023

> I got evicted, and a TikTok friend who had been in my live when the state marshal came told Papa Bear. I brought all my food over to his house and cried out in his driveway while I organized my car. After breaking the news to my aunt, I hugged him and went over to her house.
>
> Later, I wrote, "Erin told me I was being silly for not wanting to tell you any of this shit, and I said, 'I didn't want to scare him off before we were even friends.' And she said you seem like a really genuine guy and that she thought you'd help any way you can."
>
> "Well...am I a genuine guy?"
>
> "Sweetheart, I don't know if I've ever had the pleasure of knowing a more genuine guy. I keep writing things like 'I don't know what to make of you' and 'I'm scared I'm going to lose you,' but they're both not true anymore. I feel like you're an answer to multiple prayers, and if I haven't pushed you away by now, I think I'm good. So thank you."
>
> "Aw, thanks," he answered. "I can handle a lot of woman...to a point! LOL."

November 11, 2023

I received another sweet message from Shells: "So since Snap decided to not like me today, I'm going to give up and type this—maybe there's a reason. Anyway...you do deserve the love and the kindness that you are having poured out upon you right now. Whether you can see what's behind the scenes or not, you are clearly making a difference in a lot of people's lives on a daily basis; you take the time to spread positivity, light, wisdom, and experience to people who need it at just the right moments and you're not afraid to speak your mind. That's something to be admired and respected all on its own. I hear people all the time say, 'What did I do to deserve____' and the fact of the matter is—you are just you—you matter, your voice reaches to people who need to hear it the most, and you live life as a decent human being while not forgetting that others around you are also human. Your job now is to simply embrace the love that surrounds you and let it come."

At 5:55 pm, Papa Bear and I manifested the shit out of a word search mantra. He saw miracles, connection, self-care, and lessons. I saw alignment, love, self-care, and creativity.

I said, "Yay. Okay, now let's manifest the shit out of that because it's 11-11, and it's about to be 5:55 on 11-11!"

November 12, 2023

You, by Donna Ashworth: "If every single person who has liked you in your lifetime, were to light up on a map, it would create the most glitteringly beautiful network you could imagine. Throw in the strangers you've been kind to, the people you've made laugh, or inspired along the way and that star-bright network of You would be an impressive sight to behold. You're so much more than you think you are. You have done so much more than you realise. You're trailing a bright pathway that you don't even know about. What a thing. What a thing indeed."

November 13, 2023

  I posted a meme: "My only focus right now is creating the life I want for myself."
  Bank balance had 888. It means abundance, success, and financial prosperity.

November 14, 2023

  By four, I was settled in the Airbnb I'd call home for the next six weeks.

November 18, 2023

  I had a panic attack, laying in the bed in the Airbnb, I whispered, "I just want to know (sob sob) why I'm never enough."
  I posted a meme: "Biggest flex is loving yourself the way you wished they did. Be your own damn upgrade."
  I was annoyed with myself by 7:30, mostly because of how I let it affect me. He'd told me he didn't see a romantic connection with me, and it confused me. Why was I good enough for —— and not "romance?" What did I keep doing so wrong?

November 19, 2023

  I posted a meme: "She was made from November rain / Pleasure and pain / Scorpion stings, pretty things, and the flames of Phoenix wings. —Michelle Schaper
  Not to get super graphic, but this was the 13th wildly heavy day of a wildly heavy period. I was super uncomfortable not being at home, bleeding all over anything. I've been praying for menopause (in reality, I've been dealing with symptoms for years) to start so I can just go through as much shit as possible before the new year. But the way I was bleeding, I got scared I might be miscarrying, so I

made a doctor's appointment. She said I was behaving like any normal 42-year-old under immense stress. She gave me a drug that gave my body a trick, and I stopped bleeding. For two weeks.

November 23, 2023

I was watching FRIENDS in my FRIENDS Thanksgiving shirt at 7:30 in the morning. I had holiday coffee from Dunkin', I'd woken up in a great mood; it was still a holiday even if I was by myself. I invited everyone on TikTok to come hang out, tell me what they're thankful for. To find that small thing to be thankful for and come see me.

I ordered Cracker Barrel Thanksgiving dinner and watched Hallmark movies all day, like usual.

At 4:44 PM, I was listening to music, and the Cranberries sang "I thought nothing could go wrong / But I was wrong, I was wrong."

Reading those now shines a whole new light. First of all, the Cranberries on Turkey Day (again, those funny guardian angels)? Secondly, I'm sure that was also for Papa Bear.

November 24, 2023

"Let them go. If you feel unloved, let them go. If you feel like a burden, let them go. If you feel unappreciated, let them go. You have to stop chasing people. If they block you, ignore you... let them go. Let those who naturally gravitate towards you, enjoy your energy. We spend too much time clinging onto people so they don't leave. Cherish those who want to see you, who want to talk to you, who are there by choice. Do they make time for you; don't make time for people who don't make time for you."

I posted a meme: "Her entire life led to the moment when she said, 'This is the life I want' & she never again wasted time on anything that wasn't that."

"So I'm sitting here writing my life story, and something that I've said since the beginning on

TikTok is I'm a mirror, right? I reflect back the energy that you put off. Reading this journal? I am a mirror of my mother." I made a face. *"I echo her every...move almost. I am not bipolar. But I act like I am when she's sick. And it's scary. And I am going to get out of it. This will be the last time I let anybody"*—I nodded on the emphasis—*"determine my mood."*

It's only been a month since I made that one, but it's become glaringly apparent that I have to somehow cut the metaphysical cord. I don't know if she's aware of the control she's had over me, but it ends now.

November 27, 2023

Ruby and Cookie somehow managed to pick up fleas. In the 40 degree weather. I'm pretty sure I manifested that shit (the yard at the Airbnb scared me), and I was pissed. I bombed the room and my car, washed all their blankets, medicated and bathed the dogs, and still didn't cure them. So four weeks later, at the vet, we found out they were still badly infested, but the vet assured me fleas were terrible this year. So they got a pill "that worked," another bath, will be professionally groomed, and if that doesn't work... We hate fleas. I literally am still itching.

I posted a meme: "Pay attention to your patterns. The way you learned to survive may not be the way you want to continue to live. Heal and shift." — Dr. Thelma Bryant-Davis.

"A wise woman once packed all her stuff and said 'This fucked up shit will not be my story,' then she left and lived happily after."

November 30, 2023

4:44 PM: We were downtown to watch the Tree Lighting in New Haven, and Leona Lewis "Bleeding Love" was the song. I got out of my car, leaving the dogs, to go see a show that didn't really start until nearly three hours later. But I stayed, I was patient, and it was beautiful. It was my first time seeing a tree being lit in person.

December 1, 2023

"I'm going to be taking a break from lives for a little while. Um, few days. I don't know how long. So it's just gonna be videos. I'm plugging through this writing, and I really want to get it done. And the faster that happens and the quicker I can get out of this Airbnb, the faster we can get back to lives as normal. So I'm super excited for what this year, this month, is gonna bring, but more so for what next year is going to bring. So 2024...will be awesome."

I started my Hallmark Christmas movie checklist with The Most Colorful Time of the Year, which was about a color blind Christmas teacher. I asked TikTok to think about what it would be like to see the world in black and white. "It would be so sad," I said. "The Christmas tree lighting last night alone was...magical."

December 3, 2023

A good friend sent me snaps of her car, which was overrun with kids and looked quite similar to mine. My first reaction was "oh my gosh, girl, you'll feel so much better if you clean your car!" and then I asked myself why I couldn't do the same for myself when I preach self-care all day, every day. "Do you know how much unhealth we're inhaling when we get in our car?" I asked her. "You'd say the same to me if you saw my car, 'Coco, clean your car, oh my God!' It's so easy to say to someone else, someone we care about, but why can't we do it for ourselves, when we supposedly care about ourselves?"

As a matter of fact, Papa Bear had told me the same thing, "You have a nice car, you shouldn't have anything in it except for a blanket for the dogs in the back." As if reading my mind, at 11:10, he sent me a "good morning" video from Instagram.

"Ooh, I love," I wrote, "but I don't know how to access the sound. If you want to use it that is. If it was just for me, then thank you."

"It was just for you," he replied, sweetly, "Straighten that crown and be super creative today."

Of course that made me cry, because our relationship had already dwindled down to being about TikTok only. But I would have been okay with that if he'd continue to do things like that. But my anxiety got the better of me, for the last fucking time, and I ruined it, as I do all good things.

December 4, 2023

"I took the weekend to write. It was beautiful. I've had a fantastic couple of days."

Ruby growled.

"Ruby's growling again while dripping water from her face. So I'm gonna go live for an hour."

December 5, 2023

Bob Seger was on, singing "Like a Rock," "Felt like a million. Felt like number one."

December 7, 2023

On my drive home—and by home, I mean the Airbnb I'm currently residing in—today, I was angry. Typically, driving calms me, and I've managed to get my road rage under control over the past couple years. (Life is too short already, y'all. Slow down and be kind on the road.) But tonight, people seemed extra annoying, so I beeped a lot, and a couple folks even got my finger rather than my teeth. So I made myself focus and I got excited to come home and write. For once, I feel like I'm working on something that will actually benefit me and mine (or most of mine. My mother won't like it). I got excited for what the future holds (again), rather than simply living day to day.

I came home with McDonald's for dinner and wrote on my Facebook, "I got a milkshake with dinner because I have no one to cuddle my boobs after a mammogram." I may have a face in mind right now, but only God knows who will be there in the end. I have faith my ride-or-die is coming. It's my turn.

Y'all, as I plow through the old, sometimes painful memories, the "current" is taking on a life of its own. I literally feel like I'm speaking to the world, and it's mind-boggling to think I could be! God willing (universe willing, whatever your beliefs!), I'll finally be able to help as many people as I've wanted to. My entire life, I just prayed for people to love. Please let me help you. I'll be your rainbow when it's dark, I'll help you find your silver lining. One of my favorite lyrics, "let me love you until you can learn to love yourself." I have a lot of love to give.

December 8, 2023

1:11 PM: I've seen all the angel numbers as usual today. A certain man still comes to mind, but I know he's seeing them too. I had my mammogram yesterday, and my father told me he has a tumor on his kidney. I feel so oddly like I'm literally writing my life right now, that I've almost half-convinced myself that we are about to be tumor buddies. I've gotten so good at preparing for every outcome, good or bad, that it's like nothing can surprise me anymore. It's mind-blowing.

December 9, 2023

We went to see Santa at Lyman Orchards today; Cookie sat in Mrs Claus's lap, Ruby got the Big Guy. I finally made it inside the store, which is beautiful. I can't wait to look at everything properly.

So it's my second day of a fairly heavy period. Last month, I wouldn't stop bleeding, huge amounts. Thankfully, my doctor said I'm just behaving as any normal 42-year-old under immense pressure would, so she put me on a med that tricked my body into thinking I'd ovulated. Strangely (or not, I guess, because, science), my period started the day the med ended. Now it seems to be here with gusto, and I'm praying it... well, I'm praying it's the last one, so whatever needs to happen.

I've been so certain that it's "my turn" this time that I keep asking God to throw everything he can that he knows I can handle: menopause, cancer, homelessness (that's not one I'm enjoying, I'll be honest).

At 1:56 PM, I sent Papa Bear a pic of my dashboard, whose numbers were stopped at 111 and 222.4 and "Get Together" by the Youngbloods. By this time, he didn't care.

December 10, 2023

So into my third week of literally bleeding all over this Airbnb (my last one was over two weeks!!), I understand part of what's happening: you know they say God brings you out of your comfort zone? I'm way way uncomfortable. I'm lucky because I had financial help to afford an Airbnb, and I also managed to get heavy-bleeding pads at Amazon. Y'all. I can't afford that shit. If this isn't menopause for me, I'm gonna have to figure something else out, because (not to be graphic), I can't keep one of those things on for longer than an hour. So here's my idea, my prayer, which I believe is small enough to be a good starting point. I'm going to start a feminine-hygeine-product drive. I can't change homelessness yet, but I can help there, even if it's one package at a time.

Anyway, so I go to Google to see what verses talk about God bringing you out of your comfort zone, and in the top 5 is "my" verse from when I first started going to church, Jeremiah 29:11. It says "do you ever doubt yourself? Doubt your ability to succeed? Those are not your own thoughts. Those are lies from the enemy who already knows of the plans God has for you, to prosper you and to give you a future and a hope (Jer 29:11). He's just trying to make you doubt and give up short of the finish line. Don't. God is the author of your story and the finisher of your faith. The next time the enemy tries to cause you to doubt yourself or your purpose, remind him of the truth! Phew. I sure love hearing that, even when I know it. It's like hearing the person you love say they love you. I have to remember to tell myself I love you more often.

December 11, 2023

  Michelle, my dear friend Red Wagon Bakery LLC on TikTok, just spoke her three year plan. She will have enough to sell her house and get an RV and travel the country with her food trailer. Three years. In the same amount of time, I hope to be able to do the same, but I want the home base in Connecticut. After this few weeks of being "homeless," I need the assurance somehow. If that means I only have the RV, so be it. I'll find a beautiful piece of land and build a tiny house as our base. God willing. We got this.

  Watching "It's Christmas, Eve," with LeAnn Rimes and Tyler Hynes, which is one of my fave Hallmark movies. I've had a connection to LeAnn since my dad took me and my brother to Billy Bob's in Ft Worth to see her sing when she (and I) was 12. She was the only singer I picked from the start as the Masked Singer. Anyway. No reason I'm writing this particularly, other than I love both of them. If it's too late for Hallmark this time, look it up next year. It's a good one.

  I sent in for a "Cameo" From Jeremy Jordan. A little bit of Christmas magic for myself. It was…well, magical, ya know? I gotta keep that little magic to myself… It was 2 minutes and 15 seconds of him cheering for me, plus singing an "inspiring" song, and it's magic. (I ended up sharing it! Come enjoy the magic with me on TikTok!)

  But it encouraged me to look up his Instagram, which I'm never on anymore, and there was a post for a show in Boston and New York. With a meet and greet. I told myself if tickets weren't exorbitant, I'd go to Boston by myself. I'm still not ready to brave

New York. You guys, they were dirt cheap. Does no one else know the magic of this man? Or is he so humble he can continue to play smaller venues for cheaper prices and offer himself for $50?

God works, man. It's not even that mysterious anymore. I get to go see this city I've imagined for years, steeped in history, and listen to the melodious tones of one Jeremy Jordan. Maybe I'll even get to hug him!

December 12, 2023

It will never cease to annoy me that Hermione's dress isn't blue in the Goblet of Fire movie. That being said, I believe watching these movies for the umpteenth time is helping open my imagination. JK Rowling did it. Why can't I? (Although, to be honest, I never would have been able to imagine half the things she did!)

I tried to get my brother into my optimistic mindframe, but he got there before I could say anything...

Praying for the book to hit the NY bestsellers list in the first couple of weeks.

JIMMY: Just be realistic with the fact that your book won't hit The NY Times best sellers list in the first couple of weeks, and then have a plan in place in case that doesn't happen.
ME: Lmao I do. Thank you. And don't say won't please. Or I won't tell you anything.
JIMMY: But, I hope it is awesome and you become the #1 writer in the world.
ME: Thank you. That's more like it.

December 13, 2023

I've been crying all day because I'm angry with someone who was supposed to be a friend. The words "I hate you" literally keep coming to mind, and I hate that. I hate feeling angry. After a few months of sharing Angel numbers and other exciting things with him, he's turned a complete 180 on me, for no reason that he will share with me, other than I'm "too much" and he needs "easy and go-with-the-flow." This to the girl who will literally go to Walmart in pajamas and no makeup just to spend time with you and then happily get pushed out the door when it's time for your next play date.

So if instead of all the wild fun things I've been imagining for him, he's supposed to be a lesson in how to be angry, I don't like it. I keep praying that God will bring me through everything "bad" that he can while I'm homeless... everything He knows I can handle. But I don't want to be angry anymore. It makes me feel sick. Help.

December 14, 2023

Why is it so hard to say the hard stuff even when you know it's in your best interest? I'm waiting till 5:55 to go check my messages, because no matter what (if he blocked me, if he read it and didn't reply, or if he replies angrily), I'll still have my angels and God.

Do you have to prepare for every scenario before doing something? Me, I have to plan like every angle. Guard myself for every possibility. Going to check now.

He did indeed block me. So I managed to push him away, this guy who was poly, looking to be friends even if there was no spark, that I had a ton in common with. How. The fuck. Am I ever supposed to be in any kind of relationship that lasts longer than a week if no one can stand to be around me? Was my mother right when she said I'd never get married because I'm too much of a bitch? Is this extrovert with the capacity to love millions really destined to be alone? I love myself, and I love my dogs, but why am I successful at pushing every single human away?

I posted a meme: "I finally threw in the towel. But God threw it back and said, 'Wipe your face, girl. We are almost there.'"

December 15, 2023

    I already have an answer, I think. I did it on purpose. I test until I am successful. Do you know how much I hate admitting this? I might be wrong. I might need more help forgiving myself than I thought. Six weeks ago, I was hugging him, begging him to "not let me self-sabotage," not to let me ruin this. But I pushed and picked until he blocked me, which is what I needed him to do for me to stop contacting him. To give him a break, which is all he'd asked. Will I try to make amends after the new year? We will see what my gut says then. I'm confused right now. Do I miss him, or do I miss what I hoped to get from him? What I got from him wasn't made up... that's the fucking annoying part. I don't understand how the magic can exist on one side. It's not fair.

December 16, 2023

    "Hello, my lovelies. It's time to start the artwork for my book"—I shake my head, my eyes closed—"which is mind-blowing...that I'm almost to the end and ready to publish. And I have a lot of ideas..."

December 17, 2023

    So I'm crying a lot (again) because I am to blame for this one. I am unbelievably pissed at myself. I've had some revelations that I'll be sharing with him, but with no one else simply for one reason: if I get lucky enough that he forgives me, that story will be in the sequel. Yes, my ridiculous, anxious writerly brain has him forgiving me... but it's also coming to terms with him not forgiving me, and him being nothing more than a lesson. One more heartbreak that I caused myself. I'm so. Angry. At myself.

    I posted a meme: "I think I say I love you too much. It's strange how sometimes it startles people. But then I remember, that's why I'm here. To love and to startle." —jkkennedy

December 18, 2023

 Chinese fortune: Everything you are against weakens you. Everything you are for empowers you.

December 19, 2023

 Bank balance starts with 222.

December 23, 2023

 Goodness, it's been a week already. I am so thankful my time in this Airbnb is almost up. I will be home soon, the dogs will be safe, happy, and healthy, and we will begin to live again. I sent him a Christmas card with an apology, one that no one but he and I will ever read (unless he forgives me.). There's one thing I think I forgot to write while I was apologizing, and that was "thank you." The lessons I learned from going crazy on him were the final bullshit I had to figure out about myself. I'm sad that I may have lost his friendship, but I'm thankful I understand what I'm doing to ruin things for myself. Girl, from here on out, I got you. You deserve all the good things and this version of me will get them for us.

 Dinner at K&F's was wonderful. It's just so peaceful to be among people who love each other, even when you're the fifth wheel. Always.

December 24, 2023

 4:44 PM: Bank balance includes 333.

December 25, 2023

 It's Christmas morning and I've already been crying, but I'm stopping it now. I started off the morning by making my morning rounds on TikTok, and I bounced into a friend's live and was immediately blocked, before I'd even said a word. Just for being me. On Christmas. So yeah.

 Now I'm watching the Brady Bunch and trying to get back into the holiday spirit. Later, watching Magic Mike's Last Dance, I found one part very poignant (Zadie): "One of the most primal feelings human beings experience is the desire to belong, to feel connected to other beings and to be part of a tribe. In fact, brain scans have shown that social rejection creates virtually identical brain activity as physical assault."

December 26, 2023

Writing the recent stuff is really hard. Harder than writing about my mom. I'm so mad at myself for the way I fucked up. I did it on fuckin purpose, literally. Begged him several times not to "let me" self-sabotage, as if he was in charge of me, or as if he was my conscience... But he's not, he wasn't, and he was incapable of stopping me from fucking it up because that's what I do. I ruin good things for myself. Literally, the last step in my healing will be when I know I deserve the good things that are happening to me.

December 27, 2023

Writing about November 6 and watching all the footage I gathered, I'm laughing and crying. One of the things I told Papa Bear when I first started making videos for him was that he fulfilled that fantasy of a beautiful man being sweet. I'm laughing because this footage is... sweet. And sexy. And him. And I'm crying because I had him in real life (I don't mean had him as in possessed him, but had him as a friend), and I ruined it, as I always somehow manage to do.

December 28, 2023

I bought myself a ticket to see Jeremy Jordan in Boston. There's a meet and greet afterward, and you know my imagination has started spinning. In his cameo, he said if I get on the NY bestseller list, I better give him a shoutout. I say, I'm giving you a shoutout in my book, how about giving me one to help get me to that list? New Yorkers love JJ. ("I say, that what you say...is what I say." Not JJ's role, but his musical.)

My rent check cleared today and left my balance at $2.22. (Don't worry, I have other accounts.)

January 6, 2024

Wow. Good Lord, that was weird to write. I saw a lot of Angel numbers today (nearly every time I looked at the clock!!), and I know it's time to send this book off. I'm excited and terrified and so many more emotions. It's my turn, right, God?

My friend Squirrelly took a test on FB that said the real story of her life was "A Phoenix rising from the ashes." Excited, I commented "That's me!!!" and went to take the test myself. Squirrelly's said, "She is beautiful on the inside and out, with her heart as big as the Galaxy and unbreakable fighting spirit. Her life has not been easy, but she has turned the sorrows of her past into her unfailing strength. It would be a mistake to underestimate this stubbornly independent woman. She will always fight for her loved ones, no matter how exhasuted she is from her own responsibilities. She is a woman you will always want by your side."

Mine said, "The silent storm returns. She faces many battles alone, doing everything she can to make sure those she cares about don't suffer the same. She's not a sweet talker, and her brutal honesty often confuses people, but she's the most loyal friend anyone could have. Smart, stubborn, and independent, always sincere, she's the person worth fighting for. But never take advantage of her kindness, because once her trust is broken, she will leave. She is like the sun, absolutely capable of shining alone."

January 8, 2024

I went to pick up my first draft of this book at Staples, then I went to Walmart, where I told the

> cashier and the man in line behind me that I was about to publish my book. As I was realizing the date, one of my guardian Angel's birthday (Elvis lol), my total ended at $48.88. Angel numbers in abundance forever, but those eights are hard to come by.

January 12, 2024

> "I love it when you call me big poppa" has been stuck in my head all day. My book was approved at the publisher's... we are on our way. So, tomorrow is the 13th, which is my lucky number. It will be the last "day" of this book... and of course I'll see what memories there are. I'm happy.

January 13, 2024

In "The Weight Loss Diaries" on this day fourteen years ago, my goal was to get to 170 by July 4, as I was trying to go to Cali and wanted to be super cute. I just wrote in the vision board page of my journal, a suggestion from my therapist, whom I loved, all my goals for the year. I am going to also write them here, where staying accountable to even one hundred people—I told my therapist I could sell one hundred copies of this book in my sleep!—seems like it will really work. So here we go.

1. Publish my autobiography.
2. Get my tattoo.
3. Go to karaoke.
4. Cali in July for Joc and Greg's wedding.
5. *Gilmore Girls* fest in October.
6. Texas State Fair in October.
7. Get under two hundred

Addendum: get to 170 fourteen years after making the goal.

Writing that, my blood pressure keeps rising. I have a very specific set of lyrics stuck in my head, a song by Joe Iconis for the show *Smash* and performed by the illustrious Jeremy Jordan. It gives me chills every time I hear it: "And the last thing I hear / As the impact grows near / Is it a scream or a cheer? Well, never mind, I'll never find out / 'Cause Broadway, I am here!"

I always hear a splat as the music cuts off. It's kind of a depressing song, I'm not gonna lie, but when JJ sent my cameo, he sang from *Newsies*, which is much more cheerful:

"Now is the time to seize the day / Stare down the odds and seize the day / Minute by minute, that's how you win it / We will find our way / But let us seize the day."

So remember, no matter what you believe in, if it's God or Buddha or Zeus or Santa Claus, make sure you believe in yourself. My story is about to get so good. Know how I know? I hold the pen. In the immortal words of my favorite Bruno, "Don't believe me? Just watch."

About the Author

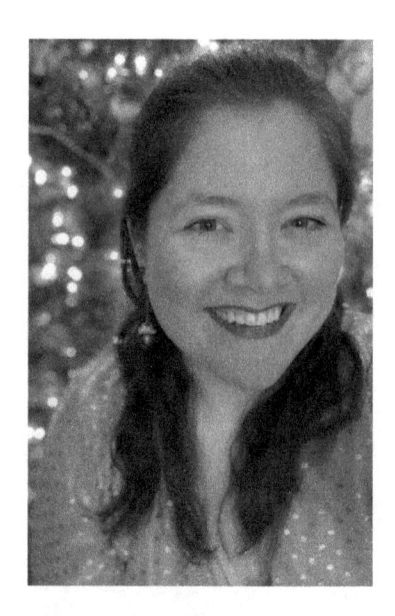

Courtney, a.k.a. Coco, was admired her entire life for her perseverance, strength, and bravery. She dreamed of New England, Connecticut, in particular, since she was a kid, spurred on by *Gilmore Girls* and Hallmark movies. She's thrilled to finally call it home, and she's excited to see what magic can happen here. Even when there are freeze warnings in April.

www.ingramcontent.com/pod-product-compliance
Lightning Source LLC
LaVergne TN
LVHW040741170125
801530LV00018BA/73/J